HERMAPHRODITES IN RENAI

Women and Gender in the Early Modern World

Series Editors: Allyson Poska and Abby Zanger

In the past decade, the study of women and gender has offered some of the most vital and innovative challenges to scholarship on the early modern period. Ashgate's new series of interdisciplinary and comparative studies, 'Women and Gender in the Early Modern World', takes up this challenge, reaching beyond geographical limitations to explore the experiences of early modern women and the nature of gender in Europe, the Americas, Asia, and Africa. Submissions of single-author studies and edited collections will be considered.

Titles in the series include:

Childbirth and the Display of Authority in Early Modern France
Lianne McTavish

Salons, History, and the Creation of Seventeenth-Century France
Mastering Memory
Faith E. Beasley

Literary Circles and Gender in Early Modern Europe
A Cross-Cultural Approach
Julie Campbell

Women's Letters Across Europe, 1400–1700
Form and Persuasion
Edited by Jane Couchman and Ann Crabb

Masculinity, Anti-Semitism and Early Modern English Literature
From the Satanic to the Effeminate Jew
Matthew Biberman

Hermaphrodites in Renaissance Europe

KATHLEEN P. LONG
Cornell University, USA

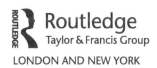

Routledge
Taylor & Francis Group

LONDON AND NEW YORK

First published 2006 by Ashgate Publishing

2 Park Square, Milton Park, Abingdon, Oxon OX14 4RN
711 Third Avenue, New York, NY 10017, USA

Routledge is an imprint of the Taylor & Francis Group, an informa business

First issued in paperback 2016

British Library Cataloguing in Publication Data
Long, Kathleen P., 1957–
    Hermaphrodites in Renaissance Europe. – (Women and gender
    in the early modern world)
    1. Hermaphroditism in literature 2. European literature –
    Renaissance, 1450–1600 – History and criticism
    3. Hermaphroditism
    I. Title
    809.3'35266

Library of Congress Cataloging-in-Publication Data
Long, Kathleen P., 1957–
    Hermaphrodites in Renaissance Europe / Kathleen P. Long.
        p. cm. – (Women and gender in the early modern world)
    Includes bibliographical references and index.
    ISBN 0–7546–5609–8 (alk. paper)
    1. Hermaphroditism – History. 2. Hermaphroditism – Europe – History – 16th
    century. 3. Renaissance. 4. Gender identity – Europe – History – 16th century.
    I. Title. II. Series.

    RC883.L66 2006
    305.3094'0903–dc22   2005032203

ISBN 978-0-7546-5609-8 (hbk)
ISBN 978-1-138-25938-6 (pbk)

To Doug
"ita di iubeatis, et istum/nulla dies a me nec me deducat ab isto."

Contents

List of Illustrations

Acknowledgments

This book began as a thirty-page article. By the time I had put in all the background information an anonymous reader had asked for, I had a book-length manuscript. First, I must thank this reader for pointing out many other accounts of hermaphrodites for me to explore. Next, I owe a debt of gratitude to a number of my colleagues and students: to Nelly Furman, who advised me on large portions of the project; and to Marilyn Migiel, Mary McKinley, and Tom Conley, who encouraged this work and gave me advice on revision. The support of François Rigolot, Larry Kritzman, Richard Regosin, Hope Glidden, Daniel Russell, and Gisèle Mathieu-Castellani has been important not only for this project, but for my career.

I am grateful to Erika Gaffney, for guiding this project along. I thank Pat FitzGerald for making the book printable. Many students inspired my work: Duane Rudolph and Patricia Gravatt deserve particular recognition for their lively discussions with me of all things early modern.

I am indebted to the Folger Shakespeare Library, for its help in my research, and for providing me with a copy of the original edition of the *Description de l'Isle des Hermaphrodites, nouvellement descouverte*, as well as to the Houghton Library at Harvard, whose copies of Clovis Hesteau de Nuysement's works, *Poeme philosophic de la verité de la phisique mineralle* and *Traittez de l'harmonie et constitution generalle du vray sel, secret des philosophes ...* I used for this study. I wish to thank the Division of Rare and Manuscript Collections, Cornell University Library, particularly Katherine Reagan, Susette Newberry, and the rest of the staff, for helping me find early editions of the works used in this book, and for helping me locate pictures to illustrate it. Their support made my research pleasant.

Most of all, I thank Douglas Long, my technical and moral support, who has seen me through this project and many other challenges.

A version of chapter one of this book appeared as "Sexual Dissonance: Early Modern Scientific Accounts of Hermaphrodites," in *Wonders, Marvels, and Monsters in Early Modern Culture*, ed. Peter Platt (Newark and London: University of Delaware Press and Associated University Presses, 1999), pp. 145–63. This piece is reprinted with the kind permission of Associated University Presses.

A version of chapter three appeared as "Jacques Duval on Hermaphrodites," in *High Anxiety: Masculinity in Crisis in Early Modern France*, ed. Kathleen P. Long (Kirksville: Truman State University Press, 2002), pp. 107–38. This piece is reprinted with the kind permission of Truman State University Press.

Part of chapter five appeared as "The Chemical Wedding in the Works of Clovis Hesteau de Nuysement," *Dalhousie French Studies*, special issue on *Le Mariage sous l'Ancien Régime*, ed. Claire Carlin 56 (Fall 2001): 27–35.

A version of chapter eight appeared as "Hermaphrodites Newly Discovered: The Cultural Monsters of Sixteenth-Century France," in *Monster Theory: Reading Culture*, ed. Jeffrey Jerome Cohen (Minneapolis: University of Minnesota Press, 1996), pp. 183–201.

Introduction:
Sex and Gender Wars

In Renaissance France, long before the debates over sex and gender, there was *sexe*, a term which largely encompassed both those postmodern concepts. In an era obsessed with the (re-)establishment of "natural law," the distinction between the natural/biological and the cultural was not evident; in fact, theologians and jurists often deliberately effaced the line that separated the two.[1] In medical and alchemical treatises, the instability of the term *sexe* becomes apparent, particularly when hermaphrodites and other individuals "change" their sex. The very existence of the hermaphrodite challenges the neatly delineated dual-sex system, according to which one has to be either male or female. Still, jurists and medical authors alike try to impose one sex, male or female, even on the hermaphrodite. In so doing, they bring the concept of sex into direct confrontation with a body that does not conform to that concept. This confrontation reveals the "imaginary" nature of this culture's concept of sex, bringing it closer to our postmodern notion of gender.[2] The "imaginary" nature of early modern sex designations also leaves a space for fluidity of gender roles, at least in literary and philosophical works, the latter including not only reworkings of Platonic and Neoplatonic texts, but also what is now designated as "philosophical" alchemy. In these works, men and women change their sex at will – or against their will – or disguise it; they conjoin and share their sexed identities, to form a more perfect, hermaphroditic, whole. All this directly violates the "natural laws" separating and distinguishing the sexes, laws imposed by Church and State. Thus, the codification of sex roles seems contemporaneously accompanied by subversion of those very roles. The insistence upon the naturalness of these roles is accompanied by the suggestion that they are not natural.

It is this larger issue of authority and subversion that the hermaphrodite comes to exemplify. Not merely an image of sexual confusion or of the problematic status of the nature/culture debate in the sixteenth century, the hermaphrodite becomes an image of

---

[1]   To the point, of, as Natalie Davis points out, insisting on the existence of a "King Bee"; see *Society and Culture in Early Modern France* (Stanford: Stanford University Press, 1975), p. 126.

[2]   For this formulation of the "imaginary" in relation to sex and gender, I am indebted to Guy Poirier's work, *L'Homosexualité dans l'imaginaire de la Renaissance* (Paris: Champion, 1996); I would refer readers to this work for a more sustained discussion of *l'imaginaire* as it relates to sexuality in the sixteenth century.

social disorder and civil strife, particularly as it becomes attached to the representations of Henri III (king of France from 1574 to 1589) and his court, in political pamphlets and in Thomas Artus's novel, *L'Isle des Hermaphrodites, nouvellement descouverte* (*The Island of Hermaphrodites, Newly Discovered*, first published around 1605). In this work, the hermaphrodite becomes the image both of a country torn by its differences, and potentially unifying those differences by means of tolerance.

Thus, their country and their culture torn by civil wars caused by religious differences and resulting in new levels of political dissent, the French became obsessed with the figure of the hermaphrodite as an expression both of this internal strife and of the potential solutions to it. Across the cultural spectrum, the figure of the hermaphrodite rises again and again to prominence, dominating debates over medical practices as well as the strange alternative world of alchemical thought, recurring frequently in the poetry of the late sixteenth century, serving as an expression of social disorder in political pamphlets directed against Henri III, and appearing and reappearing in satirical novels directed at the courts of Henri III and Henri IV (king of France from 1589 to 1610). Interest in the hermaphrodite cuts across disciplinary lines, to such a degree that surgeons and professors of medicine cite popular pamphlets and literary works as sources for their ideas.

The rise of the hermaphrodite as a cultural icon coincides with a number of world-changing events, and is overtly connected with these events in a number of works. Theodor de Bry (1528–1598), in his *America*, the project of publishing all known accounts of European contact with the Western hemisphere, begun by him in the 1580s and continued by his son and other descendants until 1644, associates the hermaphrodite with the New World. The political pamphlets use hermaphrodites as an image of the disruptive effect the Reformation had on religious and social unity in France. It should be noted that the hermaphrodite also appears frequently in alchemical and medical treatises in Germany and Switzerland, two other countries profoundly affected by the Reformation.[3] This study will consider these treatises as well as those by French authors, as these works represent a coherent intellectual community that read each other's work, imitated and alluded to each other frequently, and advanced similar questions. Political pamphlets, while exploiting the figure of the hermaphrodite in order to denounce Henri III, also propose an early form of republicanism, in which the people participate in the process of governance, particularly in the selection of their king. In the works of Ambroise Paré (1510?–1590, surgeon to the French royal family) and Jacques Duval (1555–1615, a surgeon based in Rouen), the hermaphrodite becomes associated with a sustained debate concerning medical practices, one in which the surgeons, who learn their trade by observing the living body, face off against the doctors, professors who teach medicine out of the works of classical philosophy,

---

[3]   Hermaphrodites became popular in England somewhat later than on the continent; this phenomenon is well-documented and analyzed by Ruth Gilbert, *Early Modern Hermaphrodites: Sex and Other Stories* (New York: Palgrave, 2002).

particularly Aristotle. The hermaphrodite is thus associated with the rise of empirical science, and the valorization of clinical practice over bookish learning.

The hermaphrodite consequently becomes the symbol of various cultural battles being fought over the course of the sixteenth century. Political and intellectual institutions, religious and medical practices, social and legal structures, are either confirmed or called into question by this figure. For the hermaphrodite is profoundly ambiguous, as becomes its form. When used in a satirical context, its ambiguous nature confirms the importance of clear-cut social divisions. When used in more mystical and lyric works, acceptance of the ambiguities it represents becomes a way out of destructive social strife. The hermaphrodite is thus at one and the same time a profoundly conservative and a profoundly revolutionary figure; its various manifestations can be used to track the progress of innovations in medicine and social attitudes and of resistance to this progress, as we shall see from the various medical and alchemical treatises on the one hand, and the political pamphlets on the other.

The medical and alchemical treatises can be seen as offering "theories" of hermaphrodism, and thus reflect early modern thought concerning sex and gender. It must be noted that all of the medical treatises in this study do not use a word for gender; in this period, gender is purely a grammatical term (*genre*), designating whether a noun is masculine or feminine. This grammatical categorization does overlap with social constructions of what we now deem to be gender, as certain qualities, and objects or things with certain qualities, are designated as feminine, while others are designated as masculine. These grammatical gender designations are still in flux, at least to some degree, in sixteenth century France.[4]

When discussing either the human body or the social roles that men or women take on, the medical treatises analyzed in this study invariably use the word *sexe*. This is because social status and behavior and biological sex distinctions are not seen as divergent by most early modern authors; most discussions of natural law portray women's subordination to men as the natural result of their reproductive status.[5] Even in treatises that seem to question these carefully elaborated distinctions between male and female, the distinction between sex and gender is not obvious, but rather fraught with complexity. Jacques Duval's portrayal of Marin le Marcis as feminized by his captivity and lack of activity calls into question even the notion of a fixed biological sex; the body itself is affected by its surroundings. Sex and gender exist in a fluid symbiotic relationship in this portion of the treatise. Just as the categories imposed on the hermaphrodite by early modern law, to make it conform to the expectation of clear sex distinctions, are in fact unstable, so the distinction between sex and gender

---

4   See, for example, François Rigolot, "Quel 'genre' d'amour pour Louise Labé?," in *Poétique* 55 (Paris: Seuil, 1983): 303–17.

5   A complex discussion of this association takes place in Thomas Laqueur's assessment of the one-sex theory; see "The Demands of Culture," in the chapter "Destiny is Anatomy," *Making Sex: The Body and Gender from the Greeks to Freud* (Cambridge, MA: Harvard University Press, 1990), pp. 52–62.

falls apart, when our authors debate how "sex" can be established by means other than external signs. Postmodern questions concerning the sex/gender distinction reflect the more complex relationship between the biological and the cultural that emerges in the sixteenth century, and that is particularly evident in the treatises of Caspar Bauhin (1560–1624, a professor of botany and anatomy at the University of Basel)[6] and Jacques Duval.[7]

The fundamental problem posed by the existence of the hermaphrodite is that, in a world divided into male and female, the hermaphroditic body is not identical to itself. As suggested above, the coexistence of male and female in one body calls into question the one-sex theory, based on the Aristotelian notion of the female as merely a deficient male. If this theory were to hold true, then when male and female were joined in one body, the female would be subsumed into the male, as Salmacis is into the body of Hermaphroditus in Ovid's version of the myth of the hermaphrodite.

This study also proposes a modest corrective to postmodern notions of the primitive nature of early modern understandings of sex, gender, and sexuality. For example, Anne Fausto-Sterling suggests in her book, *Sexing the Body*, that sex and gender are complex and often mutable markers of bodies that are shaped both by genetic codes and social programming. She traces the dawn of explorations of sex/gender to the seventeenth and eighteenth centuries. Her view of the Renaissance is of a culture that has not yet dealt with the issues raised by intersexuality, although it is coming into an awareness of those issues: "all over Europe the sharp distinction between male and female was at the core of systems of law and politics. The rights of inheritance, forms of judicial punishment, and the right to vote and participate in the political system were all determined in part by sex."[8] In short, whether one was male or female really mattered; social groups, political power, money were all linked to what we now call gender. Intersexuality was not recognized by most legal systems, in that "hermaphrodites" (the term most frequently used for intersexuals in the sixteenth century) were designated as male or female in order to inscribe them into the social order.

Nonetheless, a variety of sexes are recognized in the medical treatises of the time. Intersexuality is in fact an almost obsessively recurrent theme in Renaissance

---

[6]　*De hermaphroditorum monstrosorumque partuum natura, ex Theologorum, Jure-consultorumque, medicorum, philosophorum & rabbinorum sententia libri duo ...* (Oppenheim: Galleri, 1614). This book, complete with illustrations taken from the work of Theodor de Bry, is a marvelous encyclopedia listing virtually every reference to hermaphrodites in works written up until the seventeenth century.

[7]　*Des hermaphrodits, accouchemens des femmes, et traitement qui est requis pour les relever en santé, & bien elever leurs enfans ...* (Rouen: David Geuffroy, 1612). These questions are presented by Moira Gatens, in "A Critique of the Sex/Gender Distinction," *Imaginary Bodies: Ethics, Power and Corporeality* (London: Routledge, 1996), pp. 3–20.

[8]　Anne Fausto-Sterling, *Sexing the Body: Gender Politics and the Construction of Sexuality* (New York: Basic Books, 2000), p. 35.

culture, from alchemical works to political pamphlets. For an identity that is effaced by the legal system, intersexuality, particularly in the form of the hermaphrodite, is one of the most visible figures of the time. The intersexual is celebrated and reviled, alternately a monster and a god, thus reflecting ambivalence towards the rigid gender roles imposed by the law as well as towards what has been declared by law and by the Church to be sexual deviance. The omnipresence of the hermaphrodite in most aspects of Renaissance culture suggests attraction towards sexual ambiguity as well as fear of transgression of sexual roles. In particular, the medical treatises of the period reflect the complexity of these attitudes, as well as the variety of sexual bodies that are to be found in nature. When a range of evidence, in the form of documents from various realms of culture, is examined, a complex view of sex/gender is revealed.

Many articles have been published on intersexuality/hermaphrodism in the Renaissance. These studies tend to focus on the hermaphrodite either as an object of scientific study, or as a literary figure, thus perpetuating a division between the disciplines that was not so pronounced in the Renaissance. This study of the figure of the hermaphrodite in Renaissance culture brings a variety of disciplines back together: medical and alchemical treatises, lyric poetry, political discourse, and satirical novels. In demonstrating the close relationship between these disciplines in their representation of sexual and gender ambiguity (that is, the ambiguity of the body as a biological entity and as a cultural/social presentation of that entity), this study proposes that sex and gender are not self-contained categories, but are crucial to our ways of knowing the world (epistemology), to social and political ordering (the hierarchy of power), and even to spiritual matters (religious debates and divisions).

The hermaphrodite is an obsessively present figure in almost all aspects of early modern culture, most of all in France, where rigid enforcement of narrowly defined gender roles was believed to be the very foundation of society. As this society seems to crumble under the weight of religious strife and social disorder, these rigid gender divisions are being called into question. The hermaphrodite becomes both an icon of political disorder and one of the potential unity that could arise from an acceptance of diverse religious views. These mutually contradictory uses of the hermaphrodite signal political and social shifts, as well as a deeper epistemological crisis: how does one distinguish the true from the false (or the self from the other, the Catholic from the Protestant) if deceptive appearances are all that we have to guide us? The hermaphrodite, often appearing male or female in order to conform to social norms, does not necessarily have a body that matches this appearance. Seeing is not always believing.

This, then is the importance of maintaining an interdisciplinary approach in the discussion of sex and gender in the early modern period: the imaginary aspect of sex, which can be seen as an early form of gender, is as significant to early modern authors as direct observations of the body. This imaginary aspect not only drives social responses to the sexed body, but, as Duval will argue, can transform the body itself. In a nation where one must be male to govern, the sexual imaginary thus had a profound impact on politics.

The introduction and the first five chapters of this book survey some of the major sources for Renaissance images of the hermaphrodite. The introduction reviews some classical versions of the myth of the hermaphrodite, representative of a range of attitudes towards intersexuality – from the monstrous to the divine – as well as the presentation of homosexuality in Petronius's *Satyricon*, a text influential for late Renaissance representations of the hermaphrodite.

The first chapter, "Sexual Dissonance: Early Modern Scientific Accounts of Hermaphrodism," analyzes the work of Ambroise Paré, in particular its relationship to literary and popular sources, in order to demonstrate the extent to which medical treatises of the period might have been guided by cultural attitudes towards sex and gender. The second chapter, "The Cultural and Medical Construction of Gender: Caspar Bauhin," continues the analysis of the relationship between medicine and cultural attitudes through a study of the work of an influential professor of anatomy and botany, but views it in the light of sixteenth century skepticism, which allows some authors to reject classical authorities in favor of more empirical approaches to sex/gender designations. "Jacques Duval on Hermaphrodites," the third chapter, traces the further rise of empirical science over more traditional and conservative medical practices, and how this transformation of the discipline creates the opportunity for a more nuanced understanding of the body (particularly in relation to sex and gender). Nonetheless, medical discourse remains trapped in the traditional division of the sexes into two clear-cut roles, male and female, even though this traditional view is contradicted by actual observation of the complexly gendered hermaphroditic body.

As the fourth chapter, "Hermetic Hermaphrodites," and the fifth chapter, "Gender and Power in the Alchemical Works of Clovis Hesteau de Nuysement," suggest, alchemy offers an alternative to the somewhat more conservative and more mainstream medical tradition, even as it echoes that tradition. The mutability of forms represented by alchemical discourse echoes the potential mutability of gender roles. In alchemical treatises, the doubly-gendered hermaphrodite is a symbol both of dissolution and of divine power; it is also the monster depicted in popular pamphlets of the time. Still, philosophical or spiritual alchemy can be seen as offering a more positive and inclusive alternative to the rigid religious, political, and social hierarchies of the day; it is therefore profoundly subversive and often declared heretical in this period. The role of alchemy in the creation of a nuanced representation of sex and gender has been largely ignored by scholars until this moment. Yet alchemical works were widely published and read, by women and men. Our postmodern view of alchemy as a trivial pursuit, rather than as a widespread practice involving preparations of medicines and dyes, spiritual contemplation, and an even wider range of practices that brought the physical and the spiritual together, obscures its importance in the early modern period. Thus, a major body of work concerning sex and gender roles is generally ignored in studies of gender in the early modern period. Given that this work provides a striking alternative to the notions promulgated by academic medicine of the time, this omission tends to distort scholar's views of the early modern period. This study proposes to remedy this oversight.

The more positive, almost Neoplatonic, hermaphrodite of the alchemical tradition is adopted by court poets and others, as is evident in the sixth chapter of the book, "Lyric Hermaphrodites." This figure serves to define the king's power as at once divine and almost supernatural. Unfortunately, these ambiguous images of Henri III are almost immediately turned against him and against his agenda of religious tolerance, as the conservative Catholic League links his divine hermaphrodism to accusations of homosexuality and bisexuality (a propaganda campaign analyzed in the seventh chapter, "The Royal Hermaphrodite: Henri III of France"). Once again, at the end of the sixteenth century, the view of hermaphrodism as monstrous dominates the more positive view of it as a symbol of divine power.

In the final chapter, "Hermaphrodites Newly Discovered: The Cultural Monsters of Sixteenth-Century France," Thomas Artus's novel, *L'Isle des Hermaphrodites*, is studied as a summary of the cultural anxieties elicited by the figure of the hermaphrodite and by its effacing of neat, hierarchical gender divisions. According to the narrator of this work, without the assumption of male superiority over the female, the family, all laws, the army, religion, the government, and all other social institutions crumble into utter chaos. Yet the hermaphrodites are depicted as not only amusing, but somewhat alluring and highly sexualized, which suggests that the society that cannot hold fast in the face of such charming creatures is fragile indeed.

For the figure of the hermaphrodite evokes all of the crises of the Renaissance: the discovery of "new" cultures that had flourished without the benefit of Christianity, the Reformation itself and the violent religious conflicts it engendered (echoed by the sacrificial hermaphrodite of the alchemical treatises), the consolidation of royal power at the expense of traditional feudal power structures. It is an always changing figure that reflects the turbulent times in which it was so frequently invoked.

Platonic and Neoplatonic Sources

The hermaphrodite's dual nature, at once divine and monstrous in the more menacing sense of that word (from *monstrare*, meaning to show, but also to indict or condemn), stemmed from long philosophical and religious traditions, already well-established by classical times. The hermaphrodite's central role in early gnostic thought, as Creator of the universe, is the most striking example of divine hermaphrodism. The hermaphrodite as a subhuman or weakened figure dominates Greek and Roman depictions. Although Marie Delcourt argues that in pre-historic cults, the hermaphrodite was a figure of divine power, of fertility and procreation, of the union of mother and child,[9] written accounts, even Aristophanes' tale in the *Symposium*, are ambiguous at best. The hermaphrodite, while designated as one of the original beings from which men and

---

[9]   Marie Delcourt, *Hermaphrodite: Mythes et rites de la bisexualité dans l'antiquité classique* (Paris: Presses Universitaires de France, 1958), pp. 30–39.

women are descended, is also described in comic terms. In his account, Aristophanes balances distinction with dissolution of difference; "in the beginning," there were three sets of double beings, male, female, and hermaphrodite.[10] At once sublime and ridiculous, Aristophanes's hermaphrodites represent a pre-verbal and pre-Oedipal undifferentiated state (and yet, not completely, since they are at once male and female – thus, they remain at the limits of distinction). They threaten to revolt against the gods, and they are bisected and subjected once more to the laws of the gods by further categorization and distinction. This imposition of distinction nearly kills them, and the hermaphrodites (of all genders) seek constantly to efface the gap between themselves.

This myth of idealized dissolution is further subjected to categorization in a theological sphere, when Leone Ebreo reconciles the Aristophanic version to the account of the Creation of Man (and coincidentally, Woman) in *Genesis* in his *Dialoghi d'amore*, first published in 1535 in Rome.[11] Leone also cleverly explains the contradictions in the Biblical version, thus subjecting *Genesis* to Aristophanic hermaphrodism:

> ... that Adam, that is the first man, whom God created on the sixth day of the Creation, being a human individual, combined in himself male and female without division; and therefore the text says that God created Adam in His own likeness, 'male and female created He them.' And at one time it speaks of Adam in the singular as a man, at another in the plural – male and female created He them – to denote that, being one individual, he contained in himself both male and female. Wherefore the ancient Hebrew commentators in their Chaldean commentary here say, 'Adam was created of

---

10 Plato, *Symposium*, trans. Michael Joyce, in *The Collected Dialogues of Plato*, eds Edith Hamilton and Huntington Cairns (Princeton: Princeton University Press, Bollingen Series, 1963), pp. 542–3 (189e–190b).

11 Edgar Wind points out, in his chapter on "Pan and Proteus" in *Pagan Mysteries in the Renaissance* (New York: Norton, 1958), p. 211, that Philo and Origen gave this interpretation of the original human, which Pico then adopted, as did Agrippa von Nettesheim in his *De occulta philosophia* (Wind, *Pagan Mysteries*, pp. 3, 8). Thus, the notion of the original, unfallen man as a hermaphrodite was quite widespread in the Renaissance. This information follows Wind's discussion of the hermaphroditic Venus figure in Spenser's *Faerie Queene* (IV, x, 41):

> ... she hath both kinds in one,
> Both male and female, both under one name:
> She sire and mother is herself alone,
> Begets and eke conceives, nor needeth other none.

This female version of the hermaphrodite seems unusual, but might well stem from early versions of an Earth-goddess who produces life independently (for example, Ovid, *Metamorphoses*, bk 1, l.157).

two persons, the one part male the other female.' Moreover, the last text, which says that God created Adam male and female and called their name Adam, they interpret as meaning that Adam alone contained both sexes, and that there was first an individual called Adam, because the woman was never called Eve until she was separated from the male, Adam. And this was the source of that ancient androgyne of Plato and the Greeks who was half man and half woman.[12]

According to Leone, the creation of Eve was the source for the Platonic myth of bisection of the androgyne. Leone carefully ignores the double men and women of the original Aristophanic myth, since his goal is to glorify heterosexual, marital, love.[13] Leone portrays the division into male and female, resulting in categorization, as the cause of sin (by weakening the hermaphroditic being) and of the Fall of man.

Leone conflates the spiritual androgyne with the monstrous hermaphrodite; this association of the monstrous with the divine is characteristic also of the alchemical texts, and takes on particular strength by the end of the sixteenth century.[14] Thus, Leone can be seen as offering a valuable alternative to Marsilio Ficino's more spiritual reading of the Aristophanic myth, one that proves fruitful for French lyric poetry.[15] Ficino eliminates any possible corporeal referent from the text, saying that the hermaphroditic form is a figure for two forms of intellect, one natural and

---

[12] Leone Ebreo (Leo Hebraeus), *The Philosophy of Love*, trans. F. Friedeberg-Seeley and Jean H. Barnes (London: The Soncino Press, 1937), pp. 348–50.

[13] Naomi Yavneh, "The Spiritual Eroticism of Leone's Hermaphrodite," in *Playing with Gender: A Renaissance Pursuit*, eds Jean Brink, Maryanne C. Horowitz, and Allison Coudert (Urbana and Chicago: University of Illinois Press, 1991), p. 86, discusses Leone's hermaphrodites as a symbol of heterosexual union.

[14] As Yavneh notes, Carla Freccero, in her essay "The Other and the Same: The Image of the Hermaphrodite in Rabelais," from the collection *Rewriting the Renaissance: The Discourses of Sexual Difference in Early Modern Europe*, eds Margaret W. Ferguson, Maureen Quilligan, and Nancy J. Vickers (Chicago: University of Chicago Press, 1986), pp. 145–58, distinguishes the term "androgyne" from that of "hermaphrodite," relegating the former to the spiritual realm, and the latter to that of the purely monstrous. This distinction becomes less and less operative with the rise of medical treatises towards the end of the sixteenth century. For an excellent study of the history of the androgyne in this period, see Marian Rothstein, "Mutations of the Androgyne: Its Functions in Early Modern French Literature," *Sixteenth Century Journal* 34, 2 (2003): 409–37.

[15] See Gisèle Mathieu-Castellani, *Les Thèmes amoureux dans la poésie française, 1570–1600* (Paris: Klincksieck, 1975), pp. 98–9; but note that whereas Mathieu-Castellani states that Leone's *Dialoghi* did *not* justify carnal love, his work was in fact used quite often for that purpose (since he does seem to justify physical love within the context of marriage). See also Guy Demerson, *La Mythologie classique dans l'oeuvre lyrique de la "Pléiade"* (Geneva: Droz, 1972), pp. 169, 175, 181; 194, 208–9, 213, 240, 243, 355.

one supernatural.[16] In fact, the hermaphroditic device on Gargantua's medallion[17] can thus be seen as a humorous extension of Leone's version of the myth, rather than of Ficino's philosophy.[18] At any rate, whether effaced in an image of purely spiritual love, as in Ficino's commentary on the *Symposium*, or held by the bonds of marriage, the hermaphrodite (although powerful) remains tamed in the context of Neoplatonic philosophy, an image of harmony. The perfect, masculine aspect controls the feminine; and thus, within the Neoplatonic hermaphrodite, the feminine is effaced.[19] But this was not the only version of the hermaphrodite to dominate the Renaissance. The medical assessment of the hermaphrodite was still as an anomaly; alchemy joined the image of fruitful union with that of death and decay. And the Ovidian hermaphrodite, in its various Renaissance manifestations, expressed a fear of castration by means of insatiable female sexuality, a fear of loss of male identity.

---

[16] *Marsile Ficin: Sur le Banquet de Platon ou de l'Amour*, ed. and trans. Raymond Marcel (Paris: Les Belles Lettres, 1956), p. 169. For a reading of this passage, see again the essay by Freccero, cited above.

[17] François Rabelais, *Gargantua*, ed. V.L. Saulnier (Geneva: Droz, 1970), p. 60.

[18] Jerome Schwartz notes this possibility in his article, "Scatology and Eschatology in Gargantua's Androgyne Device," *Etudes rabelaisiennes*, 14 (1977): 272–4 (the section on Leone). Leone is also echoed in Barthélemy Aneau's emblem book, *Imagination poétique* (Lyon: Macé Bonhomme, 1552), p. 19, in the image of marriage. Again, as in Rabelais's image, the heads of the hermaphroditic couple face each other:

L'Hermaphrodite est icy en pincture
A double face, & a double Nature,
Lune de Masle, & l'aultre de femelle,
En un seul corps, ou l'un l'autre se mesle,
Puys deux baisers sont baillez, & renduz
Par les deux chefs l'un vers l'autre estenduz.
    Qui sont plaisirs d'Amours perpetuel
De l'un vers l'autre, en effect mutuel.

(The hermaphrodite is here in paint, with a double face and a double nature, one of male, and the other female; in one body, one and the other are mixed, then two kisses are offered and returned, by two heads, one stretched towards the other. Which are the pleasures of perpetual love of one towards the other, in effect mutual.) Unless otherwise noted, all translations of primary sources in this study are my own. This figure is also analyzed by Schwartz (269).

[19] Yavneh, p. 94: "The masculine, says Filone, is the perfect, active intellect, whereas the feminine is the imperfect, passive body; in perfect union, the sensual feminine body is obedient to masculine reason and intellect."

The Hermaphrodite as Effeminate Man: Ovid and Aristotle

In Ovid's version of the hermaphrodite, the feminine, while effaced in the union itself, presents a less obedient, tractable aspect. Heterosexuality, while it brings on a loss of identity for the woman, menaces a diminishing of identity for the man as well. Whereas, to a large extent, the Aristophanic myth represented the search for the origins of the self, as distinct from the other, the Ovidian myth expresses the fear of dissolution into the other, the fear that those boundaries created at the dawn of time may at any moment be transgressed.

Hermaphroditus, although designated as the son of Mercury and Venus,[20] is named only *puer* until his transformation in the waters of Salmacis's spring. Yet his identity is already given only as derivative and divided:

> cuius erat facies, in qua materque paterque
> cognosci possent; nomen quoque traxit ab illis. (*Met.*, bk 4, ll. 290–91)

> (In whose face, they could know [recognize] the mother and father; even his name was taken from them.)

This lack of differentiated or individual identity, of his own face (it is rather those of his mother and father), of his own name, already signals the boy's fate. He is posited at first as the subject of the story, the master of the gaze into a pool made to be looked at (and through):

> … videt hic stagnum lucentis ad imum
> usque solum lymphae. (*Met.*, bk 4, ll. 297–8)

> (He saw there a pool of water glistening with light to the very bottom …)

This spring is inhabited by the nymph Salmacis, who is also gazing at the boy: "cum puerum vidit visumque optavit habere" (l. 316: "when she saw the boy, she wanted what she saw"). She proposes her love to the boy, who seems ignorant of love ("nescit enim, quid amor," l. 330); she even begins to touch and kiss him in what is described as a threatening way (l. 335: "iamque manus ad eburnea colla ferenti" – "she already is placing her hands on his ivory neck"). He tells her to desist (*desinis*) or he will flee (l. 336); thus trying to make himself the subject of his own story, to dictate the action. Assuming his right to be where he is, and ignoring her right to be in or at her own spring, he sends her away. Her response, while conciliatory on the surface, indicates that she is not prepared to relinquish her own power as subject: "Loca … haec tibi

---

[20] Ovid, *Metamorphoses*, ed. William S. Anderson (Leipzig: Teubner, 1985), bk 4, l. 288. All references to Ovid are to this edition (and give book and line number); all translations are my own.

libera trado,/ hospes" (ll. 337–8: "I leave this place free to you, my guest"). He is her guest; she *allows* him to be there.

Hermaphroditus seems intent upon retaining and creating distinctions. He cuts himself off from Salmacis by his refusal; he sees the pond as a distinct entity from the nymph herself, when in fact the two exist in a sort of symbiotic relationship, different and yet the same. His mania for categorization and separation leads to a blindness towards the effacement of distinction that is already operating in the water. This blindness leads to a permanent dissolution of his separate identity (if that identity ever existed). As he dips into Salmacis's water, she cries victory ("meus est!" at line 356); she surrounds him ("circumfunditur", l. 360) and wraps around him like a serpent (l. 362) or ivy around a tree (l. 365). Still, the boy resists union with the nymph, and so she wishes for permanent union, which the gods grant in a seemingly perverse way:

> ... 'ita di iubeatis, et istum
> nulla dies a me nec me deducat ab isto.'
> vota suos habuere deos: nam mixta duorum
> corpora iunguntur faciesque inducitur illis
> una; velut siquis conducat cortice, ramos
> crescendo iungi pariterque adolescere cernit,
> sic, ubi conplexu coierunt membra tenaci,
> nec duo sunt sed forma duplex, nec femina dici
> nec puer ut possit, nec utrumque et utrumque videtur. (*Met.*, bk 4, ll. 371–9)

('So the gods grant me this, that no day take him from me or me from him!' This wish had gods to grant it. For the mixed bodies of the two were joined, and one face formed out of them; as if someone grafted a branch onto the bark of a tree and saw them in growing joined and maturing together, so the limbs came together in a tight embrace, and they were not two, but a dual form, and it could not be said that it was either woman or boy, but it seemed to be neither and both.)

It is here, after the transformation (at line 383) that Hermaphroditus is finally named. In an attempt to retain his position as subject (even though he is now both subject and object), the boy wishes that the pond have the same evil power over any man who steps into it: "quisquis in hos fontes vir venerit, exeat inde/semivir ..." ("whoever may come to this spring, may he leave here half a man").

This hermaphrodite is quite different from the Aristophanic version, in which male and female remain distinct within the hermaphroditic whole. Here, it could be said that Ovid is echoing the "one-sex" theory suggested in parts of Aristotle's work (particularly the *Generation of Animals*):[21]

---

[21] In *The Complete Works of Aristotle*, ed. Jonathan Barnes (Princeton: Princeton University Press, Bollingen Series, 1984), vol. 1, pp. 1111–218; particularly p. 1113 (716b 5), pp. 1128–32 (726b 1–729a 30), hereafter cited as *GA*. For the reception of Aristotle in the Renaissance, see Ian Maclean, "Medicine, Anatomy, Physiology," in *The Renaissance*

If, then, the male stands for the effective and active, and the female for the passive, it follows that what the female would contribute to the semen of the male would not be semen but material for the semen to work upon. This is just what we find to be the case, for the menstrual blood has in its nature an affinity to the primitive matter. (*GA*, p. 1132; 729a 30)

The woman, as material on which the male works, is inferior:

Again, as the first efficient or moving cause, to which belong the definition and the form, is better and more divine in its nature than the material on which it works, it is better that the superior principle should be separated from the inferior. Therefore, wherever it is possible and so far as it is possible, the male is separated from the female. For the first principle of the movement, whereby that which comes into being is male, is better and more divine, and the female is the matter. (*GA*, p. 1136; 732a 1–10)

Or more clearly: "For the female is, as it were, a mutilated male, and the menstrual fluids are semen, only not pure; for there is only one thing they have not in them, the principle of soul" (*GA*, 737a 25). Aristotle cites Empedocles as attributing gender to greater or lesser heat (*GA*, p. 1182; 764a 1–30); heat being considered a refining and perfecting factor in generation (see Laqueur, cited above).[22] He modifies this theory somewhat: "For when the first principle does not bear sway and cannot concoct the nourishment through lack of heat nor bring it into its proper form, but is defeated in this respect, then must the material change into its opposite, Now the female is opposite to the male ..." (*GA*, p. 1185; 766a 15–20). Thus, the female is not only an inferior male, but a sort of genetic defect, a monster: "If then the male is a principle and a cause, and the male is such in virtue of a certain capacity and the female is such in virtue of an incapacity ..." (*GA*, p. 1186; 766a 30); "For even he who does not resemble his parents is already in a certain sense a monstrosity; for in these cases nature has in a way departed from the type. The first departure indeed is that the offspring should become female instead of male; this, however, is a natural necessity" (*GA*, p. 1187; 767b 5). Aristotle repeats these concepts with insistent frequency: "If the generative residue in the menstrual fluids is properly concocted, the movement imparted by the male will make the form of the embryo in the likeness of itself"

Notion of Woman: A Study in the Fortunes of Scholasticism and Medical Science in European Intellectual Life (Cambridge: Cambridge University Press, 1980), pp. 28–46, as well as Evelyne Berriot-Salvadore, *Un Corps, un destin: la femme dans la médicine de la Renaissance* (Paris: Champion, 1993). See also Thomas Laqueur, "Destiny is Anatomy," in *Making Sex*, pp. 25–62.

22   This theory of gender as "heat-related" is echoed by Galen and then by many Renaissance theorists, such as Jacques Ferrand. See Thomas Laqueur, *Making Sex* ("Destiny is Anatomy," p. 29), and Constance Jordan, *Renaissance Feminism: Literary Texts and Political Models* (Ithaca, New York: Cornell University Press, 1990), pp. 135–6. Jordan links this issue to occasional "transsexuality" and thus to hermaphrodism.

(*GA*, p. 1188; 767b 15). If the movement, or first principle, fails, then a female or a monster will result; Aristotle gives the same explanation for both phenomena: "If the movements relapse and the material is not controlled, at last there remains what is most universal, that is to say the animal" (*GA*, p. 1191; 769b 10). That which is female or monstrous escapes from the father's control, from the divine organizing, categorizing, dividing principle, and wallows in its own chaos. It is in this context that Aristotle introduces his discussion of monstrous and multiple births, a discussion which includes the hermaphrodite:

> Sometimes animals are born with too many toes, sometimes with one alone, and so on with the other parts, for they may be multiplied or they may be mutilated. Again, they may have the generative parts doubled, the one being male, the other female; this is known in men and especially in goats. (*GA*, pp. 1192–3; 770b 30–33)

Aristotle finds the explanation for such deformities of excess as hermaphrodism in the quantity of material provided by the mother. Aristotle denies the possibility of the "perfect" hermaphrodite, in which both male and female characteristics are complete. He is somewhat vague as to the cause of this double, yet different, nature:

> In certain cases we find a double set of generative organs [one male and the other female]. When such duplication occurs the one is always functional but not the other, because it is always insufficiently supplied with nourishment as being contrary to nature; it is attached like a tumour (for such growths also receive nourishment though they are a later development than the body proper and contrary to nature). If the formative power prevails, both are similar; if it is altogether vanquished, both are similar; but if it prevail here and be vanquished there, then the one is female and the other male. (*GA*, p. 1195; 772b, 26–33)

In short, if the formative power of the male seed should prevail, then a male offspring will result. If the material supplied by the maternal womb overcomes the male seed, then a female will be born. But if the male seed should only dominate in part, and the material maintain some power, then a hermaphrodite will result.[23] If the material produced by the female has some power in the determination of gender, then perhaps the female's role in generation is not, after all, insignificant. The existence of hermaphrodites embarrasses Aristotle's neatly ordered system of male self-generation.

---

23 Jacques Duval in particular criticizes what he sees as silly argumentation, *Des Hermaphrodits*, ch. 41, x7v.

Men Rule, Women Drool: Livy, Petronius, and the Political Uses of Intersexuality

The classical image of the hermaphrodite embraces more than the subversion of categories such as sex; it also unites the idea of sex with notions of race and species, and with the question of what is natural. According to Livy, the hermaphrodite is a more horrifying portent than even a river of blood or a meteor shower, and the rite for cleansing society of this threat to its very existence is elaborate:

> Relieved of their religious scruples, men were troubled again by the report that at Frusino there had been born a child as large as a four-year-old, and not so much a wonder for size as because, just as at Sinuessa two years before, it was uncertain whether male or female. In fact the soothsayers summoned from Etruria said it was a terrible and loathsome portent; it must be removed from Roman territory, far from contact with earth, and drowned in the sea. They put it alive into a chest, carried it out to sea and threw it overboard. The pontiffs likewise decreed that thrice nine maidens should sing a hymn as they marched through the city.[24]

The boundaries of gender are re-established by ritual incantations made by virgins, in some ways the ultimate symbol of sexual difference and of maintenance of those boundaries.

So, the fear of dissolution of categories reached beyond this basic question of sexual difference, to the problematic difference between human and animal, natural and unnatural. In another passage of Livy, the human hermaphrodite is even listed as an animal:

> Further, dread forms of animals were reported in several places: among the Sabines, a child of uncertain sex was born, while another was found whose sex, at the age of sixteen, could not be determined. At Frusino there was born a lamb with a pig's head, at Sinuessa a pig with a man's head, on the public land in Lucania, a colt with five feet. All these disgusting and monstrous creatures seemed to be signs that nature was confusing species; but beyond all else the hermaphrodites caused terror, and they were ordered to be carried out to sea, as had been done with a similar monstrosity not long before in the consulship of Gaius Claudius and Marcus Livius.[25]

The insistence on using the masculine form *natus* for the birth of the hermaphrodite, and later the word *semimares*, indicates the difficulty ancient Romans experienced when faced with gender ambiguity. This refusal even to recognize on an intellectual level what nature presents to them, is accompanied by a ritual of repression, in which

---

[24] Livy, *Historia naturalis*, bk 27, translated by Frank Gardner Moore (Cambridge, MA: Harvard University Press, Loeb Classical Library, 1963), ch. 37, pp. 356–9.

[25] Livy, *Historia naturalis*, bk 31, translated by Evan T. Sage (Cambridge, MA: Harvard University Press, Loeb Classical Library, 1961), ch. 12, pp. 38–9.

the infant cannot even be killed or buried, but must be drowned far out in the sea. This annihilation of ambiguity seems designed to deny its existence. Ironically, the repressed returns quite insistently, as hermaphrodite after hermaphrodite is born and destroyed. Livy gave multiple accounts of these births, thus indicating fascination with as well as repulsion towards these beings.

The fact that the Romans are more horrified by a hermaphrodite than by a man-faced pig reveals something about the status of women in the Republic. But the conjunction of these two forms of "monstrosity" also reveals a fear of effacement of difference between species. If man can be monstrous, then he is no more than an animal; and perhaps he is even worse. If man's identity is based on division between himself and others who are placed on a lower social or "natural" plane by the very act of separation, then effacement of that division and the intrusion of the other, whether animal or female, into the masculine domain of the self, form a threat to man's status and even to his identity. This is as true of early modern France as it is of Livy's Rome; and the alternating fascination and horror with which early modern hermaphrodites were greeted reflect this cultural source.

The biological and epistemological problems that the hermaphrodite poses cannot be separated from the political issues that link sexuality and class. Although the overlapping nature of these issues is suggested in the passages from Livy and Ovid, they are pushed to the forefront of Petronius's *Satyricon*. Ambiguity in gender roles and in physical appearance is linked to the homosexual romance of the novel, thereby creating a cluster of issues that reappear in Thomas Artus's novel, *L'Isle des Hermaphrodites*, which in fact alludes to this romance.[26] Gender, particularly gender roles as expressed through sexuality, is linked to questions of class and power. In his mordant satire, Petronius seems to take on Roman sexual mores, which are defined by and define social status. The young man Giton is described in feminine terms, and although the description is sexually charged, it is also derogatory: "An adolescent sullied by all sorts of pleasure and by his own confession worthy of exile, free except from debauchery, freeborn but only for debauchery, whose years (youth) are worth only a token, hired as a girl even by one who thought he was a man."[27] In clothing and behavior, the antihero Encolpius and his cohorts, especially Giton, destabilize the distinctions between masculine and feminine.

---

26 Thomas Artus, *Description de l'Isle des Hermaphrodites, nouvellement descouverte*, republished as part of Pierre de l'Estoile's *Journal de Henri III* (the edition cited here is Paris: La Veuve de Pierre Gandouin, 1744; this is a reprint of the 1724 Duchat edition), p. 30: "... ils envoyerent querir quelques-uns qui chantoient des mieux, & quelques joueurs de luth, lesquels commencerent à jouer & chanter un air, le suject des paroles duquel me sembloit avoir ouï dire autrefois être dans *Petronius*, aux amours de *Trimalcion* ...". The modern edition was prepared by Claude-Gilbert Dubois, *L'Isle des Hermaphrodites* (Geneva: Droz, 1996).

27 Petronius, *The Satyricon*, eds Evan T. Sage and Brady B. Gilleland (New York: Irvington, 1982), p. 76 (section 81).

It is no wonder, then, that in the Renaissance, fragments of the Satyricon were published along with other pieces of poetry that emphasized various forms of gender ambiguity. There was a cluster of editions of the fragments towards the end of the sixteenth century, particularly the collections made by the classical scholars Henri Etienne (1563) and Pierre Pithou (1565, 1587).[28] One fragment in particular, from the later Pithou edition, and attributed to a C. Maecenatis Cilnii, is significant because of its later history:

> Dum dubitat natura marem faceretne puellam,
> Factus es, ô pulcer, paene puella puer. (Petronius, *Satyricon*, Pithou edition, p. 152, G4v)

> (When nature was hesitating whether to make a boy or a girl, you were created, o beautiful almost girl almost boy.)

Pithou includes this fragment because of its similarity to some of the material in the *Satyricon*. Caspar Bauhin, in his treatise on hermaphrodites, attributes a similar but expanded version of this poem to a very ancient poet "Pulicis":

> Cum mea genitrix gravida gestaret in alvo
>   Quid pareret, fertur consuluisse Deos.
> Mas est, Phoebus ait, Mars foemina, Junoque neutrii.
>   Cumque forem natus, Hermaphroditus eram,
> Quaerenti letum, Juno sic ait, occidet armis,
>   Mars cruce, Phoebus aquis, sors rata quaeque fuit,
> Arbor obumbrat aquas, ascendo decidit ensis,
>   Quem tuleram casu, labor & ipse super:
> Pes haesit ramis, caput incidit omne, talique
>   Foemina, vir, neutrum: flumina, tela, crucem.[29]

> (When my pregnant mother bore me in her womb, she was compelled to consult the Gods as to what would be born. A male, Phoebus said, Mars a girl, Juno, neither. So when I was born, I was a Hermaphrodite. Seeking to know my death, I was told by Juno that I would be killed by arms, Mars said by the cross, Phoebus by water, and so my fate was settled. A tree shaded the water. While I was climbing, my sword fell, thrown by the fall, I slipped and fell on it; my foot caught in a branch, my head fell [into the stream]. Thus by all, river, sword, cross, did I die, woman, man and neither.)

---

[28] Henri Estienne, ed., *Fragmenta poetarum veterum latinorum, quorum opera non extant: Eunii, Accii, Lucilii, Laberii, Pacuvii, Afranii, Naevii, Caecilii aliorumque multorum* (n.p.: Fuggeri, 1563); ed. Pierre Pithou, *Petronii Arbitri Massiliensis Satyrici Fragmenta Restituta et aucta* (Antwerp: Plantini, 1565); *Petronius Arb. Satyricon* (Paris: Patissonium, 1587).

[29] Caspar Bauhin, *De hermaphroditorum monstrosorumque partuum natura* ... B7v.

The popular attribution of this poem to "Antonio Panormitano," although mocked by Bauhin, is probably more likely than to some ancient Latin poet. Bauhin's source is apparently Angelo Poliziano (Politian), who also quotes a Greek version and offers a Latin translation (cited by Bauhin, B7v–B8). At any rate, this poem is circulating in the Renaissance as a classical work, and is loosely associated with the Satyricon. It is imitated frequently in French, first by Pierre le Loyer,[30] then by Jean Loys, and finally by Tristan l'Hermite.

This piece seems occult, as it would make sense only in the context of some strange sacrificial ritual. Each gender – male, female, and neuter (neither) – is killed off by a different form of death. One could argue that the male is castrated, since his sword slips and he is cut by it at the same time. The female is dissolved in water, the element with which she is associated, thus recalling the myths of Byblis, Cyane, and Arethusa.[31] The word *crux* could also designate a rack on which those to be executed were torn to pieces, thus splitting the neuter into its component parts. Or, since the hermaphrodite is hung upside down, this death could recall the reversal of nature that this being was thought to represent. But in fact, each death seems to apply to each and all of the genders. The absolute annihilation by multiple forms of death, crucifixion, drowning, and scission seems to recall Livy's horrendous hermaphrodites which must be destroyed completely in order to cleanse Rome of some impurity. In fact, the hermaphrodites mentioned in Livy are destroyed by drowning. The Aristophanic beings are cut in two. Crucifixion, although not historically linked to hermaphrodites, is the favored Roman mode of execution, eventually inflicted on homosexuals. If this is a classical epigram of a later date, by 390, the death penalty had been prescribed for passive homosexual intercourse (male sexual aggressivity obviously remained an ideal in the early Christian period, as it had been in ancient Rome). This penalty was later extended to all forms of homosexuality.[32]

To some extent, it can be argued that the early Roman social hierarchy was further enforced by free men who imposed their sexual will on others; women, slaves, and sometimes men of lower standing had no recourse in the case of sexual assault, and were expected to accept it. A free man who practiced the passive role (that is to

---

30   In his *Sonnets politiques ou meslanges*, from *Les Oeuvres et meslanges poetiques de Pierre le Loyer, Angevin* (Paris: Jean Poupy, 1579), pp. 98–9.

31   Ovid, *Metamorphoses*, bk 9, ll. 450–665; bk 5, ll. 409–37; bk 5, ll. 577–641.

32   See also Amy Richlin, *The Garden of Priapus: Sex and Aggression in Roman Humor* (New Haven: Yale University Press, 1983), and "The Meaning of *irrumare* in Catullus and Martial," *Classical Philology* 76 (1981): 40–46; as well as T.P. Wiseman's study of Catullus, *Catullus and his World: A Reappraisal* (Cambridge: Cambridge University Press, 1985), especially pp. 10–14. These works were signaled to me by Philip Covitz, in his undergraduate thesis for Brandeis University, *Catullus and Lesbia: A Biographical Approach to the Poems* (1990). Justinian made this prohibition even more repressive, and included all forms of homosexuality in 538/39 and in 559, according to James Brundage, in *Law, Sex, and Christian Society in Medieval Europe* (Chicago: The University of Chicago Press, 1987), p. 121.

say, allowed himself to be penetrated) in intercourse would be deprived of certain rights (Brundage, p. 49); Giton, because of his feminine looks and demeanor, is assumed to be a slave (Petronius, *The Satyricon*, p. 44). Thus, sexuality and politics were intimately linked. Petronius's novel, although a parody of Greek romance, is also obsessively about social status and various forms of power (sexual, financial, political). This constellation of concerns brings the problem of ambiguous gender from the ethereal realms of spiritual and epistemological questions of distinction (as manifested in Plato and Ovid) to the more immediate political and social effects of such concerns. *The Satyricon* thus conveys the grittier side of gender ambiguity to a late Renaissance audience. It is also clear from Petronius's novel, as from Ovid's tale, that the supposedly philosophical and spiritual discussions of gender and sexuality cannot remain outside of the realm of the political.

One final source is crucial to the development of late Renaissance theories of the hermaphrodite, and brings the political and theological realms together in the discussion of this figure. Saint Augustine, in the sixteenth book of *The City of God*, discusses various monsters, among them hermaphrodites, and asserts that not even these monsters are contrary to nature, as they are created by the will of God. For Saint Augustine, these and all creatures are the signs of God's power: "But no faithful Christian should doubt that anyone who is born anywhere as a man – that is, a rational and mortal being – derives from that one first-created human being. And this is true, however extraordinary such a creature may appear to our senses."[33] This call to acceptance is echoed in the sixteenth century by Michel de Montaigne: "Ce que nous appelons monstres, ne le sont pas à Dieu ... Nous apelons contre nature ce qui advient contre la coustume," ("Those which we call monsters are not so to God ... We call that which is not familiar to us unnatural ...").[34] Monsters are deemed such because of the ignorance of men, not because of the imperfection of nature. This view will serve throughout the Middle Ages as a counterbalance to the more negative Aristotelian view of monsters.

The Hermaphrodite and Questions of Identity

Still, the image of the hermaphrodite is most often an expression, and a powerful one, of the fear of the other. Expression of this fear is also apparent in the assumption

[33] Augustine, *The City of God*, trans. Henry Bettenson (London: Penguin, 1976), bk 16, ch. 8, pp. 661–2. For a more detailed analysis of this passage, see Lorraine Daston, "Marvelous Facts and Miraculous Evidence in Early Modern Europe," *Critical Inquiry* 18 (1991): 93–124, reprinted in *Wonders, Marvels, and Monsters in Early Modern Culture*, ed. Peter Platt (Newark, DE: University of Delaware Press, 1999), pp. 76–104.

[34] Michel de Montaigne, "D'un enfant monstrueux," *Les Essais*, ed. Pierre Villey (Paris: Presses Universitaires de France, 1978), bk 2, essay 30, p. 713.

that natives of the newly discovered world are cannibals,[35] in the obsession with monsters,[36] and with monstrous births in particular.[37] As Donna Haraway points out, monsters are implicated in the creation of individual and community identity:

> Monsters have always defined the limits of community in Western imaginations. The Centaurs and Amazons of ancient Greece established the limits of the centred polis of the Greek male human by their disruption of marriage and boundary pollutions of the warrior with animality and woman. Unseparated twins and hermaphrodites were the confused human material in early modern France who grounded discourse on the natural and supernatural, medical and legal, portents and diseases – all crucial to establishing modern identity.[38]

Seen as the ground against which "normal" identity is delineated, these monsters also problematize the notion of human identity by their effacement of boundaries between animal and man and between male and female.[39] Fear of this indistinction is apparent in the severe legal sanctions imposed on hermaphrodites who do not live within the gender decided for them by doctors and the state, sanctions that are linked to a clear phobia concerning homosexuality and an obvious misogyny, according to Lorraine Daston and Katharine Park.[40]

These images of the other, often clustered together in medical treatises (Bauhin associates all types of monsters with hermaphrodites) and alchemical works suggest a fear of the dissolution of the self as an individual identity and voice. There is a fear in these images of the hermaphrodite of cannibalism as well as of gender blurring and monstrosity, a fear of being subsumed or replaced by the other, or worse, of being

---

[35]	See Michel de Montaigne, "Des Cannibales," in *Les Essais*, bk 1, essay 31, pp. 202–14; and Michel de Certeau, "Montaigne's 'Of Cannibals': The Savage 'I'," in *Heterologies: Discourse on the Other*, trans. Brian Massumi (Minneapolis: University of Minnesota Press, 1986), pp. 67–79.

[36]	See Jean Céard, *La Nature et les prodiges* (Geneva: Droz, 1975).

[37]	Montaigne, "D'un enfant monstrueux," *Essais*, 2, 30, pp. 712–13; Ambroise Paré, *Des Monstres et prodiges*, ed. Céard (Geneva: Droz, 1971); as well as Pierre Boaistuau, *Histoires prodigieuses les plus memorables qui ayent esté observes depuis la nativité de Jesus Christ, jusques à nostre siecle ...* (Paris: Vincent Sertenas, 1560).

[38]	Donna Haraway, "A Cyborg Manifesto: Science, Technology, and Socialist-Feminism in the Late Twentieth Century," in her *Simians, Cyborgs, and Women: The Reinvention of Nature* (New York: Routledge, 1991), p. 180.

[39]	The breaching of boundaries between human and animal is seen by Haraway as a twentieth-century event ("Cyborg Manifesto," p. 151), yet the permeability of such boundaries, and their artificial (that is, culturally created) nature was explored early on by Classical and Renaissance philosophy. Montaigne, in his "Apologie de Raimond Sebond," explores animal language and technology (particularly in medical matters) to shatter the illusion of human uniqueness.

[40]	"Hermaphrodites in Renaissance France," *Critical Matrix* 1 (1985): 1–19.

the other. To further complicate matters, the hermaphrodite is associated in virtually all of the alchemical literature and some of the satirical materials with incest and human sacrifice (the cutting of the body into tiny pieces). Thus, dissolution of the family and of the body itself seems to be a menace related to that of the elimination of gender distinction.

To some extent, these fears must be placed within their historical context, as I have suggested above. The French countryside and its people were continually ravaged, over the course of more than forty years, by the Wars of Religion. Catholicism as a crucial element of French identity had been cast into doubt by the presence of the Huguenots, who were at once French and not French, the self and yet other. The fact that this presence was menacing is proved by the vehemence with which many French Catholics undertook the annihilation of their Protestant countrymen, during the massacres of Saint Bartholomew's Day in particular, but also over the course of several centuries.[41]

The hierarchy of French society also depended critically on the model of domination of man over woman. This model in turn depended on a large body of scientific and philosophical knowledge, as well as theological doctrine. As intellectuals such as Paré[42] and later Bauhin began to question the Aristotelian view of the woman as the mere field of generation, to propose a more egalitarian view of conception (based to some degree on Hippocrates), the distinction between male and female, usually made simply on the basis of the assumption that men were superior, and women inferior or underdeveloped men, was destabilized. Many of the early cases of revisionist theories of generation, in which the woman as well as the man provides the seed for the embryo, revolve around the figure of the hermaphrodite, a being whose conception cannot in fact be explained by the male-dominated theory. Yet other authors, such as Duval, use the hermaphrodite to maintain a more conservative discourse on gender (and on race).

The importance of maintaining the distinctions, arbitrary or not, upon which the culture was based is expressed in every discipline. Thus, scientific discourse seems to respond to deep-seated cultural needs – the need of a nation or of a particular group to protect and perpetuate itself by maintaining those boundaries between the self and the other – rather than discovering some sort of absolute empirical truth upon which the culture would then base itself.[43] What we want to find through scientific observation, we find by structuring the observation itself in certain ways. Of course,

---

[41]   Pierre Miquel, *Les Guerres de Religion* (Paris: Fayard, 1980).

[42]   Paré only mentions this theory in relation to the generation of hermaphrodites in *Des Monstres*; as Laqueur quite rightly points out, he is still somewhat trapped in the one-sex theory in a later chapter of the same book, and in his surgical treatise (*Making Sex*, pp. 126–7).

[43]   Judith Lorber notes this tendency even today, in her chapter "Believing is Seeing: Biology as Ideology," in *Paradoxes of Gender* (New Haven: Yale University Press, 1994), pp. 37–54.

early modern theories of knowledge were more openly oriented towards culture, often including what was "possible" or believable, and even popular tales, as valid forms of knowing. Truth was not an absolute entity for most early modern intellectuals, but rather what was commonly accepted. Nonetheless, enforcement of certain "truths" seems particularly vehement at the end of the sixteenth century, just as these truths seem to be losing their hold. And science becomes an important tool in the defense against the breakdown of categories or against the realization that these categories bind as well as separate.

For example, to the early modern imagination, monsters link the human with the animal, not only because of children born with horns or fur, or the dog with the face of a boy, but because both the human and animal realms are divided into "natural" and "unnatural" by these means.[44] That which is "natural" stays within assigned boundaries, that which is "unnatural" crosses them. Hermaphrodites link the female with the male in a problematic relationship, where the female no longer exists only as a negative reflection of male superiority, but as a sex that is at once different from and connected to the male. The female is obviously not male (not even an inferior male), or the hermaphrodite would be identical to itself, which it is not. Yet in the hermaphrodite, the female is not entirely divided off from the male, either. The feminine is not subsumed into the masculine; both are subsumed into a problematically differentiated whole. According to early modern norms, which associate the natural with clear distinctions between genders, races, and species, the hermaphrodite is not natural. Thus, one can see in the figure of the hermaphrodite, and in the fearful response to this figure, the potential dissolution of sixteenth-century French social structures based on the early modern notion of "natural" law.

As Bauhin's treatise in particular makes clear, there is a distinction between the biological functions and characteristics of the hermaphrodite, and the political functions of the hermaphrodite. When accepted as an interpretable given, that is, when its body is observed, the hermaphrodite cannot have a specific value assigned to it, cannot be condemned by or assimilated into society; it is merely a fact. When interpreted, this figure is invariably politicized, and subsequently effaced by the text created around it. This is to say, the hermaphrodite is overtly read rather than described, treated as an allegory of some event. Thus, its specificity is destroyed and its difference erased by the meaning imposed upon it. The ridiculous nature of such interpretation is underscored by the story Bauhin appends to his version of the monster

---

[44] See, for example, Paracelsus, in *Concerning the Nature of Things* (*De Natura rerum*; trans. Arthur Edward Waite, in *The Hermetic and Alchemical Writings of Aureolus Philippus Theophrastus Bombast of Hohenheim, called Paracelsus the Great*; London: James Elliott and Co., 1894), bk 1, p. 123, compares animals' refusal of monstrous offspring to the human response: "... know that monstrous growths amongst animals ... rarely live long, especially near or amongst other animals, since by their engrafted nature, and by divine arrangement, all monsters are hateful to animals duly begotten from their own likeness. So, too, monstrous human growths seldom live long."

of Ravenna, one in which a German Archbishop is accused of being a hermaphrodite by his rival, the Duke of Brunschweig. Although the Archbishop tries to counter this accusation by revealing his body to all who are willing to observe, language overcomes physical presence and creates the meaning of the body, and the rumors of his dual condition persist (Z6v). For Bauhin, the body expressed is the body repressed, made to conform to a system that effaces it in favor of performative roles. As a professor of anatomy, he struggles with the problematic need to discourse upon the body. For him, the hermaphroditic body, which resists such interpretation, becomes the ultimate figure of any body, and of all that which cannot or should not be controlled by means of language. Such resistance makes the hermaphroditic body the site of subversion of the very political institutions it has been enlisted to support.

The result of this attempt to represent hermaphroditic ambiguity is a diverse group of polymorphous texts. Bauhin's treatise vacillates between a scientific establishment of clear-cut categories and a careful undermining of those categories by means of contradictory specific examples. The alchemical works offer a variety of images and styles of discourse (poetry, parable, emblem, fugue) which break down supposedly rigid chemical formulae into meaningless and yet evocative groups of words. These texts beg for a meaningful reading of some sort, yet also frustrate that imposition. Artus's novel, *L'Isle des Hermaphrodites*, in its odd and lengthy lists of laws (the ultimate site of social meaning, one might expect), plays with polyvalence as both a destructive and endlessly reconstructive force. Hermaphroditic texts offer a cornucopia of words, images, and categories, which in the end defy all systematization, particularly binary. What binds all of the texts analyzed in this study is their paradoxical use of signs in order to demonstrate the resistance of the body to signification, and in order to subvert the politics of interpretation, which is the inevitable result of any system of discourse. Such politics create an insuperable gap between theory and any possible "reality." If theory is the crystallization of discourse, and if discourse is a supplement, which covers over or replaces the body, then the body, and the hermaphroditic body in particular, demonstrates the inefficacy of theoretical discourse. This is the trap that Bauhin and the alchemists find themselves facing.

Gender is the most obvious, most discussed manifestation of this politics of interpretation. Contemporary critics and sociologists have recognized gender as at once a product of society and a self-creating process which underlies most (if not all) social structures:

> As a social institution, gender is a process of creating distinguishable social statuses for the assignment of rights and responsibilities. As part of a stratification system that ranks these statuses unequally, gender is a major building block in the social structures built on these unequal statuses.[45]

---

45   Judith Lorber, *Paradoxes of Gender*, p. 32.

In their article "Fetishizing Gender: Constructing the Hermaphrodite in Renaissance Europe," Ann Rosalind Jones and Peter Stallybrass establish that Renaissance intellectuals already recognized gender as a precarious distinction, one produced by the accoutrements of culture such as clothing, gesture, and language.[46] The threat that the recognition of the factitious nature of gender represented, above all when combined with the realization that gender was so basic to many social structures, created a backlash, particularly in France. This backlash is most evident in the political pamphlets decrying Henri III of France's public display of ambiguous gender. But these pamphlets convey the paradox that the "crisis of gender" in Renaissance France reveals: the call for a return to clearly defined gender roles stands also as an admission that these roles can be created and recreated. Even though much of seventeenth century French culture (particularly the legal system) covers over this flaw in gender-based social structures, the questions about these roles have been raised and remain active in many genres considered marginal or subversive by our standards: alchemical treatises, personal memoirs, satirical pamphlets reveal an ongoing discussion of gender ambiguity.

Sixteenth century France, and the court of Henri III in particular, afford an exceptional opportunity to study how a culture creates, defines, and questions gender at various levels and in various disciplines. At and around the Valois court, medical experts, alchemists, philosophers, lyric poets and political polemicists circulated and conversed. Ambroise Paré was the court physician; Philippe Desportes and Clovis Hesteau de Nuysement were court poets (Henri in fact gathered a large circle of literati around him). The figure of the hermaphrodite, as monstrous and/or divine, held a place of prominence in the works of these authors. In political pamphlets and Artus's satirical novel, *L'Isle des Hermaphrodites*, Henri is associated with the hermaphrodite, and is invariably denigrated or disempowered by this association. Undoubtedly, the hermaphrodite was studied at the Valois court in alchemical and Neoplatonic treatises as a figure of transcendent power. This figure was then twisted by critics of Henri into a monstrous form. Still, this monstrosity was not simply horrifying, but, as the etymology of the word suggests, it points to broader questions concerning knowledge and power.

The concerns surrounding the issue of sex as expressed in classical and medieval texts are embodied in three figures that recur persistently in Renaissance culture. The monster of Ravenna, with its blurring of boundaries between natural and supernatural (as well as between natural and unnatural), between animal and human, and between male and female, is frequently discussed in medical treatises and popular pamphlets of the sixteenth century. This creature recalls the absolute horror and cruelty with which Romans greeted hermaphroditic children, and thus suggests the menace to Renaissance society that dissolution of distinctions represented: this monster is often

---

[46] In *Body Guards: The Cultural Politics of Gender Ambiguity*, eds Julia Epstein and Kristina Straub (New York: Routledge, 1991), p. 87. It should be noted, however, that even a concept that more closely resemble our own notion of gender is always designated in Renaissance texts by the term "sex."

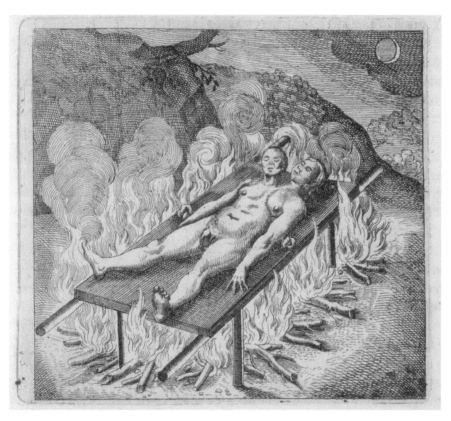

Figure 1   **Plate 33, the hermaphroditic rebis being sacrificed, from Michael Maier's *Atalanta fugiens* (Frankfurt: Andreae, 1687). Courtesy of the Division of Rare and Manuscript Collections, Cornell University Library**

interpreted as an Apocalyptic figure. The alchemical rebis, on the other hand, can be read as a vestige of the divine hermaphrodite, through whom destruction becomes transcendence. The rebis is the direct heir of Neoplatonic and Gnostic traditions. Strangely, both figures serve the purpose of the Reformation: the monster of Ravenna, as a symbol of excess, was read as a condemnation of the Papal court; the rebis, destroyed, purified, and reborn by means of fire, was co-opted by French and German Protestants as a consolatory figure. The corrupt Roman emperor Heliogabalus is the sterile reverse of the hermaphroditic coin. Neutered by surgery in the attempt to become a woman, Heliogabalus is adopted by late Renaissance authors (particularly the polemicists of the reactionary Catholic League) as a symbol of the emptiness created by excess, particularly an excess of religious toleration. The simultaneous existence of two contradictory or conflicting religious "truths" calls into question the existence of any truth whatever, just as the coexistence of two sexes in one body neutralizes at least the reproductive power of the body in question.

Thus, the resurgence of the figure of the hermaphrodite in Renaissance France represents not merely a re-evaluation of sex roles, but a profound epistemological crisis. If such distinctions as those between the sexes (as well as between class, race, and species) are largely created by society, and if our ways of knowing are founded upon these distinctions (in the form of classifications of observable objects and language), then all knowledge is provisional and factitious. In the realm of language, the hermaphrodite can be seen as a figure of the paradoxical necessity of linkage and disjunction between the signifier and the signified. The hermaphroditic body itself is categorized obsessively by Paré, Bauhin, and Duval; yet this body remains unavailable to our scrutiny, the categories merely covering over, writing away, an unacceptable problem of distinction. The medical treatises become ineffectual supplements which lead the reader away from the hermaphroditic body and into a proliferation of imposed distinctions. Of greater interest are the moments in these treatises when the gap between bodily reality and medical discourse becomes apparent; this occurs most frequently in the works of Caspar Bauhin, laden with references to myth, to lyric poetry, to folk beliefs. Here, the arbitrary tyranny of gender roles is made manifest, even if the author retreats back into these roles.

The body remains the focus of the alchemical texts studied in this book; it is omnipresent yet ungraspable, the hidden but manifest truth constantly alluded to. For this reason, the hermaphroditic body is frequently associated with water, particularly water as that element from which all of creation was formed. This focus represents a departure from Neoplatonic sources and some earlier alchemical works; perhaps the obsessive attempts in these works to ground themselves in the body should cause them to be categorized as baroque. But this obsession also recalls certain gnostic traditions. These attempts to "think through the body," as fruitless as they also may be, represent a rejection of the spiritual/material, mind/body, male/female dichotomies that informed Western European culture. Well into the eighteenth century, alchemical texts remained the richest sources of this potentially subversive form of gnosticism.

It should be noted that classical and Renaissance sources associate hermaphrodism with transvestism, homosexuality, and bisexuality. This association underscores the "fetishistic" nature of gender that Jones and Stallybrass observe in early modern texts. But even as transvestism plays with sex and gender roles, and bisexuality seems to subvert them: "Paradoxically, then, bending gender roles and passing between genders does not erode but rather preserves gender boundaries" (Lorber, p. 21). The emphasis on passing from one gender to another, on the incongruity of one's dress, reaffirms the belief that there is an essential sex underneath. The hermaphrodite can participate in society only after it has been surgically or at least imaginatively recreated as male or female.[47]

---

[47]   Suzanne J. Kessler, "The Medical Construction of Gender: Case Management of Intersexed Infants," *Signs* 16 (1990): 3–26. Reprinted in her book, *Lessons from the Intersexed* (New Brunswick, NJ: Rutgers University Press), pp. 12–32.

Because the hermaphrodite was and is inconceivable within social boundaries, its mere existence calls these boundaries into question. The bodily reality of the hermaphrodite, obliterated by social norms, remains the ungraspable truth which calls all of these gender-based norms into question. It is the only truly subversive figure, standing in the margins, mocking the construction of gender.

Thus we are presented, even in the sources for the image of the hermaphrodite as received by the Renaissance, with a cluster of overlapping concerns and issues. The hermaphrodite is a figure of divine strength and of self-sufficiency. And yet again, it is an effeminate man, a woman, a lesser being, sub- rather than supernatural. The issue of monstrosity, of what is or is not natural, is embodied in the bimorphous being. The problematic issue of gender is also summarized here; and thus the hermaphrodite is linked to bisexuality and transvestism. This issue enlarges within the hermaphroditic body to throw into confusion all notions of identity (self as opposed to other, subject as opposed to object, definition by family relations). The confusing amorality of the hermaphroditic image raises questions about ancient, medieval, and Renaissance notions of good and evil; it seems to rest just beyond those two realms. It can be read as a descent into the chaos that lies outside of carefully categorized culture; yet it is also a symbol of harmony, of generation, of corruption, and of renewal. The Renaissance mind is forced to question not only what it knows, but its ways of knowing, because of this figure; and yet it can hope for something greater beyond its own limiting and divided culture. The hermaphroditic figure, like the alchemical *euroboros*, becomes a symbol of the end of an order, an era, and of the beginning of a new era. It is the perfect figure for troubled times.

Chapter 1

Sexual Dissonance: Early Modern Scientific Accounts of Hermaphrodism

The Body in Culture

The medical treatises published in late sixteenth-century France and Switzerland offer a clear indication of the significant shift being prepared in the medical profession from reliance on classical sources to more empirical methods of inquiry; those treatises on sex, sexuality, and childbearing show that these shifts are significant for the early modern elaboration of sexual difference and of gender roles. Publishing in France was dominated by the faculty of theology at the Sorbonne, the prime censoring body in this period, which also dictated the teaching of medicine, as the faculty of medicine was subordinated to the faculty of theology. The Sorbonne vehemently, and sometimes violently, advocated Aristotelian and Thomistic thought over any other. But, by the end of the sixteenth century, the control the Sorbonne wielded was slipping: a number of influential surgeons such as Ambroise Paré and Jacques Duval published treatises that either subtly or openly called into question its conservative approaches. More progressive universities such as Basel and Montpellier supported faculty (Caspar Bauhin at Basel) and produced students (François Rabelais) who published innovative works on sex and sexuality. The following chapters, on medical treatises in Continental Europe, will trace this shift from scholastic and rigidly categorical discussions of sex to more skeptical and flexible presentations of sexual difference.

As Thomas Laqueur demonstrates in his book *Making Sex*,[1] the Renaissance was at first still dominated by dualistic, primarily Aristotelian, notions of sex and of generation, privileging the male as the superior, that is to say active, force in reproduction. A significant movement away from these notions can be traced towards the end of the century, one that, as Lorraine Daston and Katharine Park have demonstrated, is linked to the revival of Hippocratic medicine in the second half of the sixteenth century.[2] Furthermore, alternatives to this simply dualistic worldview already existed in alchemical treatises of the time, and in other forms of mystical thought. In many alchemical treatises, the body is seen as part of a larger (in fact,

---

[1]   Particularly in the chapters, "Destiny is Anatomy," pp. 25–62, and "New Science, One Flesh," pp. 63–113. See also Ian Maclean, *The Renaissance Notion of Woman*.

[2]   Lorraine Daston and Katharine Park, "The Hermaphrodite and the Orders of Nature: Sexual Ambiguity in Early Modern France," *Gay and Lesbian Quarterly* 1 (1995): 419–38.

potentially infinite) whole that is represented as the Divine. One can see in this view of the relationship between macrocosm (the Divine) and microcosm (often portrayed as human) the origins of Spinoza's notion of "an absolute and infinite substance" (as summarized here by Elizabeth Grosz):

> Substance has potentially infinite attributes to express its nature. Each attribute adequately expresses substance insofar as it is infinite (the infinity of space, for example, expresses the attribute of extension), yet each attribute is also inadequate or incomplete insofar as it expresses substance only in one form. Extension and thought – body and mind – are two such attributes. Thus, whereas Descartes claims two irreducibly different and incompatible substances, for Spinoza these attributes are merely different aspects of one and the same substance, inseparable from each other. Infinite substance – God – is as readily expressed in extension as in thought and is as corporeal as it is mental.[3]

The body, then, cannot be contained by the conceptual structures that privilege the mind; as with any entity,

> … The forms of determinateness, temporal and historical continuity, and the relations a thing has with coexisting things provide the entity with its identity. Its unity is not a function of its machinic operations as a closed system (i.e., its functional integration) but arises from a sustained sequence of states in a unified plurality (i.e., it has formal rather than substantive integrity). (Grosz, *Volatile Bodies*, p. 12)

As Moira Gatens notes, the Spinozist body is "a productive and creative body which cannot be definitely 'known' since it is not identical with itself across time."[4] Similarly, in many alchemical treatises, the body is seen as dissolving and reconfiguring its own boundaries.

By the end of the sixteenth century, influential medical authors recognize the intractability of the body in the face of dualistic legal, theological, and philosophical discourses. Theoretical discussions of hermaphrodism focus on the imagined monstrosity, easily contained within a dualistic mode of thought, because it does not in fact exist (or is at least believed by the very authors who describe it not to exist). The "biological" hermaphrodite, on the other hand, can only be defined by a legal determination of its status or by extreme medical intervention (usually deadly in the early modern period), but can never be adequately described, since, in the early modern scheme of things, the hermaphroditic body is never identical with itself even in a specific time frame.

---

[3] As summarized by Elizabeth Grosz in *Volatile Bodies: Toward a Corporeal Feminism* (Bloomington: Indiana University Press, 1994), p. 10.

[4] "Towards a Feminist Philosophy of the Body," in *Crossing Boundaries: Feminism and the Critique of Knowledges*, eds Barbara Caine, E.A. Grosz, Marie de Lepervanche (Sydney: Allen and Unwin, 1988), p. 68.

Thus, the evolution of theories of sex and sexuality is linked to the figure of the hermaphrodite, particularly in the works of Paré,[5] Bauhin, and Duval. Duval and Bauhin use the figure of the hermaphrodite to reveal the significant differences between male and female, rather than arguing for one sex (male). Although they still repeat some Aristotelian notions about the superiority of the male (more so Duval than Bauhin) and although the innovations in these works remain unfulfilled until much later (Laqueur would argue that the seventeenth and eighteenth centuries form the period of real change in general attitudes towards sex or gender),[6] they re-open the question of sex and sexuality in significant ways, and help to shake the stranglehold of Aristotelian theories of generation. Thus, we will read these three works as precursors to an important shift in the representation of sexual difference in medical texts.

This shift in the representation of sex and sexuality is accompanied by a shift in the modes of scientific discourse. In the works of Bauhin in particular, a tension between theoretical explanations and actual case studies becomes quite evident. The theory, stemming from Aristotelian and Hippocratic philosophical medicine, cannot be reconciled with empirical evidence. While the importance of empirical data is increasingly recognized in the late sixteenth century, the sheer force of the humanist revival of classical sources carries the authority of Aristotle and Hippocrates well into the seventeenth century, thus maintaining this uneasy contradictory coexistence of outdated theory and contemporary observation. The inhuman hermaphrodite, such as the monster of Ravenna, being almost totally inscrutable, is more easily placed within a theoretical framework; that is to say, a reading can be imposed on a figure which is not remotely human. But a human hermaphrodite with no other "monstrous" characteristics, such as Marie-Germain (although she is more a transsexual than a hermaphrodite), seems to jar with longstanding constructs of gender (as the social or imaginary manifestation of sex), as we shall see. This tension is evident in Paré's *Des monstres*, in the juxtaposition of the Marie-Germain story with the chapter on hermaphrodites. It is even more apparent in Bauhin's repeated attempts to theorize about the cause and nature of hermaphrodites while drawing from real case studies that defy any coherent explanation. Jacques Duval manages to crystallize case studies within clear rules of sex distinction, returning to essentially Aristotelian models; his work signals the return in the seventeenth century to orderly and hierarchical notions of gender, at least in the medical profession. Nonetheless, some of the cases he cites reveal the gap between cultural notions of gender, and actual manifestations of ambiguous sex. In this contention, I might seem to be contradicting an argument made by Daston and Park that what postmodern theorists now deem "cultural" rather than natural was not so clearly distinguished in the early modern period. Indeed, distinctions between natural and cultural were not so clear in the legal or medical works of the time, and the revival

---

5   *Des monstres et prodiges*, from the *Deux livres de chirurgie* (Paris: Dupuys: 1573, 1575); the modern edition consulted is that of Jean Céard (Geneva: Droz, 1971).

6   In his chapter, "Discovery of the Sexes" in *Making Sex*, pp. 149–92.

of the work of Sextus Empiricus, and particularly of his accounts of cultural relativism in *The Outlines of Pyrrhonism*, problematized the acceptance of "active" and "passive" sexual roles as natural categories. Duval's insistence on the importance of language for the designation of gender, and his retreats at crucial moments into mythological or literary examples, underscores the problematic relationship between theories of sex inherited from classical philosophy and the empirical evidence the dual-sexed body offers to the contrary. Clearly, the imaginatively created or the far-distant monstrous hermaphrodite serves as a better example for proponents of Aristotelian models, since it is in essence a blank sheet on which anything can be written. But the blankness of the monstrous hermaphrodite, the possibility it offers for manipulation of the body into any form, put into question any of those theories which might depend upon it. Thus, the monstrous hermaphrodite is at once fundamental to established theories of sexual difference and destructive of them, showing them as purely imaginary constructs that create their own evidence in circular fashion.

The Monster of Ravenna

Ravenna, 1512. A hermaphroditic monster is born, which, due to its mixture of sex and species, remains indecipherable. Because it does not fit into neat categories of male or female, man or animal, it must be made to conform to some type. Thus, the monstrous form becomes a blank page onto which a highly politicized text is inscribed. In fact, this monster has an illustrious and long iconographic genealogy, traced by Ottavia Niccoli in her book *People and Prophecy in Renaissance Italy*.[7] It also metamorphoses, from a two-legged creature to a monopede, from bearing the letters YXV to simply a Y and a cross, from bat-wings to bird-wings, from no sexual characteristics to hyper-masculine to hermaphroditic, as these various forms suit the interpretations placed upon them. Niccoli points out that these readings are politicized from the first manifestations of the creature; first clerical abuse is suggestion, then the corruption of the Papal Court (*People and Prophecy*, pp. 46–51). Nearly a half-century later, Pierre Boaistuau, author of the *Histoires prodigieuses*, offers a version of this text. Boaistuau seems particularly concerned with monsters and with monstrous births, and clearly places hermaphrodites in this category (as does Tesserant, who augments his collection of tales). His story of the hermaphroditic monster of Ravenna is taken from Rueff's version of the story; he also credits Lycosthenes, Multivallis,[8] and Hedio, and

---

[7] Princeton: Princeton University Press, 1990, ch. 2, "Monster, Divination, and Propaganda in Broadsheets," pp. 30–60.

[8] According to Céard, in his edition of *Des monstres*, pp. 153–5, this is the first account of the monster, written by Joannes Multivallis in a continuation of Eusebius' *Chronicon* (Paris: H. Estienne, 1512). Multivallis also offers the allegorical interpretation used by Lycosthenes (Conrad Wollfhart, *Prodigiorum ac ostentorum chronicon*, Basel: H. Petri, 1557), Boaistuau, and Bauhin (Céard, p. 175).

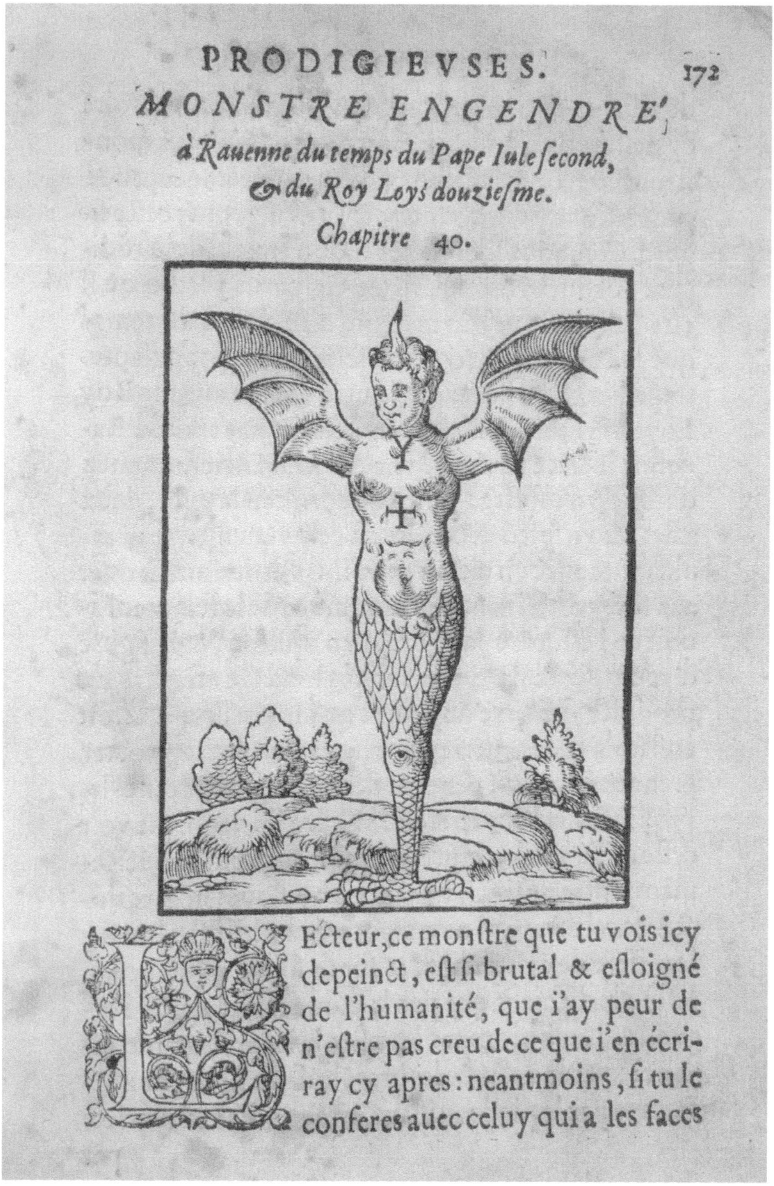

PRODIGIEVSES.   172
MONSTRE ENGENDRE',
à Rauenne du temps du Pape Iule second,
& du Roy Loys douziesme.

Chapitre 40.

L Ecteur, ce monstre que tu vois icy
depeinct, est si brutal & esloigné
de l'humanité, que i'ay peur de
n'estre pas creu de ce que i'en escri-
ray cy apres : neantmoins, si tu le
conferes auec celuy qui a les faces

Figure 1.1   Monster of Ravenna, from Pierre Boaistuau and Claude de
Tesserant, *Quatorze histoires prodigieuses, adioustées aux
precedents* ... (Paris: Jean de Bordeaux, 1567). Courtesy of
the Division of Rare and Manuscript Collections, Cornell
University Library

the interpretation of the monster is virtually identical to that of Multivallis, with the negative references excised. This monster seems to represent a fear of the confusion between human and animal, as well as between male and female. This confusion is represented as a threat to political and authorial authority: "Lecteur, ce monstre que tu vois icy depeinct, est si brutal & esloigné de l'humanité, que i'ay peur de n'estre pas creu de ce que i'en écriray cy apres …" ("Reader, the monster which you see pictured here, is so brutal and distant from humanity, that I am afraid of not being believed when I write what I am about to write").[9] Rather than offering a scientific explanation alleging the problems and risks of generation, as he does in other stories, Boaistuau offers the usual allegorical reading of the creature:

> … il fut engendré à Ravenne mesme (qui est l'une des plus anciennes citez d'Italie) un monstre ayant une corne en la teste, deux aesles & un pied semblable à celuy d'un oyseau ravissant & avec un oeil au genoil, il estoit double quant aux sexe, participant de l'homme et de la femme, il avoit en l'estomac la figure d'un ypsilon, & la figure d'une croix, & si n'avoit aucuns bras … par la corne estoit figuré l'orgueil & l'ambition: par les aesles, la legereté & inconstance: par le default des bras, le deffault des bonnes oeuvres: par le pied ravissant, rapine usure & avarice: par l'oeil qui estoit au genoil, l'affection des choses terrestres: par les deux sexes, la Sodomie: & que pour tous ces pechez qui regnoient de ce temps en Italie, elle estoit ainsi affligée de guerres: mais quant à l'Ypsilon & à la Croix, c'estoient deux signes salutaires: car l'Ypsilon signifioit vertu, & puis la Croix, qui denotoit que s'ilz vouloyent se convertir à Iesus Christ, & songer à sa Croix, c'estoit le vray remede. (Boaistuau, *Histoires prodigieuses*, pp. 172–3)[10]

> (… there was born at Ravenna itself (which is one of the most ancient cities in Italy), a monster with a horn on its head, two wings, and one foot similar to that of a bird of prey, and one eye on its knee, double as to its sex, participating in both male and female natures, it had on its stomach the sign of a Y and the sign of a cross, and yet it had no arms … the horn was the symbol of pride and ambition: the wings, lightness and inconstancy: the lack of arms, the lack of good works: by the raptor's foot, pillage, usury, and avarice: by the eye that was on the knee, the attraction to earthly matters: by the two sexes, Sodomy: and that because of all of these sins that reigned at this time in Italy, this country was thus afflicted by wars. But as for the Y and the Cross, those were two signs of salvation: because the Y signified virtue, and then the Cross, which conveyed that if they would convert to the laws of Jesus Christ, and think of his Cross, that was the true remedy …).

---

[9]   Pierre Boaistuau, *Histoires prodigieuses les plus memorables qui ayent esté observes depuis la nativité de Jesus Christ, jusques à notre siecle …* (Paris: Vincent Sertenas, 1560), p. 172.

[10] This reading is in fact not entirely original, and taken mostly from the Multivallis version of this tale. For a comparison, and complete history of this monster, see Céard's edition of Paré's *Des monstres*, note 18, p. 153. For whatever reason, Paré has chosen to cite Boaistuau as his source ("Preface," p. 3). All translations of this text are my own.

The moral message that Boaistuau inscribes into his reading of this body is quite clear. It should be remembered that, even through the Renaissance, the term sodomy was used to designate a wide range of behaviors considered to be vices, from male homosexuality to bloodshed.[11] The Y and the cross symbolize potential salvation through repentance. The whole "text" is a critique of Julius II and his corrupt circle (as it is in Paré's treatise, *Des monstres*). This monster cannot merely be described, it must be read, and to a large extent, the reading creates the monster. A "normal" body would simply enter at birth into an already established system of meaning known as culture. A monstrous body remains outside of any such system, being exceptional, and must have a new system created to integrate it into the established culture. This body must be controlled by language, by being "read" (and thus written) in an acceptable fashion. Thus, this "brutal" monster is read allegorically as a call to return to the Christian (and heterosexual) system. Those who do not follow the dictates of Christianity are equated with the monster, and thus also silenced or effaced by the neatly inscribed allegory which controls it.

The narrative thus becomes a means of expulsion of that which is unusual, therefore unreadable and unacceptable. The hermaphroditic/monstrous body is simply *forced* to fit, as it will be later by the surgeon's knife[12] and by the insistence upon its legal definition as male or female. That aspect of creation which does not fit easily into the classifications and categories created by language, is at once tamed and effaced by

---

[11]   See John Boswell, *Christianity, Social Tolerance, and Homosexuality. Gay People in Western Europe from the Beginning of the Christian Era to the Fourteenth Century* (Chicago: University of Chicago Press, 1980), p. 93, n. 2: "Wherever possible the term 'sodomy' ('sodomia') has been excluded from this study, since it is so vague and ambiguous as to be virtually useless in a text of this sort. Its etymology is probably a misprision of history, and it has connoted in various times and places everything from ordinary heterosexual intercourse in an atypical position to oral sexual contact with animals. At some points in history it has referred almost exlusively to male homosexuality and at others almost exclusively to heterosexual excess." Boswell points out that interpretations of the destruction of Sodom are still debated, and that the range of possible sins at the cause of this annihilation are great (pp. 93–5). See also Boniface's definition of sodomy as incest or adultery (Boswell, p. 203). Gregory W. Bredbeck also deals at some length with the ambiguity of this term in the Renaissance, and its evolution towards a more specific meaning, in his book *Sodomy and Interpretation, Marlowe to Milton* (Ithaca: Cornell University Press, 1991), pp. 10–19: "The point here is not that sodomy during the early Renaissance was asexual but rather that its lack of sexual specificity allowed the term to be used in unspecified ways ..." (p. 11). In fact, one broadside against the French court, cited by Pierre de l'Estoile in his *Registre-Journal du Regne de Henri III* (Geneva: Droz, 1997), vol. 3, p. 17 (entry for January 1579), calls the King and his followers "princes de Sodome," and then enumerates murders and massacres rather than sexual acts ("sacrifices," "le sang des agneaux innocens," "l'holocauste ardent des moutons," "vos mains ... Sont trop plaines de sang").

[12]   See Suzanne J. Kessler, "The Medical Construction of Gender," pp. 3–26.

language, to serve the purposes of the structures it defies. In this case, the monster serves French political interests, justifying Louis XII's incursions into Italy as punishment of inordinate vice.[13] Thus, the near-destruction of Ravenna is ascribed not to the French invasion, but to Julius's own warlike nature, which stirred up divisions within the city-state. Such is the clever, self-protective nature of culture.

Paré's account of this hermaphrodite from Ravenna as an example of a monster created by the wrath of God evokes some discomfort at the politicized use of this figure; he describes it but does not explain it, except as a result of the bloody battle in that city:

> Autre preuve. Du temps que le Pape Jules second suscita tant de malheurs en Italie et qu'il eut la guerre contre le Roys Louys douziesme (1512), laquelle fut suyvie d'une sanglante bataille donnee pres de Ravenne, peu de temps apres on veit naistre en la mesme ville un monstre ayant une corne à la teste, deux ailes et un seul pied semblable à celuy d'un oyseau de proye, à la joincture du genoüil un oeil, et participant de la nature de masle et de femelle, comme tu vois par ce pourtraict. (*Des monstres*, pp. 7–8)

> (More evidence. At the time that Pope Julius the second gave life to so many misfortunes in Italy, and when he had his war against the King Louis XII [1512], which was followed by a bloody battle held near Ravenna, a short time after, a monster was seen born in the same town, having a horn on its head, two wings and one foot similar to that of a bird of prey, at the knee an eye, and partaking of both male and female natures, as you see in this portrait.)

In spite of the lengthy descriptions that form the subtexts with which he is working, and to which he clearly alludes in his preface (he mentions "Boistuau" and Claude de Tesserant, who continued the *Histoires prodigieuses*, along with Saint Augustine), Paré gives short shrift to this monster, concentrating rather on the historical context. In fact, a certain skepticism creeps in over the course of the entire work, as Paré includes chapters on beggars' frauds, such as the one who used the arm of a hanged man to counterfeit a diseased one of his own, or the woman who feigned a tumor on her breast, the man who feigned leprosy, and several other such devices. Paré devotes five chapters to such tricks, and follows these stories with accounts of demons and witches. Unlike Bauhin, who later expresses some doubt about the possibility of discerning the truth, Paré evokes through these stories the sense that careful observation will lead to a revelation of the truth. Nonetheless, the juxtaposition of stories of fraud with those concerning witches and demons does give pause.

Clearly, Paré is more concerned with the medical and scientific issues concerning hermaphrodism, even if these issues are still bound with legal and political concerns. In

---

13 See Jean Céard's note on this monster in his edition of *Des monstres* (p. 154, note 18); clearly both Boaistuau and Paré are thinking of Louis XII of France's 1512 campaigns in Italy, and perhaps the later campaigns of François Ier as well.

earlier editions of *Des monstres*, Paré had included this creature in his commentary on hermaphrodites, but had moved this reference perhaps because it might have confused his comparatively straightforward discussion of the causes of hermaphrodism.[14] Although he does mention one monstrous birth in relation to a political event in his chapter on hermaphrodites (a double-bodied, one-headed male is born the day the Genevans and Venetians reconcile), this infant is not hermaphroditic. Paré thus tries to distance any political or allegorical reading of hermaphrodites from descriptions of the natural causes and manifestations of hermaphrodism. He treats hermaphrodites much more as oddities of nature than as supernatural portents of evil, offering a more scientific explanation for their existence: "c'est que la femme fournit autant de semence que l'homme" (p. 24: "it is that the woman contributes as much seed as the man"). Thus, while Boiastuau and Tesserant recoil in horror when faced with these examples of unstable sex, Paré favors actual examination of the hermaphroditic body ("Les Medecins et Chirurgiens bien experts et advisez peuvent cognoistre si les hermafrodites sont plus aptes à tenir et user de l'un que de l'autre sexe …" p. 25: "Doctors and surgeons who are expert and well-advised can recognize whether hermaphrodites are more likely to pertain to and use one or the other sex …"), and some form of scientific investigation, and avoids at least to some degree superstitious condemnation.

In 1600, Bauhin repeats the description and reading of the monster of Ravenna.[15] Once again, the hermaphrodite is associated with homosexuality, as well as with innumerable vices (greed, usury, inconstancy, pride, worldliness). This reading is again identical to that of Multivallis, except that Bauhin declines to interpret the cross and the Ypsilon. Thus, although this body is read as a critique of Julius II (as in Paré), Bauhin declines to place this monstrous sign in a religious context. The monstrous body, emptied of "natural" existence and denied a place in the "natural" order of things, becomes the instrument of political narrative.

Bauhin further underscores the purpose of this secularization of a well-known figure by means of a more contemporary counter-example he attaches to the traditional description. He cleverly ends this chapter with a tale of false accusation of hermaphrodism, made for political reasons by the Duke of Brunschweig against the Archbishop. The poor Archbishop repeatedly displays his attributes, to no avail:

> Albertus Dux Brunswicens. referente Crantzio Archiepiscopo Bremens à Joanne diacono suae Ecclesiae traductus erat, quod esset Hermaphroditus, & in utramque venerem aeque promptus. Archiepiscopus inspiciendum se praebuit in balneis, multis

---

[14] See Céard's note on this subject, *Des monstres*, p. 153.

[15] "An. Dom. 1512 Ravennae monstrum natum est, quod habebat cornu in capite, alas duas, brachia nulla, pedem unum ut avis rapax, oculum in genu, sexum utrumque, in medio pectore Ypsilon & crucis effigiem." (Z5: "In the Year of Our Lord 1512 a monster was born in Ravenna, which had a horn on its head, two wings, no arms, one foot like that of a bird of prey, an eye in its knee, the organs of both sexes, and the image of a Y and a cross in the middle of its chest.")

militaribus, consularibus & civibus Bremae: nec tamen quievit ortus semel rumor. (*De hermaphroditorum*, Z6v)

(Albert, the Duke of Brunschweig was reported to have told Johann, the deacon of his Church, that Crantzius, the Archbishop of Bremen, was a Hermaphroditus, equally capable of either form of pleasure (sex). The Archbishop offered himself for inspection in the baths to many soldiers, magistrates, and citizens of Bremen: nonetheless, he could not calm the rise of this rumor ....)

Clearly, hermaphrodism is being used in this case as a political tool, not only as a portent, but as a sign of male deficiency. In this context, the tale becomes a critique of the political uses of the hermaphrodite, as propaganda holds greater force than any observed "reality." This example foregrounds the purely discursive nature of politicized or socialized hermaphrodism, as well as the dependence of gender roles on representations of gender that have nothing to do with any essential physical characteristics. In the end, the Archbishop's body is irrelevant, written over as it is by political propaganda. Henri III's body is similarly written and rewritten by the propagandists of his time; eventually, in his case, discourse effectively and actually destroys his body, leading to his assassination.[16] Thus, although the gap between discourse and any possible bodily reality is already apparent to Renaissance intellectuals, the power of discourse cannot be denied, since it leads to actions that transform the body.

Science and Culture

It must be recognized that science often served the cultural discourse of the body rather than observing the natural body or transforming deep-seated cultural attitudes, and that the more imaginative aspects of culture were not easily separated from scientific discourse in the sixteenth century. Paré in particular owes a great debt to, and acknowledges, texts that modern readers would not necessarily consider scientific, associating Boaistuau and Tesserant with St Paul and St Augustine, ancient prophets and philosophers, and finally with classical authorities in the realm of medicine.[17] The inclusion of Boaistuau in particular in this list indicates a very

---

[16] For background on this polemical campaign against Henri III of France, see David A. Bell, "Unmasking a King: The Political Uses of Popular Literature Under the French Catholic League, 1588–89," in *The Sixteenth Century Journal* 20 (1989): 371–86.

[17] "... comme nous monstrerons cy apres par plusieurs exemples d'iceux monstres et prodiges, lesquels j'ay recueillis avec les figures de plusieurs autheurs, comme des Histoires prodigieuses de Pierre Boaistuau, et de Claude Tesserant, de sainct Paul, sainct Augustin, Esdras le Prophete, et des anciens Philosophes, à sçavoir d'Hippocrates, Galien, Empedocles, Aristote, Pline, Lycosthene, et autres ..." *Des monstres* ("Preface," p. 3: "... as we shall demonstrate after this by means of numerous examples of these monsters and

different notion of authoritative – what we might now call academic – discourse than is held today. Boaistuau's *Histoires prodigeuses* links scientific knowledge with the popular pamphlet, and underscores the lack of clear distinction between these two fields of endeavor.[18] The material in his stories resembles that found in the *canards*, or popular "news" pamphlets, of the day.[19] The format of his stories also resembles that of the pamphlets; they are short, and always preceded by a brief descriptive title and a (usually) shocking picture. In fact, Jean de Bordeaux, publisher of the 1567 edition of the *Histoires*, produced *canards* as well.[20] And although Boaistuau quotes authoritatively from classical and humanist authors such as Augustine, Jerome, and Jacob Rueff,[21] this technique was common even in the pamphlet literature of the day.[22]

Tesserant more closely links the realm of popular pamphlets and that of scientific discourse in his accounts of hermaphrodism, and seems even more concerned with the link between ambiguous sex and monstrosity in his fourteen *histoires*, especially in the second and third stories. Although Boaistuau does mention the Hippocratic treatise

---

prodigies, which I have collected, with the illustrations, from several authors, such as the *Histoires prodigieuses* of Pierre Boaistuau, and of Claude Tesserant, from saint Paul, saint Augustine, Esdras the Prophet, and from the ancient Philosophers, such as Hippocrates, Galen, Empedocles, Aristotle, Pliny, Lycosthenes, and others ...").

[18] I am citing the 1560 edition of the *Histoires prodigieuses* (Paris: Sertenas), as well as the 1567 edition of fourteen stories added by Claude de Tesserant, *Quatorze histoires prodigieuses adioustées aux precedentes* (Paris: Jean de Bordeaux). For an excellent analysis of the *Histoires*, see Jean Céard, *La nature et les prodiges*, "Les débuts d'un genre: L'histoire prodigieuse," pp. 252–72.

[19] Boaistuau's subjects include: the devil (ch. 1), comets (chs 2, 19), the deaths of kings (ch. 3), monstrous births (chs 5–7, 31, 35, 40), other monsters (chs 14, 17, 22, 24, 27, 28, 29, 32, 34), cannibalism (chs 5, 33, 36), thunder and lightning (ch. 8), floods (ch. 10), earthquakes (ch. 12). See, for comparison, the list offered by Jean Céard at the end of *La nature et les prodiges*, pp. 480–83. See also Jean-Pierre Seguin's list of *canards*, *L'Information en France avant la periodique* (Paris: Maisonneuve et Larose, 1964).

[20] For example, many years later, *Monstres prodigeux advenus en la Turquie, depuis l'année de la Comette, iusqu'en l'an present 1624. Menaçans la fin, & entiere ruyne de l'Empire turquesque ...* (Paris: Jean de Bordeaux, 1624).

[21] Author of the influential *De conceptu et generatione hominis*, Rueff was a doctor from Zurich, and his work is one of the founding pieces of teratology, serving as the inspiration for Paré, Bauhin, Duval and others. In particular, his discussion of monstrous births, rather more enlightened than that of Paré or Bauhin in its treatment of these as similar to other genetic anomalies, has to be considered part of the origin of a decided trend in scientific discourse. See Céard, *La nature et les prodiges*, pp. 293–4; Céard cites the Frankfurt (1580) edition of Rueff's work.

[22] Céard explores the problematic relationship between scientific inquiry and popular literature in his section on "Les histoires prodigieuses et les *canards*," *La nature et les prodiges*, pp. 468–79.

De genitura, Tesserant seems even more concerned with the causes of monstrous or hermaphroditic births than his predecessor; he begins his "Histoire de deux enfans Hermaphrodites lesquels s'entretiennent, & de la cause de telle conionction" with that Hippocratic argument taken from Rueff and later echoed by Paré, that monsters are the result of too much or too little "seed."[23] Tesserant links hermaphrodites to cases of multiple births, particularly of children of both sexes. Like Boiastuau, he reads such unusual cases as presages more than as medical anomalies, pointing out that:

> ... un Hermaphrodite, on l'a prins non seulement pour un monstre, mais aussi pour un grand malheur, tellement que anciennement aussi tost que tels monstres naissoient, tant les Romains que les Grecs les faisoient precipiter en la mer ... (Tesserant, *Quatorze histoires*, p. 222)

> (... a hermaphrodite has been taken not only as a monster, but as a great misfortune, so much so that in ancient times as soon as such monsters were born, the Romans as well as the Greeks had them thrown into the sea ...)

He traces the evolution of ancient attitudes towards an acceptance of these beings, in a passage also echoed by Paré:

> ... on s'est contenté de leur faire eslire duquel sexe ils vouloient user, avec defenses sur peine de la mort, de n'user de l'autre pour les inconveniens qui en pourroient advenir. Car autrefois, comme sainct Augustin au mesme chapitre escript, quelques uns en abusoient de telle sorte, que par un usage mutuel & reciproque, ils paillardoient l'un avec l'autre, servans chacun à son tour tantost d'homme, & tantost de femme ... (Tesserant, *Quatorze histoires*, p. 223)

> (... later, the people limited themselves to making these beings choose which sex they wanted to use, with prohibition upon pain of death of use of the other because of the inconveniences that could result. Because in earlier times, as St. Augustine writes in the same chapter, some abused in such a way, that by means of mutual and reciprocal usage, they debauched each other, serving each in turn sometimes as the man, sometimes as the woman ...)

The threat implied by ambiguity of sex to a society based so fundamentally on distinctly gendered roles is formidable. Later, Thomas Artus' novel, *L'Isle des Hermaphrodites*, would satirize not only the court of Henri III but the fragility of a society based on

---

[23] "Mais ce que nous avons touché en passant, Des monstres, lesquels ou la trop grande abondance de semence, ou le defaut d'icelle a faict naistre ou avec moins ou avec plus de membres que la composition parfaicte de l'homme ne requeiert nous invite à l'histoire de quelques monstres ..." ("But that which we have touched upon in passing concerning monsters which are born either because of too great abundance of seed or from lack of it with fewer or more members than the perfect composition of man requires leads us to the story of several monsters," p. 222).

such normative views of sex and gender roles. It is no wonder, then, given the threat that blurring of gender roles represented, that the most vehement moralizing occurred in relation to those roles.

Although there were compelling precedents for a more tolerant approach to such "anomalies," even these precedents could not bypass hierarchized notions of gender, but in fact inscribed the hermaphrodites comfortably within the hierarchy. Augustine, using Pliny's *Historia naturalis* (7.2) as his main source, does not use such moralistic discourse. In his discussion of various monstrous races, he mentions the Androgyni: "... others have the characteristics of both sexes, the right breast being male and the left female, and in their intercourse they alternate between begetting and conceiving."[24] Augustine suggests that for the anomalous hermaphrodites born in every era, sex is already assigned from birth:

> As for *Androgynes*, also called Hermaphrodites, they are certainly very rare, and yet it is difficult to find periods when there are no examples of human beings possessing the characteristics of both sexes, in such a way that it is a matter of doubt how they should be classified. However, the prevalent usage has called them masculine, assigning them to the superior sex; for no one has ever used the feminine names, *androgynaecae* or *hermaphroditae*. (*City of God*, bk 16, ch. 8, p. 663)

Linguistic usage, perhaps dictated by mythology (the male Hermaphroditus being the original hermaphrodite), in turn dictates scientific categories. This tendency for scientific investigation to be language-driven becomes even more evident in Bauhin's treatise, with its two opening chapters on the Greek and Latin names for hermaphrodites ("De nominibus Hermaphroditorum, quibus eos Graecis donarunt," and "De Hermaphroditorum appellationibus Latinis," A7–B3) and its subsequent chapters on the definitions and classifications, as well as the literary manifestations, of hermaphrodism (chs 3–5).

It is within the atmosphere of rigid enforcement of sexual roles that the medical treatises of the time must be considered. As enlightened as Paré, Bauhin, and Duval may have been for their time, and as much as they struggled to bring empirical evidence and anatomical observation to the study of the human body, they worked within theological, legal, and political frameworks that dictated specific and unmoving roles for men and women in society, that dictated ideal bodily forms and rejected all that fell outside of the norm. Their work reflects their culture as much as it reflects the struggle of early modern science to reach beyond cultural constraints, when confronted with the results of direct observation of bodies.

It is thus not surprising that the *Histoires prodigeuses* of Boaistuau and Tesserant is the first source mentioned by Paré in *Des Monstres*.[25] The combination of received

---

[24] Augustine, *City of God*, p. 661.
[25] The best introduction to this work remains Jean Céard's analysis in *La nature et les prodiges*, ch. 12: "Ambroise Paré Tératologue," pp. 292–314.

culture and scientific observation in this work is revealed by the list of causes of monstrous births, in which God's anger, the work of Demons and Devils, and beggars' tricks hold as important a place as heredity or the condition of the mother.[26] Nonetheless, Paré's more tolerant view of hermaphrodites is in keeping with the inclusive definition of monsters and prodigies that arises not so much from his preface as from the work as a whole.[27] For Paré, that which is monstrous is not necessarily unnatural; the term changes meaning in the various contexts he creates for it.[28] The quotidian meets with the supernatural in this treatise, and Paré's designation of that which is marvelous excludes condemnation, except in the cases of beggars, witches, and demons. In essence, that which is not harmful to others is not subject to harsh moral judgment. While this may not seem exceptional to the modern reader, this refusal to condemn that which is simply anomalous was in fact unusual in the early modern period. More often than not, monstrous children were viewed with suspicion and fear; if not killed, they were ostracized and treated as freaks, as Montaigne's appeal

---

[26] "La première est la gloire de Dieu. La seconde, son ire. La troisiesme, la trop grande quantité de semence. La quatriesme, la trop petite quantité. La cinquiesme, l'imagination. La sixiesme, l'angustie ou petitesse de la matrice. La septiesme, l'assiette indecente de la mere … La huictiesme, par cheute, ou coups donnez contre le ventre de la mere … La neufiesme, par maladies hereditaires ou accidentales. La dixiesme, par pourriture ou corruption de la semence. L'onziesme, par mistion ou meslange de semence. La douxiesme, par l'artifice des meschans belistres de l'ostiere. La treiziesme, par les Demons ou Diables." ("The first cause is the glory of God. The second, his wrath. The third, the too great abundance of seed. The fourth, a too small amount. The fifth, the imagination. The sixth, the narrowness or smallness of the womb. The seventh, the inappropriate posture of the mother … The eighth, by a fall or by blows against the belly of the mother … The ninth, hereditary or accidental illnesses. The tenth, from rotting or corruption of the seed. The eleventh, by mixing or confusion of the seed. The twelfth, by the artifice of evil con-men. The twelfth, by Demons or Devils," p. 4).

[27] Janis Pallister's translation of the word *prodiges* as "marvels" is quite apt in the context of the treatise as a whole; Ambroise Paré, *On Monsters and Marvels*, trans. Janis L. Pallister (Chicago: University of Chicago Press, 1982). Although I consulted Pallister's translation while writing this article, I did not use her version, as she based her work on an edition of *Des monstres* other than that used by Céard, and as there are significant differences between these editions.

[28] Paré includes natural deformities in children and animals; gallstones and other medical anomalies (chs 15–18); beggar's tricks (which were hardly unusual, but were often monstrously disgusting; chs 20–24); the horrifying effects of witchcraft and demonic powers (chs 25–33); marine "monsters" observed and imagined (from crocodiles to giant geese, ch. 34); monstrous birds like the ostrich, of which he has a skeleton (ch. 35); and monstrous species of animals, including the giraffe, the unicorn, the elephant, the bison, the rhinoceros, and various animals that have human faces and live on air (ch. 36). This list of marvels ends with "celestial monsters" (ch. 37), comets, battles in the sky, rains of blood, as well as the planets and stars.

for tolerance in his essay "D'un enfant monstrueux" reveals: "Ce que nous appellons monstres, ne le sont pas à Dieu … Nous apelons contre nature ce qui advient contre la coustume …" ("Those which we call monsters, are not so to God … We call that which is not familiar unnatural …").[29] He is inspired to these statements by the sight of a deformed child being presented as a freak at a carnival.

In fact, in the chapter following that on hermaphrodites, "Histoires memorables de certaines femmes qui sont degenerees en hommes," Paré rejects divinatory use of sex changes and offers a more "scientific" explanation that would not demand ostracism of the people involved. Formerly, prophets would order monstrous creatures exiled or destroyed, because they believed that such creatures were evil omens. Paré's explanation links the "monstrous" to the norm, rather than excluding it; he tames that which is threatening:

> La raison pourquoy les femmes se peuvent degenerer en hommes, c'est que les femmes ont autant de caché dedans le corps que les hommes descouvrent dehors, reste seulement qu'elles n'ont pas tant de chaleur ny suffisance pour pousser dehors ce que par la froidure de leur temperature est tenu comme lié au dedans. (*Des monstres*, p. 30)

> (The reason why women can degenerate into men is that women have as much hidden in the body as men offer to be seen on the outside, except only that they do not have enough heat or strength to push outside that which by the coldness of their temperature is held as if tied within.)

Thus, all women are potential men. But Paré is careful to assure his male readership that the reverse is not true, and that they do not risk the loss of status that would accompany metamorphosis into the female sex:

> … nous ne trouvons jamais en histoire veritable que d'homme aucun soit devenu femme, pour-ce que Nature tend toujours à ce qui est le plus parfaict, et non au contraire faire que ce qui est parfaict devienne imparfaict. (*Des monstres*, p. 30)

> (… we never find a true story in which any man becomes a woman, because Nature tends always towards that which is more perfect, and does not on the contrary make that which is perfect become imperfect.)

This theory echoes the Galenic notion that heat causes the male genitalia to become externalized,[30] as well as echoing the Aristotelian assertion that women are merely imperfect or defective men. Thus, although Paré rejects the more exclusionary notion of monsters as portents of evil (thus to be destroyed), he still works within the cultural assumptions of his time in matters of sex (or gender) distinction.

---

[29] Montaigne, *Essais*, bk 2, essay 30, p. 713.
[30] See Laqueur, *Making Sex*, pp. 26–8.

Although cited by Laqueur as a proponent of the one-sex theory,[31] Paré recognizes the medical and epistemological problem that the hermaphrodites represent. In his treatise on monsters, he gives the woman an equal (not passive) role in generation when he explains hermaphrodites:

> Or, quant à la cause, c'est que la femme fournit autant de semence que l'homme proportionnément, et pour-ce la vertu formatrice, qui tousjours tasche à faire son semblable, à sçavoir de la matiere masculine un masle, et de la feminine une femelle, fait qu'en un mesme corps est trouvé quelquefois deux sexes, nommez Hermaphrodites … (*Des monstres*, p. 24)[32]

> (So, as for the cause [of hermaphrodites], it is that the woman provides as much of the seed as the man, in the same proportion, and for this reason the conceiving force, which is always impelled to create that which resembles itself, that is, from masculine matter a male and from feminine matter a female, works so that in one body are found the two sexes, named Hermaphrodites …)

Here, Paré seems to be on the verge of the two-sex system. This is reflected in his descriptions of the hermaphrodites themselves, which he places in four categories. The first is the male hermaphrodite, in whom only the male organs are functional. The second is the female hermaphrodite, in whom the female sexual organs function, but the male do not. The third sort of hermaphrodite is neither male nor female (neither set of organs functions in any way). The fourth category is the hermaphrodite that is both male and female; that is, in whom the organs of both sexes function. Paré obviously simplifies his definitions by using only reproductive capacity as his guide. The last category of hermaphrodite, which can perform sexually either as a male or as a female, poses serious legal and social problems, according to Paré, who echoes Tesserant's account:

> Hermafrodites masles et femelles, ce sont ceux qui ont les deux sexes bien formez et s'en peuvent aider et servir à la generation: et à ceux cy les loix anciennes et modernes ont fait et font encore eslire duquel sexe ils veulent user, avec defense, sur peine de perdre la vie, de ne servir que de celuy duquel ils auront fait election, pour les inconveniens qui en pourroyent advenir. Car aucuns en ont abusé de telle sorte, que par un usage mutuel et reciproque paillardoyent de l'un et de l'autre sexe, tantost d'homme, tantost de femme … (*Des monstres*, pp. 24–5)

> (Hermaphrodites which are at once male and female, are those who have both sets of sexual organs well-formed and can use either to conceive: and these, ancient and modern laws force to choose which sex (set of organs) they want to use, with the

---

31 *Making Sex*, pp. 126–7, particularly in relation to the story of Marie-Germain, which Paré sees as evidence that women contain, internalized, all the same organs as men.

32 This is a clear departure from the Aristotelian model, perpetuated by Renaldus Columbus, according to which the man gives all the elements of human life in conception, and the woman merely receives this life and nourishes it (Laqueur, *Making Sex*, pp. 135–6).

prohibition, upon pain of death, against using those which they did not choose, because of the inconveniences that could result. This is because some have misused their sexual organs in such a way that by mutual and reciprocal use they have debauched those of either sex, sometimes men, sometimes women …)[33]

The fact that Paré takes most of this text directly from Tesserant's *canard*-like work reveals the extent to which popular belief drives his analysis. No more than his source does Paré explain why this "double pleasure" is so harmful, but insists that a choice must be made. There is something potentially disruptive about this unstable sexuality. This choice that must be made is based purely on physical, mostly external, evidence, and, as Julia Epstein says: "… cultural ideas about gender-appropriate behavior have equal importance with genitalia."[34] Laqueur echoes this view in his section on "Sex, Gender, Doctors, and Law" in *Making Sex*, but Paré himself takes the issue further:

> Les Medecins et Chirurgiens bien experts et advisez peuvent cognoistre si les hermafrodites sont plus aptes à tenir et user de l'un que de l'autre sexe, ou des deux, ou du tout rien. Et telle chose se cognoistra aux parties genitales … pareillement par le visage, et si les cheveux sont deliez ou gros; si la parole est virile ou gresle; si les tetins sont semblables à ceux des hommes ou des femmes; semblablement si toute l'habitude du corps et robuste ou effeminee, s'ils sont hardis ou craintifs, et autres actions semblables aux masles ou aux femelles. (*Des monstres*, pp. 24–5)

> (Doctors and Surgeons who are expert and informed can recognize whether the hermaphrodites are more apt to have and use one or the other sex, or both, or neither. And this can be told from the genitals … and equally, by the face, and whether the hair is coarse or fine; whether the voice is low or high; whether the teats resemble those of a man or a woman; similarly, whether the whole makeup of the body is robust or effeminate, if they are bold or fearful, and other actions which pertain to males or females.)[35]

---

[33] See above, Boiastuau/Tesserant, second story of the fourteen-story continuation of the *Histoires prodigeuses*, p. 223.

[34] In "Either/Or – Neither/Both: Sexual Ambiguity and the Ideology of Gender," *Genders* 7 (1990): 108.

[35] Any critic who is skeptical about the possible impact of culture upon early "scientific" views on gender might wish to compare Paré's text to the transformation of Iphis from girl into boy in Ovid's *Metamorphoses*:

quam solita est, maiore gradu; nec candor in ore
permanet, et vires augentur, et acrior ipse est
vultus et incomptis brevior mensura capillis,
plusque vigoris adest, habuit quam femina …

(ll. 787–90: "S/he took longer steps than usual; and the same fairness was not to be seen in the face; her/his strength grew and the features of her/his face were not so soft [sharper]; the tousled hair was shorter; and there was more vigor than was normal for a woman; bk 9, ll. 666–797; translation mine).

The problem of unstable sex is solved by highly stereotypical external signs, interpreted by the observer. Thus, scientific "objectivity" is driven by a sort of collective cultural subjectivity that uses circular reasoning to justify the conclusions it wishes to make. Ovid declares vigor to be a manly characteristic, and then defines Iphis as a man because of this vigor. Similarly, Paré says that if a hermaphrodite is of womanly aspect (with female breasts and feminine body), then it is a woman; yet he does not really describe what a "feminine" body is. Once again, language fails to portray an actual body, and the legal prescriptions that govern gender designation fall far short of any viable description of the sexed body. This silence is somehow appropriate in response to the hermaphroditic body, which remains on the margins of discourse. This silence also leaves room for determination of individual cases as such, rather than, say, the blanket assumption that all hermaphrodites are male. Paradoxically, this silence in the face of that which defies dualistic discourse creates the space for reinclusion of the hermaphroditic body within such discourse, by means of a legal determination of an individual's gender, even if that individual does not have a particular sex.

Paré also links gender determination to reproduction in his discussion of how to determine the masculinity of a hermaphrodite: if the male member is the right size, if it can become erect and ejaculate, then the hermaphrodite should be designated a male. Paré humanely suggests that the hermaphrodite itself should make this determination, and that the doctors should take it at its word. Bauhin and Duval will insist on invasive examinations and medical procedures. In Paré's estimation, at least to this small extent, the hermaphrodite can be self-determining. Still, this self-determination is limited by a very specific role in society, that of reproduction. Individual identity is thus established purely in relation to others – a spouse, a child, the state – rather than by means of any sense of self coming from within.

By this use of cultural stereotypes, the hermaphrodite becomes a controllable object of scientific discourse, rather than a variable and independent subject of its own life. The social norms of gender that regulate and even efface individual behavior must be protected at all costs, and in fact protect themselves with the semblance of objective reasoning that, when examined closely, seems self-justifying (she is a woman because she looks like a woman). It is the coexistence of two sexes in one person that is threatening to society because it disrupts the clear distinction and hierarchical relations between male and female.

The proliferation of discourses at the service of dualism and in response to a hermaphroditic body that must be seen as male or female creates an aporia that is the cognate of the silence standing in for any concrete description of the sexed body in early modern medical discourse. Even while endless theories of the generation of hermaphrodites are rehearsed, the female body is merely described as that which is feminine, and the male body, as that which is masculine (and thus not feminine). Thus, both the multiplicity of discourses and the silence at the center of these discourses signal an inability to deal with the specificity of bodies. Only by shaking the stranglehold of Aristotelian philosophy, as Paracelsus and other alchemists attempted in their adoption of Eastern forms of thought,[36] would medical science be able to undertake any examination of the body as a living thing. We are still in the process of performing that examination.

---

[36] See Paracelsus, in particular the treatise *Concerning the Nature of Things*, pp. 120–94, which combines Aristotelian categorizations of the monstrous (p. 173), and more innovative views of medicine (his views on resuscitation, for example, p. 147). For an assessment of Paracelsus's importance as a precursor of modern science, see Allen G. Debus, *The Chemical Philosophy: Paracelsian Science and Medicine in the Sixteenth and Seventeenth Centuries* (New York: Science History Publications, 1977).

Chapter 2

The Cultural and Medical Construction of Gender: Caspar Bauhin

Science in the Service of Culture

The end of the sixteenth century in Europe saw the publication of a number of treatises revolving around male and female anatomy, sex, sexuality, and childbirth; three of these treatises in particular use the hermaphrodite, or, more generally monsters, as an enticement to potential readers, and thus link the ambiguously sexed body to more common experiences of sex and sexuality: Paré's *Des Monstres et prodiges*, as we have seen; Bauhin's *De Hermaphroditorum monstrosorumque partuum natura*; and Duval's *Des Hermaphrodits et accouchements des femmes*. These treatises reflect a gradual evolution in thought concerning the body, sex, sexuality, and cultural attitudes towards gender. In Bauhin's treatise, unlike Paré's, the proliferation of cultural sources (literary, philosophical, theological, and legal) on hermaphrodism exists in tension with a more empirical approach to science. Bauhin was a professor of anatomy and botany at Basel in the late sixteenth and early seventeenth centuries.[1] Clearly, he was fascinated by the question of sexual difference, and wrote not only his treatise on hermaphrodites, but one on the distinguishing features of male and female human anatomy, *Institutiones anatomicae corporis virilis et muliebris historiam exhibentes*.[2] His treatise, *De Hermaphroditorum*, apparently first published in Frankfurt in 1600, and then in Oppenheim in 1614 (with engravings taken from various works by Theodor de Bry), offers the most complete evidence of the cultural status of the hermaphrodite in the late Renaissance. In his twenty-five page long list of works cited in his treatise (given at the opening of the edition), Bauhin provides the most complete bibliographical source for every type of account of hermaphrodism, and a summary of much of the material available to Renaissance intellectuals.

---

[1]   Bauhin was author of about a dozen treatises on botany or anatomy, including the *Anatomica corporis virilis et muliebris historia* ... (Lyon: Joannes le Preux, 1597); *Theatrum anatomicum* (Frankfurt: Matthaeus Becker, 1605); *De corporis humani fabrica, libri III* (Basel: Sebastianus Henricpetrus, 1588); *Vivae imagines partium corporis humani aeneis formis expressae et ex theatro anat.* (Frankfurt: de Bry, 1620); *Pinax theatri botanici* (Basel: Ludovici Regis, 1623). His brother Johannes was also a professor of botany and anatomy at Basel, and published extensively as well.

[2]   Bern: Joannes le Preux, 1604.

De Hermaphroditorum is an important document also in that it reveals a significant difference between early modern notions of knowledge and the modern mask of scientific objectivity. Bauhin does not distinguish between literary, philosophical, theological, and medical works as being of greater or lesser value, but lists Petronius and Paré equally. It is as important for him to record the collective beliefs that inform scientific inquiry as it is to convey the results of observation from nature.[3]

But this balance between culture and science reveals the fundamentally problematic nature of scientific discourse. Any record of observations made translates the bodies in question into a particular cultural/linguistic domain. The culture within which Bauhin is writing, and into which he must translate the hermaphroditic body, is based on opposition of binaries. The hermaphroditic body can only exist in this culture as a mutilated body, severed from itself. The gap between the reality of the hermaphrodite, with all the implications this reality holds for the concept of gender, and the discursive system that attempts to express it, becomes increasingly evident in Bauhin's oscillation between medical theory and the examples taken from his own observations.

This oscillation is echoed by one between fairly revolutionary views on reproduction, and more conventional Aristotelian views on the differences between the sexes. For example, in his preface, Bauhin goes beyond even his Hippocratic model in crediting both mother and father with the conception of a child, rather than portraying the mother as a passive ground in which the male seed is planted ("quia ad Foetus ortum & incrementum utriusque parentis semen ex aequo conferat," "since to the conception and growth of the foetus the seed of each parent contributes equally," A1v).[4] Yet, when it is time to account for the difference in sexes (Bauhin's term), the treatise returns to the Hippocratic view of the female as merely a weaker or deficient male:

> At in specie sexus diversitatem Hippocrates ostendens, causam in seminis praedominatibus refert, ita quidem ut mas ex semine robusto: foemina vero, ex debiliori nascatur: robustum semen, masculum: debile, foemineum vocitans ... (*De Hermaphroditorum*, A2)

> (But Hippocrates, pointing out the difference in types of sex, attributes the cause to the predominant seed, so indeed the male is born from the stronger seed; and the female, from the weaker. He calls the stronger seed masculine; the weaker, feminine ...)

---

3   In fact, as Céard points out, medical material is dominated by other cultural records: "les ouvrages de médecine n'y tiennent qu'une petite place, non pas que Bauhin, médecin lui-même, s'en désintéresse, mais parce que les historiographes et cosmographes, les juristes et les théologiens lui offrent une matière beaucoup plus abondante" (*La nature et les prodiges*, p. 439).

4   In fact, his terminology resembles the alchemical expressions of *coniunctio*: "Semen etenim duplex in unum coalescens" (A1v: "truly the double seed joins into one"). All translations of Bauhin's work are my own.

Nonetheless, this discussion of sexual difference gives rise to a range of sexes, from the very masculine male, through the more average male, then the androgyne, to viragos and "bold, strong" women, and finally to the "soft and effeminate" double females (A2v–A3). For all of its imposition of hierarchy upon gender, associating power and superiority with that which is masculine, weakness and inferiority with the feminine, this treatise is novel in its recognition of a wide range of genders and even of sexed bodies. The almost absurdly detailed examples of various sexes destabilize the clear distinctions between them, and serve to make the figure of the hermaphrodite more natural than previous representations had done. Surely there is a long journey from Bauhin's approach to sexual difference to a real acceptance of difference in all of its forms, but one can sense movement towards a less simplistic understanding of sex in the complex machinations of this treatise. In the conclusion of his summary of Hippocrates, for example, Bauhin repeats that there are thus three forms of humanity, and that even within these forms there are different degrees of sex ("quod magis aut minus tales sint," "which may be more or less so").

Most significantly, Bauhin/Hippocrates concludes that this variation in sexual presentation is also influenced by in equal measure by "temperamentum, & alimenta, & educationes, & consuetudines" (A3v: "temperament, nourishment, upbringing, and custom"). This assessment of the importance of culture to construction of what we would think of as gender provides a necessary link between the biological model and literary/philosophical/theological sources that Bauhin offers throughout his work.

An unusual revision of the Aristophanic myth of the hermaphrodite follows the biological account of generation, balancing the natural with the cultural. Like Leone Ebreo (cited in the introduction of this study), Bauhin compares the Aristophanic myth to the hint of a male/female Adam in Genesis. Following Leone's exclusively heterosexual version of the myth, Bauhin claims that there were three sexes (the word he uses is *sexus*) at the dawn of time: male, female, and both. Thus, initially at least, unlike Aristophanes's version, this account does not accept homosexuality: the male and the female are only single beings. Bauhin's original hermaphrodite is the only figure in this version of the myth that is similar to the Aristophanic being. In a further twist, Bauhin associates these hermaphrodites with the moon, since the moon intercedes between the Sun (associated, along with its heat, with the masculine) and the Earth (because it is cold and damp, considered feminine): "quia masculum Sole genitum erat: foemina, Terra: promiscuum denique, Luna: utriusque enim Luna est particeps" (A4: "since the masculine is generated by the Sun; the feminine, by the Earth; and finally, the mixed gender by the Moon, since the Moon participates in both spheres"). Thus, he introduces gnostic and alchemical notions into the Neoplatonic source material; these alternative philosophies seem to drive Bauhin's thinking, and they resurface with some frequency throughout his treatise. In contrast to the biological model, which portrays the Androgyne, like the female, as a defective male, the Aristophanic myth and Bauhin's version of it suggest that the hermaphrodites were a race of superior beings. At the end of this tale, Bauhin again links the Platonic/Aristophanic myth to Genesis by citing Ebreo. He then links the

Hippocratic and Platonic Androgynes to the dual-sexed Galenic Hermaphrodite, which has both male and female sexual organs. Thus, Bauhin announces and demonstrates in part his program of linking literary (which he calls poetic), historical, medical and legal discourse on hermaphrodites.

Hermaphroditic Discourse

While his introduction summarizes the various forms of discourse used to express the hermaphroditic body, the first two chapters, "De nominibus Hermaphroditorum quibus eos Graeci donarunt" ("On the Names the Greeks Gave Hermaphrodites") and "De Hermaphroditorum appellationibus Latinis" ("On Latin Names for Hermaphrodites"), focus on the critical importance of language itself for the shaping of that body. These terms alternate between the somewhat derogatory "half-man" (*semimar, semivir*) and the more expressive manwoman (*marifoemina*). Bauhin points out that the term *androgyne* is often used for castrated men ("quibus virilia excisa sunt"). He adds that such a name is associated with terms for debility (mental or physical) and effeminacy. The linguistic validation of that which is masculine, achieved by means of these associations, is quite thorough (A7). Bauhin also notes that Sophocles, Virgil, and Ovid also call Centaurs "half-men" (*semihomines* in Latin); thus he, like Livy, links confusion of sex to confusion of species (A8). The second chapter similarly lists Latin discussions of Hermaphrodites (also androgynes and *semivires*), which seem to emphasize the monstrous nature of these beings with even greater insistence.

In his third chapter, Bauhin summarizes the problematic nature of the hermaphrodite quite succinctly in his attempt to define the dual-sexed being:

> Hermaphroditus definimus hominem, cui membrorum genitalium conformatio est vitiosa, & in quo praeter pudendum legitimum, alterius sexus pudendum apparet ... Vel ... Hermaphroditus est commixtio masculini & foeminini sexus, simul etiam utroque genitale proprium habente. (*De hermaphroditorum*, B3v)

> (We define the hermaphrodite as a man the shape of whose genital members is deformed, and in whom in place of a proper sexual organs, appear the organs of the other sex ... Or, the Hermaphrodite is a mixture of masculine and feminine sex, having at once its own and the other genitals.)

To some extent, one definition calls the other into question; if a hermaphrodite is a *semimar* or *semivir*, that is, his effeminacy is expressed only as a lack, then a hermaphrodite containing both male and female characteristics seems to be a logical impossibility (since femininity is only a lack of masculinity). The hermaphrodite as half-man and the hermaphrodite as dual-sexed cannot coexist in the same epistemological system. The encyclopedic nature of Bauhin's work thus seems to undercut any possibility of analyzing or even of describing the hermaphrodite.

Furthermore, Bauhin conflates biological gender with its social expression, that is to say with sexual behavior, defining the hermaphrodite as a being which has both male and female sexual organs, or which is bisexual: "Qui utraque habet membra virilia & muliebria: vel, qui turpiter & agit & patitur" ("Who has both male and female members; or who wickedly takes both the active and passive roles").[5] Sex becomes performative (and thus closer to our notion of gender), as it is defined by sexual behavior. Bauhin claims that this bisexual behavior is characteristic of an African race.[6] The adverb "turpiter" (wickedly) attached to this bisexual behavior signals the opinion that it is morally monstrous. The displaced geography of these tribes seems to protect Europe from such mores; a moral map could be drawn according to Bauhin's narrative, in which clear boundaries separate the unacceptable from the western European norm.

The fact that this mapping involves the rejection of unacceptable sexual behavior from European culture becomes clear as Bauhin continues this chapter with a discussion of the marvelous fountain of Salmacis, which, according to Ovid, transforms men into hermaphrodites. Bauhin explains this transformation as an allegory of promiscuity.[7] This promiscuity can even be translated into the intellectual realm, and associated with those who "use speech with excessive ornamentation, neglecting the right reason of truth."[8] Sexuality is also portrayed as having a civilizing effect, but this effect is also one of decadence or corruption, linked closely to rhetorical excess.

In fact, this chapter evolves in a serpentine movement from a condemnation of bisexuality, to one of sexuality or desire in any form, and finally to a longer discussion of the beneficial effects of desire. Sexuality is presented as linked purely to the feminine; but in the story of the Carians and Lelegeians, masculinity is linked to violence and barbarism.[9] Bauhin, citing Ovid's description of Salmacis, discusses the leisure necessary for the cult of love (B6v), and bemoans the fact that young men

---

[5] He also cites Bacchus here as an example of bisexual behavior: "Quod posterius de Baccho ferunt, ut virum egisse, utque foeminam passum esse" (B3v: "Which was later reported of Bacchus, that he was active like a man, and was passive like a woman").

[6] "Hinc Androgynae apellabatur populi quidam in Africa utriusque naturae, inter se vicibus coeuntes ..." (B3v: "Hence, a certain people in Africa who are of both natures, copulating among themselves in alternating roles, are called Androgynes"). Bauhin also refers to Pliny's statement that the Libyans and the Machylas (a legendary tribe) exhibit similar behavior.

[7] "Est haec fabula, imago libidinem & voluptatem, quae emasculant effoeminantque" (B5: "This fable is an image of lust and desire, which emasculates and renders effeminate").

[8] "Qui veritatis ratione neglecta, sermonum ornatibus superfluis utuntur" (B5).

[9] "Ergo ea aqua non impudico morbi vitio, sed animis Barbarorum, humanitatis dulcedine mollitis, eam famam adepta est" (B5v: "So this water acquires its fame not from the disease of immodest vice but from the souls of Barbarians tamed by the sweetness of humanity"). Bauhin adds: "Hinc dictus Venereus ab amoenitate incolarum homines illecti omnem feritatem deposuerunt" ("Hence a place is said to be of Venus, due to the pleasantness of its inhabitants, where little by little men are enticed to put aside all savagery").

pass their time in such activities, citing *L'Isle des Hermaphrodites* as an example of the corrupting influence of desire.[10]

In these multiple readings, Bauhin seems to be following a common medieval method of exegesis, *in bono* and *in malo*, exemplified by Pierre Bersuire's readings of Ovid. Bersuire also read Ovidian myths literally, historically, naturally, and allegorically.[11] Bauhin emulates this pattern in his chapter on the definitions of the hermaphrodite, citing medical and historical sources as well as various allegorical readings. Yet there is somewhat less rigidity in Bauhin's system than in Bersuire's: the insistence of the former upon citing all known sources creates a complex and often conflicting depiction of sexuality and gender. Whereas Bersuire adheres strongly to a rigid moral system, the encyclopedic nature of Bauhin's work creates a system that is not completely resolved in its morality. Like many early modern alchemists, Bauhin cannot escape the cultural traditions within which he was educated, but much of his work seems to struggle within and against the boundaries of his culture.

This tension becomes increasingly evident in the treatise, particularly when Bauhin describes different types of hermaphrodites in clinical detail, as he does in the fourth chapter. When Bauhin cites cases of men with female organs and women with small penises and testicles (C1), he becomes so concerned with describing the minute details of their bodies that the individuality of these bodies undermines the very notion of "type" which he is trying to establish.[12] The insistence upon assigning a clearly distinct

---

[10]   "Hac de re legi potest libellus Gallico idiomate conscriptus, qui Hermaphroditus inscribitur, in quo de Hermaphroditorum insula nuper reperta agitur: & quomodo, quave ratione, quibus rebus in illa insula, hoc tempore mollium & effoeminatorum corpus, singulaeque eius partes ornentur & comentur, & ornati, voluptatibus & luxuriae dediti sint, lepidissime exponitur" (B6v: "One can read a book written in French about this matter, entitled *Hermaphroditus*, in which the island of Hermaphrodites newly discovered is discussed, and it is most cleverly explained how, why [for what reason], and by what means on this island and at this time their soft and effeminate bodies, and each part of these bodies, is adorned and decked out, and once adorned, they are given over to pleasure and lust"). The timing and wording would be right for this to be a reference to the novel of Artus, *Description de l'Isle des Hermaphrodites, nouvellement descouverte*; but Bauhin does not allude to the satirical matter of the book, the court of Henri III.

[11]   D.C. Allen, *Mysteriously Meant: The Rediscovery of Pagan Symbolism and Allegorical Interpretation in the Renaissance* (Baltimore: Johns Hopkins University Press, 1970), p. 171.

[12]   "… unus est, quia apparet in eo, quod sequitur spatium (intelligas inter anum & scrotum, aut in cute testiculorum, in eo quod est inter duos testiculos (in medio scroto) figura vulvae mulieris, in quo sunt pili, & quandoque exit urina ex eo, quod est in cute testiculorum. In mulieribus autem est species, & est vulva mulieris super pectinem, sicut testiculi rari, parvi, omnino eminentes ad exteriora, quorum unus est, sicut priapus viri, & duo sicut duo testiculi" (C1: "One type [of hermaphrodite], because in it appears something which is placed in the space [that is to say, between the anus and the scrotum] or in the skin of the testicles, in that which is between the two testicles [in the middle of the scrotum], in

sex is striking; even hermaphrodites must be categorized as male or female. Bauhin does continue by citing Paré's four categories (male with female characteristics; female with male; both; neither), but again elaborates with clinical details that disrupt the simple quaternity. The impulse to categorize everything according to a two-sex system is overturned by the real nuances of difference between the bodies observed. Nonetheless, he forges ahead with the categories.[13] The male hermaphrodite is defined as a person who has the appearance of a female vulva, but who can procreate only as a male, and who is missing the female internal organs. Similarly, the female hermaphrodites may have the appearance of a penis or testicles, but they cannot function as men. The neuter hermaphrodite bears signs of both sexes but can function as neither. But the fourth type of hermaphrodite has the full sexual organs of both male and female. Bauhin again adds the odd detail that these complete beings have a male breast on the right, female on the left (so that, even in the most extreme case of confusion of gender, there remains division). This is an echo of the sixteenth book, eighth chapter of Augustine's *City of God*, which begins with accounts of monstrous races, including that of the Androgyni who have such a double configuration.

These descriptions underscore several epistemological problems posed by the existence of hermaphrodites. First, Bauhin cannot seem to find the right terminology for his discussion, and must designate that which he has observed or about which he has read in either masculine or feminine terms. This difficulty reflects a larger one in the cultural tradition concerning hermaphrodites: the hermaphrodite is not perceived as a gender unto itself or part of a more complex continuity of nuanced genders, but is even named as a compound of irreconcilable dualities: *androgyne, hermaphrodite.* Among the authors Bauhin cites, there is a resistance to recognition of even this compound nature. Most hermaphrodites are described as males with female organs or females with male attributes. The hermaphrodite as such can neither be named nor described; it remains outside of the realm of rational discourse. In this exile, it joins the realm of the supernatural, of monsters and portents. The hermaphrodite's subjugation to a rational system of discourse occurs only by its designation in terms of that which it is *not*: neither male nor female, *androgyne*. In this, it resembles woman, whom Bauhin describes only in male terms, as a defective man. Yet the disorderly sexuality of the hermaphrodite surfaces again and again in its potential activity and passivity, calling into question the rationalizing move that creates gender roles.

Bauhin reassuringly observes that *most* hermaphrodites have only one functional set of genitals (C2v); or, at times, neither set functions (the true neuter). But, although

---

the form of a female vulva, on which are hairs; and urine passes from time to time from that one which is in the skin of the testicles. However in the women [hermaphrodites] is a form, that appears to be and is in the vulva of the woman over the hair of the pubes, like sparse and small testicles, completely exposed to the outside, of which one is like a man's penis, and two like two testicles").

13   This unusual physiology also appears in a plate from Ulisse Aldrovandi's *Monstrorum historia* (Bononia: N. Tebaldini, 1642), p. 42, cited by Epstein in her article "Either/Or," p. 110.

the Latin language encompasses a common gender, Bauhin and most of the authors he cites cannot accept this concept as either a biological or social fact (C2v–C3).[14] Simply put, discourse cannot encompass the hermaphroditic body.

Sex and Sexuality

The real threat is that of disruption of the sexual hierarchy of male over female; thus, Bauhin similarly cites lesbianism and female bisexuality as problematic examples[15] According to Bauhin, women whose sexuality excludes men (in that women take on both the "masculine" and "feminine" roles) are necessarily inadequate. By this means, he manages to introduce the masculine ideal even into lesbian relationships. Bauhin continues by describing *tribades, fictrices* [sic] or *subigatrices*, women with enlarged clitorises, and equates the behavior of these women with lesbianism. This association of hermaphrodism with lesbianism is significant; for Lorraine Daston and Katharine Park have already pointed out that the problematic legal status of hermaphrodites in Renaissance France is linked to the condemnation of male and female homosexual behavior.[16] Sexual roles must remain fixed, immutable. And in fact, Bauhin reiterates Paré's injunction that hermaphrodites must choose their sex, and use only that sex.[17]

---

[14] "Et ideo impossibile est, aliquem talem natum perfectè habere membrum maris et foemina, quia utraque haec membra sunt invicem contraria: quamobrem non possunt perfecta reperiri in uno corpore. Nam impossibile est, ut in uno & eodem corde copuletur forma complexionalis propria sexu masculino & forma propria foeminino: & impossibile est, reperiri in eodem corpore duo excrementa simul perfecta, scilicet semen maris & semen foeminae ..." (C3v: "And therefore it is impossible, for anyone to be born perfectly of such a nature, to have the organs of male and female, since each of these members is contrary to the other: for this reason they cannot be found perfect in one body. For it is impossible, that in one and the same body the appearance appropriate to the masculine sex and that appropriate to the feminine be joined in association: and it is impossible that two perfect excretions be found at once in the same body, that is to say the seed of the male and the seed of the female").

[15] "... quamvis enim reperiantur mulieres, quae agunt & patiuntur, id alia de causa sit, nec utrumque perfecte facere possunt ..." (C3v: "... so that however many women can be found, who are active and passive in sex, this is for another reason, and they cannot perform either role perfectly ...")

[16] "Hermaphrodites in Renaissance France," p. 2.

[17] "Has ... leges ... sexum quo uti, & in quo manere ac vivere velint, eligere jubent, capitali poena addita ... si ab electo semel sexu discessisse deprehendantur: quidam enim utroque abusi creduntur, & promiscuè cum viris & foeminis voluptuati." (C4: "These laws ... command them to choose the sex which they use, and in which they wish to remain and live, with penalty of death imposed ... if they are caught deviating from the sex first elected: in fact anyone believed to use either sex improperly, promiscuously taking pleasure with men and women ...")

In these laws to which the treatise alludes, bisexuality and hermaphrodism are conceptually linked. The situation is further problematized by the fact, which Bauhin makes very clear in the following pages, that the choice is not left to the person in question, but is made by medical and legal experts on the basis of certain stereotypical characteristics. Bauhin suggests that many cases are dubious, and that the physical attributes of a person may change, even in adolescence. Nonetheless, he lists signs by which a male hermaphrodite may be distinguished from a female:

> Nam si vulva ... pervia sit, ut virile membrum admittere possit: si menses illac profluant: si capilli promissi sint, tenues ac molles, si facies foeminea, si vox subtilis, si mammae mulieribus similes sunt, si denique ad illam totius corporis effoeminati mollitiem, animi quoque fracti & timidi parem conditiorem additam habeant, & caeteras actiones mulieribus similes, foeminei sexus potentiores, & planè foeminae judicantur. (*De hermaphroditorum*, C5)

> (For if the vulva is penetrable, so that the male member may enter: if menses flow from there: if her hair is long, fine and soft, if the face is that of a woman, if the voice is delicate, if the breasts are like those of a woman, if, then, to this softness of the whole effeminate body, they have in addition a similar condition of the soul also broken and timid, and other actions similar to those of a woman, the feminine sex predominates and they can clearly be judged women.)

Essentially, according to this passage, a person who can be penetrated is a woman; the rest of the definition operates largely by circular reasoning. Bauhin uses the terms "like a woman" and "feminine" to define what *is* feminine. Thus, the condition of being a woman is created by its own definition. Furthermore, much of this definition would now be recognized as stemming from cultural impositions, rather than from any innate characteristics. Women are trained to be timid and "feminine." Thus, if one were to analyze Bauhin's definition of a "female" hermaphrodite, one would have to conclude that she is largely, if not entirely, a cultural construct.

The definition of a male is briefer and more absolute – in fact, disturbingly so:

> Si penem convenienti magnitudine, quoad crassitiem & longitudinem compositum habeant, se valide ac alacriter erigentem, si semine manantem, virilis sexus potentiores, & planè viri pronuntiatur. (*De hermaphroditorum*, C5)

> (If they have a penis composed of the right size, with respect to thickness and length, becoming erect quickly and vigorously, if it remains erect until ejaculation, the male sex predominates and they may clearly be pronounced men.)

The quality of being male is reduced to one organ, without any reference to a state of mind, or behavior, or other physical characteristics such as strength. The male is defined purely by the existence and behavior of his penis, just as the female is contained by a set of ill-described feminine traits. But even here, seeming modesty masks an inability to define virility. Bauhin does not clarify what the "right size" is for male sexual organs, any more than he reveals what women's breasts should look like. Obviously, the system for judging sex is closed, except to initiates in the medical profession; but this atmosphere of secrecy suggests a certain ignorance about the parameters of sex (which at this point in the treatise more closely resembles gender), and where maleness ends and femaleness might begin. Bauhin summarizes by stating that men are more masculine than feminine, and women more feminine than masculine; yet again, he is using circular reasoning which does not advance understanding of sexual difference in the slightest degree, but which places the two sexes only in relation to each other. He also states this difference as a performative one: men use their male genitalia in the sexual act, women use their female organs (C5v). His difficulty in elucidating the concept of sex reveals not only the problematic relationship between science and culture, in which traditional stereotypes obscure actual observations, but the fundamental epistemological problems which any attempt to define sex by means of external signs poses.

These epistemological difficulties are placed in the context of legal and political systems when Bauhin's discussion extends to monsters. The confusion between sexes that hermaphrodites evoke is reflected by the confusion between species that most monsters embody. Bauhin, although an apologist for hermaphrodites in many ways, thus associates them with monsters to some extent.[18] The title of his treatise, *De Hermaphroditorum monstrosorumque partuum*, at once links beings of ambiguous gender with the monstrous, and distinguishes them from it. That which is unclassifiable, which remains at the edges of intellectual experience, is treated together in this book with the same mixture of fascination and horror. Women, hermaphrodites, monsters, other races and unusual species are described by European male authorities who attempt to define these beings, so as to control them.

Bauhin does reveal a certain evolution in attitudes, away from the impulse to destroy all that is different, towards an effort to integrate the other into the same. This is, nevertheless, an effort which often resembles destruction. He reviews the current legal status of hermaphrodites:

> Yet Androgynes, when they have human form, can be counted as men according to the Jurists, and they judge them to be monsters and discharge them from the ranks of humanity, only when born deprived of human form. Nonetheless, once Androgynes were among the prodigies, and St. Augustine considered them a monstrous race of men ...[19]

---

[18] For an account of Bauhin's teratology in a larger historical context, see Katharine Park and Lorraine Daston, "Unnatural Conceptions: The Study of Monsters in France and England," *Past and Present* 92 (1981): 20–54.

[19] "Quanquam Androgynes, cum forman habeant humanum, apud Jurisconsultos ... inter homines annumerari possint, & solum existiment monstra, & expungant ab ordine hominum, forma humani destitutos partus. Nihilominus olim aliquando inter prodigia fuerint Androgynes: & Hermaphroditos D. Augustinus monstruosa hominum genera ..." (C6v–C7).

Bauhin's first statement approaches the modern definition of the term *monster*; rather than a sign of Divine will (*monstrare*), a monster is that which is not human, does not fit into the parameters of its species. Hermaphrodites are considered to be a natural phenomenon that must be accepted as human when other human characteristics obtain.[20] They are not terrifying portents that must be annihilated.[21] Within the realm of scientific discourse, there was some attempt to explain hermaphrodism as a condition that remained *within* the natural scheme, even if this effort was hampered by predominant cultural attitudes.

Hermaphrodites and the Supernatural

In fact, driven by his culture, Bauhin deems it necessary to enumerate a variety of natural, unnatural, and supernatural phenomena in relation to the hermaphrodite, and asks whether it is a sign (*ostentum*), a monster (*monstrum*), a portent (*portentum*), or a prodigy (*prodigium*).[22] According to Cicero, he adds, all of these manifestations are the same, in that they all predict or present future events (C7). But a sign is something that is *praeter naturam* (beyond the normal bounds of nature but not divine or supernatural),[23] like a comet (believed to be preternatural in the Renaissance) or thunder or lightning on a clear day. A monster is an error of nature (D1: *naturae error*), such as a calf born with a human face. There are three kinds of monsters: an animal of a different species, born to another animal; an animal of confused or mixed species; or an animal born with deformities.

Bauhin devotes considerable space to portents, which he defines as things unnatural (*contra naturam*, but not necessarily of divine origin) which predict the future. All of the examples Bauhin gives are read politically. Hermaphrodites could be portents, according to some classical definitions; that is, their bodies could be read as an allegorical text about future events. Nonetheless, this notion of portents evokes an extreme use of the body as a text, to be read as the representation of something to which

---

[20] Once again, Bauhin owes his inspiration for this relative tolerance to Augustine, who makes much the same argument about "monsters" in the sixteenth book (ch. 8) of the *City of God*.

[21] It should be observed that superstitious reaction to hermaphrodites still retained a tight hold on the popular imagination in the Renaissance. Even Montaigne equates those of ambiguous gender with monstrosity in his essay on the "monstrous child," *Essais*, bk 2, essay 30, cited in the introduction above.

[22] For a detailed analysis of the differences between prodigies and miracles in the sixteenth and seventeenth centuries, see Lorraine Daston, "Marvelous Facts and Miraculous Evidence in Early Modern Europe," particularly pp. 93–100. Daston enumerates Aquinas' categories of the supernatural, natural, and preternatural, then demonstrates a complex evolution of these categories that effaces and transforms distinctions between them.

[23] Again, see Daston "Marvelous Facts," p. 97.

it is not in any way naturally related, thus resembling Sextus Empiricus's "indicative sign."[24] The deformed body is appropriated to become the site of expression of popular fears, and the means of expelling such fears through the destruction of that which is at once too different and not different enough. Conveniently, this use of the body ritualistically controls at once the situation that is genuinely the source of fear and the body itself, which is either "read" by others and thus denied its own power as speaking or silent subject, or which is destroyed outright. In short, the deformed or differently sexed body can be read much as Jonathan Dollimore reads homosexuality, that is, as symbolically central to culture even as it is legally, medically, and socially expunged from culture.[25]

Livy's Rome, for example, is dependent upon the ritualistic expulsion of that which threatens the rigid ordering of the state; but the "threat" must exist to justify that order. One senses that other monsters would have been found if hermaphrodites had been lacking; yet hermaphrodites are the ideal monsters for a society so dependent on rigid hierarchies based on sexual difference. The social or natural (as defined by Renaissance jurists) order is justified by reference to the disorder that is to be found in monsters, women, homosexuals, and foreigners. This disorder is in turn defined by its apparent deviation from the social or natural order; thus the state itself seems founded upon circular reasoning in both Livy's and Bauhin's examples.

Bauhin analyzes prodigies as portents on the level of cosmic and elemental supernatural events (primarily of divine origin). Thus all of nature, like the human body, can be read as an allegorical text, subjected to the social order through language, and can serve to uphold that order.

Bauhin tries to reject the designation of the hermaphrodite as a monster,[26] but he allows that since the hermaphrodite is an unusual natural phenomenon, it can be read as a sign (*ostentum*). He asserts that the hermaphrodite is not unnatural, merely beyond what we are used to in nature. Yet, in a broader view of that which is to be designated as monstrous, including those with defects of any sort, those too large or too small, those with too many or too few parts, those half-human and half-animal, and those of mixed animal species, then hermaphrodites would have to be considered monstrous. This admission serves as Bauhin's transition to a lengthy discussion of the causes of monstrous births, which range from divine malediction, astral influences and bad

---

24   *Outlines of Pyrrhonism*, trans. R.G. Bury (Cambridge, MA: Harvard University Press, 1976), bk 2, ch. 10, pp. 97–102.

25   Jonathan Dollimore, *Sexual Dissidence: Augustine to Wilde, Freud to Foucault* (Oxford: Oxford University Press, 1991), p. 28: "… in our own time the negation of homosexuality has been in direct proportion to its symbolic centrality; its cultural marginality in direct proportion to its cultural significance."

26   Céard discusses Bauhin's argument about the place of the hermaphrodite in this scheme of signs and portents in *La nature et les prodiges* (p. 439), but seems to miss Bauhin's acceptance of the hermaphrodite as an *ostentum*, a sign (but one which is not suitable for divination, as Céard does point out).

winds, to the quantity and quality of seed in the mother or father, to a malformation of the uterus, to copulation at inappropriate times (during the woman's period) or in inappropriate manner (with the woman on top), to hereditary diseases, to the mother's imagination or her emotional state. Bauhin also includes nutrition as a factor in birth defects, but what is clear is that the larger issues of sexual relations and gender roles are closely linked to this discussion of the monstrous.

One part of the subsequent discussion of parturition is illuminating as to the cultural bases of gender distinction. Bauhin cites Anaxagoras and Parmenides to the effect that the seed for the female comes from the left (sinister) side of both the father's and mother's bodies; thus, science justified the association of the feminine with evil, since everything on the left side was considered to be bad. This recalls the notion that females are produced from weaker seed, as well as echoing the notion, current even in the Renaissance, that the hermaphrodite was produced in a middle chamber of the uterus.[27]

The warnings of possible deformities in an infant conceived during the woman's period, or with too much pleasure (G5), recall the rigid control of sexuality by various Christian sects. A deformed child is accepted as a judgment upon the moral worthiness of the parents; the child itself is thus often seen as tainted. Most of all, female pleasure is seen as tainted and deforming (H3); her imagination may run wild and imprint all sorts of strange forms on the child.[28]

Linked to this regulatory view of sexuality is a desire to assign other ambiguous creatures than the hermaphrodite to clearly defined categories of species. Thus Bauhin, in his thirteenth chapter, debates whether Satyrs are men, monkeys or demons. The insatiable sexuality of these priapic creatures links them to the previous discussion of generation; their ambiguity as to species, neither human nor animal, links them to the whole problematic tradition of the monstrous body, which is used as an allegory of moral standards. The confusion between species must be explained away in order to be accepted. The Satyrs' inordinate desire for women, and their prodigious male members, also seem menacing (K4). Bauhin has already expressed the belief that intercourse between humans and animals produces monsters (G5v–H1v); most of his examples involve human females conceiving by animals. Thus, once again, sexuality as an expression of bestial nature is linked to the uncontrollable aspects of women. Gender ambiguity, promiscuity and monstrosity are tied in with the recurring concern

---

[27] Danielle Jacquart and Claude Thomasset, *Sexuality and Medicine in the Middle Ages* (Princeton: Princeton University Press, 1988), p. 141.

[28] Bauhin offers as an example the woman who gave birth to a dark-skinned child because of a picture of an Ethiopian hanging on her bedroom wall (H3v). A popular version of this was the tale of the hairy, bear-like child born to a woman who had similarly observed a picture of Saint John the Baptist clothed in furs (H4). For an excellent overview of this notion of the role of the imagination in parturition, see Marie-Hélène Huet, *Monstrous Imagination*, particularly the first chapter, "The Renaissance Monster" (Cambridge, MA: Harvard University Press, 1993), pp. 13–35.

for regulation of reproduction, and particularly of the female role in reproduction. It is as if a repeated, perhaps unacknowledged, realization of women's powerful role in reproduction comes close to the surface in these discussions of monstrous forms.

Satyrs are also relegated to the realm of the demonic or diabolical (M4–M8v), further conjured away as supernatural but subjugated within a theological system, along with Pans, Wild Men, Incubi and Succubi. Bauhin has departed from the medical discourse of parturition, to give examples of demonic monsters purely from literary and theological realms. Yet one consuming concern he expresses is whether women can lie with and conceive by demons (Q2–S7v), in an echo of Paré (chapter 28 of *Des Monstres*) and the *Malleus maleficarum*.[29] The concern with male sexuality and the male role in reproduction is less sustained, as if less problematic (T5v–T8). Here, the fear of independent female sexuality (masturbation or lesbianism), observed in other sources by Daston and Park,[30] and of the possibility of reproduction without men, links women to the unnatural or demonic.

The largest portion of this treatise, ostensibly on hermaphrodites, is thus about demonic causes of monstrous births. Bauhin cleverly concludes by questioning whether demonic forms even exist, which can reproduce with humans. But the force of these chapters is to associate the monstrous with the demonic or supernatural, rather than the natural realm.[31] Hermaphrodites thus continue to occupy a marginal space, between that which is natural and that which is beyond nature, problematizing these categories by their mere existence.

Yet, in a reversal of the superstition that drives the central portion of his thesis, Bauhin returns finally to the question of the hermaphrodite in order to argue for tolerance and acceptance of those of ambiguous gender as human beings. He begins his chapter "On the Causes of Hermaphrodites" with citations of previous superstitious beliefs, which link hermaphrodism specifically to mythological African tribes, thereby expressing a more general fear of the other. But, as if to underscore the ridiculous nature of these beliefs, Bauhin offers a list of details that seem extreme (and that recall the Nuremberg Chronicle): some have only one eye in the middle of their forehead; some have their feet turned backwards; some have no mouth; some are the size of Pygmies, and women of five years old can conceive, but they live no longer than eight years. Some have only one leg, and their knee does not bend. Some have no necks, and eyes in their shoulders. There are also dog-headed men (V5v). Bauhin concludes wryly: "But it is not necessary to believe in every race of man that is said

---

[29]   Heinrich Kramer and James Sprenger, *The Malleus maleficarum* (New York: Dover, 1971), part 1, question 3, pp. 21–8.

[30]   "The Hermaphrodite and the Orders of Nature," p. 431; also Park, "Hermaphrodites or Lesbians? Sexual Anxiety and Renaissance Medicine," Ninth Berkshire Conference on the History of Women, Vassar College, June 1993.

[31]   This emphasis on the demonic echoes the structure of Paré's work, *Des Monstres et prodiges*, which also devotes eight central chapters (26–33) to demonic behaviors, but which does not discuss conception by demonic means.

to exist."[32] This skepticism hints at a nascent tension between medical observations and other forms of cultural discourse. Bauhin then presents the more positive view of monstrosity:

> God is the creator of everything ... knowing the beauty of the whole, parts of which he weaves together either through similarity or difference: but he who cannot observe the whole, is offended as it were by the deformity of a part.[33]

Thus, hermaphrodites should be accepted as part of the divine scheme, which men cannot understand. Nonetheless, Bauhin attempts to understand the hermaphroditic body, and cites Paré's explanations of the causes of this "monster": either too much seed in conception, or the mother contributes as much seed as the father.[34] Parmenides, according to Bauhin, associates hermaphrodites with bisexuals, and attributes both conditions to the imperfect joining of the seed (V7). Bauhin then debates whether both male and female carry male and female seed, or whether the seed is gender specific. He also refers to Averroes, who attributes hermaphrodism and other deformities to excess of the mother's seed (V8); apparently, the cause of deformity was quite gender specific, and the father's seed could never be in excess. Other theories alluded to attribute deformities to too much heat, too much humidity, too much matter (V8v–X2). Here, Bauhin has returned to a more naturalizing view of the hermaphrodite and of its origins.

Empirical Evidence

Once again, this proliferation of theories is swept away by Bauhin's preference for more empirical forms of inquiry; he briefly mentions the theory of seven cells in the uterus (three on the right for males, three on the left for females, one in the middle for hermaphrodites), but rejects it as utter nonsense based on his own clinical work and anatomical observations (X2v–X3). He explains that there is only one "cavity" (which he has observed in dissections) with two "pockets" (*sinus*, on the left and the right). Following long-standing tradition, he seems to argue that the left pocket is for the female, the right for the male. His enumeration of all of the factors involved in the conception of a hermaphrodite displays this traditional prejudice at its extreme; yet he proposes this theory only to reject it:

---

[32] "Sed omnia genera hominum quae dicuntur esse, esse credere non est necesse" (V6).

[33] "Deus enim creator est omnium ... sciens universitatis pulchritudinem, quarum partium vel similitudine, vel diversitate contexat: sed qui totum inspicere non potest, tanquam deformitate partis offenditur ..." (V6).

[34] Paré's account is a simplification of the Hippocratic scheme, as the mother contributes only female seed, and the father contributes male seed.

Since nature always tends towards the best, and so strives always to generate a male, and never a female; since the female is a man born by accident, and a freak of nature, as Aristotle claims in his book on animals; therefore, whenever possible a male is born, as to all the principle members. But because of the bad formation of the womb, and the incorrect position of the foetus, and due to inequality of the seed, since it cannot perfectly create a perfect male, so it generates a female or a hermaphrodite: and this latter is impotent in its male member, as is clear from experience: this is what he [Aristotle] says. This is clearly a vulgar and womanly opinion ... which ought to be refuted.[35]

Although Bauhin resists the misogynistic Aristotelian attitudes towards reproduction and gender, he condemns the philosopher with the word "womanly," thus retaining some of the prejudice he wishes to dispel. At any rate, a break from Aristotelian tradition, which had a strong hold on earlier notions of reproduction, is clear at this point in the treatise.

This tendency to cite various sources at some length, only to dismiss their theories as born of ignorance, problematizes the apparent conservatism that resurfaces from time to time, for example in the discussion of sexual positions. That of the woman on top was considered unacceptable,[36] and enforcement of male sexual superiority was a priority even for Renaissance scientists. Even the woman's position after sex was crucial for proper conception (of a male).[37] Every aspect of female sexuality seems

---

[35] *De hermaphroditorum*, X3: "Quia natura semper tendit ad melius: & sic intendit semper generare masculum, & nunquam foemellam. Quia foemella est vir occasione natus, & monstru in natura, ut Aristot. in lib. de animalibus. Quare aliquando generetur masculus, quoad omnia membra principalia; sed tamen propter malam dispositionem matricis, & objecti, & secundum seminis inaequalitatem, cum non posset perficere masculum perfectum, sic generat foemellam, ut Hermaphroditen: & is est impotens in membro virili, ut patet per experientiam: haec ille. Haec sanè vulgi & mulierculam opinio est ... quam ut refutari debeat ...."

[36] "... vitiosus hic infamisque conceptus ex indecoro concubitu conflatur, cum praeter usum ac commoditatem exercendae Veneris vir supinus, mulier prona decumbit ..." (X3–X3v: "... defective and indecent conception occurs from improper sexual position, as against usage and propriety the man lies on his back in the sexual act, and the woman bends down on top ...").

[37] "in muliere posteaquam virile semen receperit in utera, positura corporis observanda: semper vitanda est, quae modo supino sit: quoniam cum maneat tunc semen in media parte uteri, non fit absolutus mas, aut foemina, sed uterque simul, qui Hermaphroditus dicitur: cum enim attrahantur tunc nutrimentum, tam à dextra uteri parte quam à sinistra, fit quod ob mixtum illum calorem cum frigore promiscuus sexus repraesentetur; ut patere potest ex mulieribus Lunensibus (ut inquit Pierius) quae nil curantes post seminis conceptum hanc posituram, plures Hermaphroditos generant ..." (X3v: "The position of the body is to be observed in a woman after she has received male semen: it is always to be avoided, that she be in the supine position: for when the semen remains in the middle part of the uterus, it does not make an absolute male, nor female, but both at once, which is said to be a hermaphrodite: for nutriments are thus drawn as much from the right part of the uterus

to be dictated by the demands of male-oriented notions of reproduction. For example, according to Avicenna, if a woman waits too long in her cycle to conceive, the child will be a hermaphrodite (conception one to five days after the period will create a male; five to eight a female; eight to twelve a male; and after that a hermaphrodite). Here, Bauhin calls simple logic to the defense of truth: "If hermaphrodites were born (conceived) the twelfth day after the flow of menses, their number would be found to be much greater."[38] Bauhin seems to present all views in the interest of thoroughness, but rarely does he declare one interpretation to be absolutely true; one begins to wonder if he believes any of the material he is presenting. Yet these chapters serve a very useful purpose; that of dispelling misinformation and superstition, which prepares the way for a more direct observation of nature.

Bauhin even cites astrological theories of the generation of hermaphrodites (X6–X7v); most obviously, the influence of Gemini, or the conjunction of Mercury and Venus might account for the birth of such double creatures. A hermaphrodite born during a total eclipse is clearly a portent of evil, and must be destroyed. Other astrologers have contended that Mars must be present at the conjunction of Mercury and Venus in order for a hermaphrodite to be born; still others credit other stars or planets. If the Moon is present at this conjunction, the men destined to castrate themselves, the Archigalli (priests of Cybele) will be born. Here, Bauhin pauses to undercut these prolific yet mutually contradictory theories; clearly, he asserts, some form of insanity is responsible for such self-mutilation.

The conjunction of theory and reality is seen at its extreme at this point in the treatise; and although the clinical and cultural seem to mesh at various points, Bauhin reveals increasing difference and tension between these two forms of discourse in his work. The chapter following that on astrological explanations is a discussion of the internal anatomy of various actual hermaphrodites, observed during dissection. Here, the wondrous (*admirabilia* and *rara*, Y1v) becomes real. Bauhin recalls seeing a woman with a penis in place of her vulva. The feminine ovaries (which Bauhin calls *vasa praeparantia*) were doubled, so that each sent seed (eggs and sperm) to the uterus and the penis (Y1v–Y2). The cervix and the "neck" of the uterus were like those in most women, but the "vessel" itself was thicker than in most women. The penis was not connected to any scrotum, and was thinner than normal; it contained two *spongiosa corpora*, with two arteries.

Bauhin seems to prefer to talk about two living hermaphrodites he observed, dismissing the dissection with "haec sint satis de Hermaphrodito quem mortuum secui"

---

as the left, and this is done so that the mixture of this heat with cold creates the mixed [promiscuous] sex; as can be made clear from the women of Lunens [as Pierus says] who not caring about their position after conception, gave birth to many hermaphrodites ...").

[38] "Si nascerentur Hermaphroditi, post duodecimum fluoris mensium diem, copiosior eorum numerus reperiretur" (X5).

("this is enough about the dead Hermaphrodite I dissected," Y2). He categorizes the living hermaphrodites as male and female. The female was Ethiopian, and imperfect in either sex, having a short, thin penis and a narrow vagina. She asked for an operation to be made a woman outright, but was refused because of the risk to her life (Y2v). The male had a penis and two testicles, and a small opening where a vagina would be (but not penetrable, and therefore he was male).

Bauhin also cites his brother Johann, who saw the body of an eighteen-year-old girl, clothed and coiffed in feminine fashion, who had died of the plague, and who had a large penis and two testicles. But because the body had a small opening for urination "more mulierum," she was judged to be female. Yet no uterus was found, and the internal organs seemed like those of a male ("aliis masculis similis erat," Y3). She had no female breast tissue, but the penis was defective, having no urinary duct. Bauhin concludes that the girl may in fact have been a *Hypospadaeus*, a semi-eunuch, that is, a sterile male. Bauhin demonstrates some reluctance to accept the predominant medical attitude that that which is not perfectly male is female. What is clear from these descriptions is that a range of different body types exists, and that designation of sex as male or female is problematic in the face of these bodily realities.

As if to underscore the problematic nature of this distinction, Bauhin cites historical examples of the difficulty of determining sex in the next chapter. For example, in 1601, one Daniel Burckhammer, who had been married to a woman for seven years, gave birth to a girl conceived in an adulterous affair with a Spaniard (Y4–Y4v). The baby was baptised Elisabeth in a public ceremony attended by various officials and nobles (Y4v).[39] Bauhin tells a similar story of a Hungarian solder, who gave birth in 1598 (Y4v–Y5). There are also several stories of pregnant monks: one from 1478, one from earlier (Y5). A story from Basel tells of a peasant who became suspicious of a servant-girl of whom his wife seemed overly fond; and, indeed, the proper authorities, once alerted, found the servant to be much more a man than a woman. The servant in question confessed to adultery, made it clear that he had taken the male role, was punished and forced to change clothing and name (Y6). In these stories, the distinction between sexual ambiguity and sexual fraud is also unclear; Daston and Park have pointed out that this was a particular obsession in France in the late sixteenth century.[40] This fear of fraud echoes Paré and Tesserant's injunctions against "double paillardise" or bisexuality, which was seen as particularly threatening to French society. Yet Bauhin does not speak in detail of the punishment in any of these cases; it is not clear from his work how harsh the Swiss, Germans or Hungarians were, although they do not seem to react as vehemently as the French.

---

[39] This story is also told in *The Fugger News-letters: Being a Selection of Unpublished Letters from the Correspondents of the House of Fugger during the Years 1568–1605*, ed. Victor von Klarwill, trans. Pauline de Chary (London: John Lane, 1924), pp. 242–3. My thanks to Konrad Eisenbichler for this reference.

[40] "The Hermaphrodite and the Orders of Nature," pp. 426–7.

Yet Bauhin should not be read as a revolutionary researcher who accepts such ambiguity; this much is clear when he returns to the discussion of whether Adam was a hermaphrodite, with which he opened his book. Bauhin argues that the hermaphrodite is merely the image of Adam and Eve joined by God as a couple (once again echoing Leone Ebreo), and points out Church doctrine condemning the belief that the original man was a hermaphrodite (Z1–Z2). He believes that the image is meant to be an allegory of human nature, in which man and woman were meant to depend upon each other. The anti-homosexual implications are made evident in Bauhin's citation of this story as a condemnation of sodomy (Z2v). In the delicate balance between science and theology that most Renaissance intellectuals strained to achieve, in a society where procreation is mandated, a sterile being cannot be portrayed as the ideal. Even when fertile, hermaphrodites do not seem to procreate within the accepted parameters of heterosexual marriage. Science, at the service of society, must thus condemn them, and cast them aside. Under these circumstances, the marginalization of hermaphrodites seems to take on crucial importance for the political scheme of things, as is evident from the historical examples Bauhin gives in chapter thirty-five. A hermaphrodite was born during the second Punic War, fifteen others at various points in the history of Rome, for example preceding the death of Claudius, whose reign was followed by that of Nero. In almost every case, the hermaphroditic child was carried out to the deep ocean and drowned. Similarly, the more contemporary monster of Ravenna is read as reflecting general corruption and ruin in society (Z5). The inevitable result of this politicized reading of the hermaphroditic body is the use of accusations of hermaphrodism in order to discredit political rivals; such are the accusations leveled against the Archbishop of Brunschweig and against Henri III of France.

Cultural Questions

Bauhin chooses to contrast this derogatory use of the hermaphrodite not with science, but with mythological accounts in which hermaphrodism is associated with some supernatural force. Cecrops, original king of Athens (and reputedly of Egyptian origin) is alternately portrayed as hermaphroditic or as half-man, half-dragon. He was known for his wisdom and generosity (Z8v). Bauhin, in his usual recourse to reason, points out that the myth of his sexual ambiguity may have arisen from his enactment of matrimonial laws. His monstrous form may have been a figure of early Greek civilization, half-savage and half-human (Z8v–Aa). Tiresias's switch from male to female and back again results in his prophetic powers (Aa–Aa2). As Delcourt contends, the mythic hermaphrodite is revered; the bodily hermaphrodite is rejected.

This marginalization is clear from Bauhin's enumeration in chapter thirty-seven of the treatment various cultures (*Ethnicos*) mete out to hermaphrodites: the Romans, of course, drowned their ambiguous infants. According to Bauhin, who cites le Moyne, the "Indians" of Florida use their hermaphrodites as beasts of burden, particularly to carry

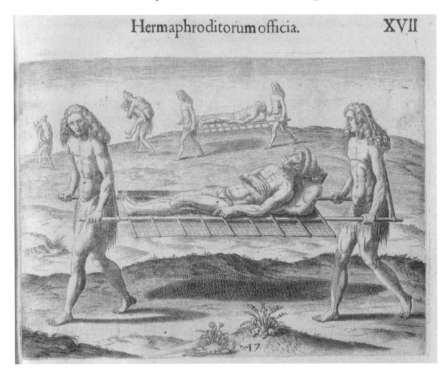

Figure 2.1   **"Floridian" hermaphrodites (probably berdaches), from Theodor de Bry, *America, Brevis narratio eorum quae in Florida Americae provincia Gallis acciderunt* ... (Frankfurt: de Bry, 1591). Courtesy of the Division of Rare and Manuscript Collections, Cornell University Library**

the dead and wounded off of the field of battle (Aa6v).[41] Thus, the hermaphrodites are associated with death and with various animal species. The hermaphrodites must also bear those afflicted with disease to the hospital: it is not clear whether they are given this role because they are considered subhuman or superhuman. They must gather all sorts of wild animals, fish and crocodiles, and carry baskets of supplies to the storehouse (Aa6v). Bauhin also uses this incredible tale to demonstrate the superiority of Christian (Western European) culture; speaking of Saint Augustine, he points out that: "He states that God above is the creator of all things" (Aa7). Bauhin argues that hermaphrodites

---

[41]   This description was originally to be found in the account of René Goulaine de Laudonnière, *L'Histoire notable de la Floride* (Paris: Auvray, 1586), A5, but was also taken up and expanded by Theodor de Bry in his collection, *America* (*Brevis narratio eorum quae in Florida americae provincia Gallis acciderunt* ... 1591), plate 17, "Hermaphroditorum officia."

should be baptized and should be allowed to enter into marriage contracts; they should be able to inherit domains and other property (Aa7). He quotes Eusebius who criticizes the Roman law condemning hermaphrodites to death (Aa7v). Thus, Bauhin uses the argument of tolerance to further the mistrust of the inhabitants of the Western hemisphere, who themselves mistreat hermaphrodites; this "tolerance" is used to further racism, as the "Indians" are equated with the ancient, savage Romans.

This tolerance has its limits, however, and the ongoing condition of hermaphrodism is deemed unacceptable, even by Bauhin, who in his thirty-eighth chapter discusses the "cure" of hermaphrodites. Male hermaphrodites who do not emit urine from the false feminine opening or vulva, can be surgically corrected to eliminate any feminine aspects. Any unnecessary organs are cut away: from a female hermaphrodite, the "false" penis and testicles; from a male, any vulva (Aa8v). Thus, the beings described as created by God in the previous chapter must be corrected by man in order to fit cultural standards of gender. Yet there was no means of "correcting" a "female" hermaphrodite in the sixteenth century, if her vagina was not sufficiently large. However, if only the opening to the vagina was too small, it could be dilated or perforated (Bb). Bauhin also suggests dilation of the cervix or even uterus, if upon examination by means of a speculum, the cervix or uterus exhibits no adhesion (Bb1–Bb1v). He describes this process in detail, but warns that only very clever surgeons should attempt it; in fact, the only attempt he made does not seem to have been successful. The woman died, although he claims that a delay in seeking medical help was the real cause of her demise. Nonetheless, some of the operations suggested by Bauhin were potentially lethal, and one might wonder if there was really a difference between drowning hermaphrodites at birth and using painful, often deadly surgery to impose contemporary notions of gender distinction upon their bodies.

Just as medicine divides hermaphrodites into male and female, and in essence refuses to recognize a hermaphroditic entity, so law delineates boundaries between male and female almost without exception. Under Judaic law, according to Bauhin, male hermaphrodites are subject to the same restrictions as any men (Bb3–Bb3v: Bauhin lists the ones regarding sexuality and dress). Female hermaphrodites are subject to the restrictions normally imposed upon women (Bb3v). They are all beneficiaries of the same protections; if they are killed, the murderer is to be punished as for any murder (Bb4). Male hermaphrodites, if they are of a holy family, are allowed to participate in religious ceremonies (this is more than hermaphrodites are allowed under Christian doctrine). They can inherit. But if a hermaphrodite is considered neither male nor female, it is treated in some cases as a non-person, in some cases as a singular person, who must be "judged" by the "priests" (Bauhin uses the Christian term *sacerdotes*) on an individual basis. There seems to be some flexibility in the Talmudic tradition concerning humans of indeterminate gender.

Christian attitudes are somewhat less flexible, as is apparent from the list of duties and of denied rights (Chapter 40). Hermaphrodites must be baptized either as male or as female, according to the sex which predominates in the individual in question. If neither sex seems to predominate, one must be assigned (Bb5). Hermaphrodites are thus made to fit uneasily into the society at large; rules are not made flexible to accommodate them, as in the Judaic system, but they are forced to conform to rigid rules (and roles) already in existence. Hermaphrodites must behave like any man or woman; for example, they must confess like any man or woman, and as often (Bb5). They may marry, but only in the role dictated by the predominant gender. This gender is to be judged (Bauhin does not clarify by whom, but as Duval's accounts make clear, designation of gender was usually performed by doctors). In the case of equal presence of both sexes, Bauhin claims that the individual in question is allowed to choose; but from the cases previously cited in other chapters, the impression arises that such freedom of choice was rare. Male hermaphrodites did enjoy some privileges over and above those of women, since apparently the consent of their parents was not required for entering into a marriage contract (Bb5v). In fact, the list of the rights of hermaphrodites merely underscores the lack of these rights among women. Female hermaphrodites, like women, could not be witnesses in a trial or to a will; in short, they had the same legal status as women (Bb6).

Hermaphrodites of any sort were bereft of certain rights. They were not supposed to enter holy orders. They could not be the rector of a university, or a judge, or a lawyer. For the purposes of these positions, hermaphrodites were considered to be *infames*, that is, disreputable. Thus Christian tolerance apparently had its limitations. Nor could a hermaphrodite be a master over others (Bb6v–Bb7: that is, in the master/apprentice relationship); its place in the social hierarchy was quite restricted. Deprivation of rights was not accompanied by a similar easing of responsibilities. Male hermaphrodites were simply punished as men; females as women.

Here, Bauhin indicates some disagreement in the civil tradition as to inheritance laws (Bb7v). A mostly male hermaphrodite – and here Bauhin refers vaguely to *virtues* as well as to physical qualities – usually should inherit, according to one jurist. Another legal expert claims that only males should inherit, not hermaphrodites. Bauhin interprets a similar pronouncement as applying only to predominantly female hermaphrodites. He adds that to the extent that women could inherit and take on responsibilities, so should female hermaphrodites. Bauhin may have, in this case, recognized the changing, in many instances declining, status of women in the early seventeenth century, and thus kept his discussion of women's rights a bit vague.[42] He does suggest that a female hermaphrodite should select one of her brothers to administer the property, if only because of the very small chance of an heir being born (Bb8–Bb8v).

It is of no small significance that Bauhin does not discuss actual cases of hermaphrodites and their legal status, even though modern scholars such as Laqueur, Park and Daston have discovered several such cases, and even though Duval, practicing medicine as a contemporary of Bauhin's, wrote shortly after about several

---

[42]　For the increasing restrictions on women, see Natalie Zemon Davis, *Society and Culture in Early Modern France* (Stanford: Stanford University Press, 1975), "City Women and Religious Change," p. 94; and "Women on Top," p. 126.

such cases.[43] For the most part, as Park and Daston suggest, the material of actual legal cases does not make the case for Christian tolerance.

Hermaphrodites in Nature

The second book of Bauhin's treatise, on hermaphroditic animals, takes a course somewhat different from that of the first. In the animal realm, hermaphrodism is seen sometimes as natural, sometimes as monstrous. Entire species of animals, like the hyena, were believed to be hermaphroditic, so that the phenomenon considered so ominous in humans is considered almost natural in animals. Still, these dual-gendered animals are portrayed as inherently menacing and evil, in a manner reminiscent of Paré's presentation of both real and imaginary beasts as monstrous. The animal realm is most often presented as a threat to various aspects of human civilization. For example, the hyena is described as a wolf-like creature (Cc2v–Cc3) that feeds on human corpses (Cc3v–Cc4). It is described as a horrifying monster (Cc3); and its eyes change color (Cc3v). Bauhin goes on at some length about the hyena's avidity for human flesh.[44] Hyenas seem to have the demonic role of harassing the spirits of the human dead (Cc4v). Bauhin cites authorities such as Pliny, Aristotle and Albertus Magnus, to the effect that hyenas can imitate human voices (Cc4v–Cc5). Thus, the demonic and supernatural are once again linked with the hermaphroditic. In fact, Bauhin seems much more interested in the predatory habits of the hyena than in its ambiguous sex: "In short, the hyena is the type [model] of frequent mutation, of severe hatred, of pernicious adulation, and of fertile tyranny ...."[45] The hermaphroditic and animal body is read as an allegory of human vice and frailty, of human failure, and suggests the abjection of the human being into an animalistic form.

The accounts of the hyena's sex are, however, conflicting: "Some affirm, others deny that hyaenas have male and female genitalia" (Cc8v). Other sources state that hyenas can change from one sex to another over the course of a year or of several years (Cc8v). Bauhin quotes Aristotle , who states that the male and the female of the species may simply resemble each other closely (Dd1v). The real justification for the accusation of hermaphrodism seems to be the hyena's lascivious behavior: "The hyena is a most libidinous animal ... this itself [their lust] increases the number of male and female hyenas, because of their immoderate desire" (Dd3). Essentially, hyenas are portrayed as bisexual (Dd3). Bauhin also claims, quoting Scaliger, that hyenas can

---

43   Laqueur, *Making Sex*, p. 136; Park and Daston, "Hermaphrodites in Renaissance France," cited above.

44   "... extrahitque cadavera, portatque ad suam speluncam, juxta quam videre est ingentem cumulum ossium humanorum ..."(Cc4: "... it pulls out the corpse, and carries it to its cave, next to which you can see a huge mound of human bones ...").

45   "In summa, Hyaena typus est crebrae mutationis, gravis inimicitiae, pernitiosae adulationis, & frugiferae tyrannidis ..." (Cc5).

conceive by animals of other species, such as dogs and wolves, leopards, panthers, and lions. The cross between a hyena and a lion is a monster called the Crocuta, mentioned by Pliny (Dd4v–Dd5). The animal kingdom seems generally monstrous in Bauhin's scheme of things; there is no order, no distinction between species in the process of reproduction. Hermaphrodism becomes symbolic of confusion of species as well as other forms of monstrosity.

Yet this monstrous being is of great medical use. Bauhin lists recipes for various remedies using parts of the hyena's body (Dd5–Ee4). When sacrificed, this body has a salubrious effect on humans; the animal kingdom is thereby subjected to the service of humanity. A live hyena boiled in oil cures arthritis or helps the digestion. If the animal is skinned alive by the right hand of a man and the skin is hung over one's entryway, one will be successful (Dd5v). The hyena's marrow can cure pains in the spine and nerves (Dd6). Its brain mixed with its heart can cure palpitations. It was believed that the eyes of a hyena were precious stones; if placed under the tongue, these would grant the gift of prophecy (Dd6v). Parts of its mouth cure canker sores (Dd7). Its tongue and spine can cure gout (Dd7). In short, the animal has almost magical properties when torn to pieces, whereas it is diabolical when living.

At this point, Bauhin decides to discuss lycanthropy (as a form of monstrosity, perhaps), considered in his time to be an extreme form of melancholy, in which a man thought he was a dog or wolf. Bauhin summarizes this condition as a division between body and soul (Ff4). This animal-like behavior may be accompanied by cannibalism or collection of corpses (Ff7–Gg); thus confusion of species is related to a primitive form of sacrificial incorporation (which Bauhin in fact mentions in relation to early Greek and Roman rites, Ff7v). In chapters nine and ten, Bauhin continues the discussion with hypotheses (some from Bodin's *Demonomanie des sorciers*) about the demonic nature of this behavior; perhaps the victims of lycanthropy are possessed or enchanted (Gg3–Hh5v).[46] Or perhaps lycanthropy is merely a demonic illusion (Hh5v–Ii7v). At any rate, this perceived degeneration is seen as brought on by a degraded soul ("vitia animarum," Gg3).

---

[46] "Bodinus in sua daemonomania, Lycanthropon sic definit: Lycanthropos nil aliud est, quam homo à diabolo in lupum transmutatus, qui plerumque quemadmodum naturales lupi pecudes persequitur: quorum aliquid postquam unguento se oblinivere, lupi facti sunt, & subinde in homines versi, lupique specie lupos inivere, eadem voluptate, qua cum mulieribus rem habere erant soliti: sic & lupinis pedibus & dentibus, aliquibus mortem intulere." (Gg3–Gg3v: "Bodin, in his *Demonomanie*, defines a Lycanthropos in this manner: a Lycanthropos is nothing but a man transformed into a wolf by the devil, most of whom chase herds of sheep in the manner of natural wolves: some of whom after they have smeared themselves with ointment, have been made into wolves, and immediately after have returned to human form, and they have had coitus with wolves in the manner of wolves, with the same pleasure which they had been accustomed to have during sex with women: and so with wolflike feet and teeth, they have inflicted death on some").

The confusion of human and animal species is once again connected to sexuality and death, as well as to the demonic. Bauhin gives enough examples of this condition to make a reader believe that it was widespread in the sixteenth century (Gg–Gg2v; Gg7–Gg8v). He also quotes numerous classical sources from Ovid and Virgil to Herodotus, as if to extend the history of this condition through time as well. He alludes to the tale of Ulysses and Circe as an example of species shifting. Bauhin reads this phenomenon on a literal and allegorical level: such transformation reflects the "degeneration of the soul," yet he assents that the wolf-man or Lycanthropos is not an imaginary creature (Ii7v). What is clear from the chapters on Lycanthropy is that the supernatural was as rightfully the object of "scientific" investigation as the natural. Science and theology were still not clearly distinct fields of inquiry. The positive effect of the mixture was the admission that certain problems or conditions were beyond human control; the negative effect was the doctrinal stranglehold the Church held on medical inquiry, whereby the ill were often associated with the diabolical, and therefore not offered the humane treatment they might otherwise have received.[47]

In a return to more pedestrian examples from the animal kingdom, Bauhin explores the characteristics of hares at some length, particularly the sexuality of this species, which has the reputation of being extremely libidinous (Chapter 14, Ll4v–Mm3v). Needless to say, their fecundity leads to the question of whether they are hermaphroditic or not, and whether the female can conceive without a male; Bauhin denies this belief (Mm6–Nn2). A truly natural animal, unlike the monstrous hyena, cannot always be of mixed sex. Yet hermaphrodites do seem more frequent in the animal than in the human world. Goats, according to Aristotle, frequently give birth to hermaphroditic kids. Bauhin cites examples of hermaphroditic oxen, dogs, deer, horses, and mules. One mule gave birth during the reign of Nero (Nn4); thus, once again, the monstrous body serves as a politicized text.

The book closes with several engravings by Theodor de Bry of hermaphrodites and of other monstrosities or deformities, thus refocusing the issues on the human form. The wide-ranging discussions in this treatise have the effect of at one and the same time universalizing and marginalizing hermaphrodism, just as the title at once divides hermaphrodism off from and links it to monstrosity. It becomes clear that the main concern is with the "purity" of humanity, and that the Roman custom of drowning hermaphrodites in order to annihilate any possible impurity is not so distant from the early modern insistence on sex distinction by all medical and legal means available. If nature abhors a vacuum, culture seems to abhor confusing and potentially "impure" plenitude.

Nonetheless, Bauhin represents a step away from Aristotelian categories, so clearly accepted and enforced by early Renaissance intellectuals such as Paracelsus (see the following chapter). Although his argument for tolerance of hermaphrodites is thin at best, and accompanied by the assertion that they must be assigned a clear-cut sex, it

---

47   Several of the wolf-men are executed (Gg7–Gg7v; Hh1v).

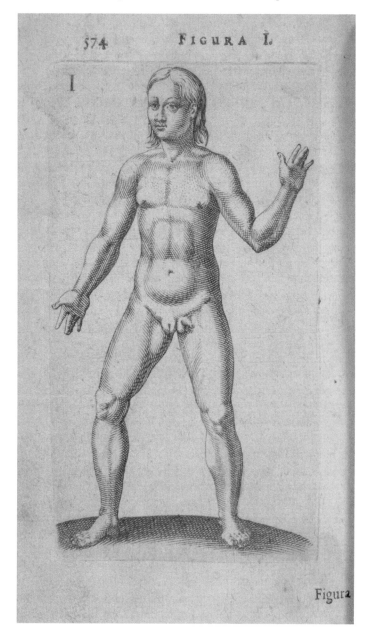

Figure 2.2   Male hermaphrodite, from Caspar Bauhin, *De hermaphroditorum monstrosorumque partuum naturae ...* (Oppenheim: Galleri, 1614). Courtesy of the Division of Rare and Manuscript Collections, Cornell University Library

suggests the potential for progress beyond the traditional intellectual justifications for superstitious attitudes towards sexual difference. His skeptical presentation of much of the cultural material cited frames vivid and complex discussion of clinically observed bodies, thus suggesting the possibility of new approaches to the issue of sex distinction. The proliferation of materials suggests almost infinite possibilities, which strain against the narrow limitations imposed on socially expressed sexual identity. Bauhin is struggling within a rigid intellectual system, but he is struggling.

Chapter 3

Jacques Duval on Hermaphrodites: Culture Wars in the Medical Profession

The early years of the seventeenth century saw a continuation of the rivalry between professors of medicine and surgeons who were increasingly literate and publishing their own treatises. This rivalry had already revealed itself in the court case concerning publication of Ambroise Paré's works. Professors at the Sorbonne felt that Paré had exceeded his limits, and had written on matters beyond the scope of a mere surgeon.[1] Increasingly, surgeons were presenting themselves as authorities on matters of medicine, with their power based on practical experience rather than knowledge of ancient texts (one point of criticism of Paré was that he did not know Greek). Thus, in this court case, in exchanges of vituperative pamphlets and medical treatises, an early version of empirical science was vying with the old, bookish ways of understanding the human body. For the professors of the Sorbonne, the issue was no less than potential loss of power over the profession itself.[2]

During this contentious period, control of childbirth was transferred from the hands of midwives to those of male surgeons.[3] Even as the surgeons began to succeed in

---

[1]   For a brief discussion of this case, see Jean Céard's edition of *Des monstres et prodiges*, pp. xiv–xix.

[2]   For an excellent discussion of the Sorbonne and medicine in this period, see Iain M. Lonie, "The 'Paris Hippocratics': Teaching and Research in Paris in the Second Half of the Sixteenth Century," in *The Medical Renaissance of the Sixteenth Century*, eds A. Wear, R.K. French, I.M. Lonie (Cambridge: Cambridge University Press, 1985), pp. 155–74.

[3]   Duval's treatise on childbirth seems to indicate that this shift was already occurring by the end of the sixteenth century, somewhat earlier than in England, and earlier than some historians of medicine have noted. See Andrew Wear, "Medicine in Early Modern Europe, 1500–1700," in *The Western Medical Tradition, 800 BC to AD 1800*, ed. Lawrence Conrad et al. (Cambridge: Cambridge University Press, 1995), pp. 234–5. For a general history of childbirth, see Jacques Gélis, *History of Childbirth: Fertility, Pregnancy, and Birth in Early Modern Europe*, trans. Rosemary Morris (Boston: Northeastern University Press, 1991). This shift from midwives to surgeons and doctors is apparent in the works of Louise Boursier (published in the early modern period as Louise Bourgeois). See her *Apologie de Louise Bourgeois, dite Bourcier, Sage femme de la Royne Mere du Roy, et de feu Madame. Contre le Rapport des Medecins* (Paris, 1627). For a modern edition of another of her works, see the *Récit veritable de la naissance de Messeigneurs et Dames les enfans de France...*, ed. François Rouget (Geneva: Droz, 2000). For an excellent study of Louise Bourgeois, see Wendy Perkins, *Midwifery and Medicine in Early Modern France: Louise Bourgeois* (Exeter: University of Exeter Press, 1996).

defining themselves as dignified practitioners of medicine, they took over tasks formerly assigned to women. Their treatises argue the necessity of control of the disruptive and disrupted female body by more rational male doctors. Jacques Duval's treatise, *Des Hermaphrodits, accouchemens des femmes, et traitement qui est requis pour les relever en santé, & bien élever leurs enfans* (*On Hermaphrodites, Childbirth, and the Treatment That Is Required to Return Women to Health and to Raise Their Children Well*, 1612) is illustrative both of this rivalry between professors of medicine and practicing surgeons and of the concomitant impulse toward men's control of all medical practices. Duval was a well-educated surgeon who practiced at Paris and Rouen, and who contended with Jean Riolan, a well-published professor of medicine from an established academic family, over the celebrated case of Marin le Marcis, the Rouen man who had been raised as a girl. Duval's work represents a sort of "fault line" in the history of science in France, privileging empirical observation and clinical examination over traditional academic modes of training based primarily on the works of Aristotle. Strikingly, he also privileges the sense of touch over sight, since in childbirth, the crucial information is unavailable to view. This shift in emphasis represents a clear break from the treatises that present copious illustrations of the infant's position in the womb, and a clear turning away from the lecture hall to the hospital ward.

While asserting the importance of the male doctor's control over the woman's body in the process of childbirth, inconsistencies in Duval's text reveal that this control is not complete, as we shall see, and that female anatomy remains something of a mystery to the men writing about it. Duval seems particularly concerned with the unruly quality of female sexuality, and although he links the power of naming with power over the body, his own assertions are unconvincing in the light of the clinical cases he discusses. He also focuses on cesarean sections, which provide the opportunity for doctors to control the process of childbirth, but his failure to save his own wife signals the limited success of this control. The issue of power hovers over the entire treatise: power over the body, control of women, power within the profession of medicine. But this power is continually asserted precisely because it is at risk, because one must contend for it. Intertwined with this contention is the status of masculinity itself, now scrutinized in detail in passages on the excellence of the penis and the perfection of sperm, now protected against the dangers which women present, whether in illness or in professional rivalry.

Although reminiscent in many ways of the work of Ambroise Paré and Caspar Bauhin,[4] Duval's work represents a turning away from Bauhin's relatively skeptical and pluralistic views in particular, towards Hippocratic models of sexual difference and generation,[5] and towards positivistic belief in the power of empirical science.

---

[4]   Whom Duval cites rather far along in his discussion (Z3 for Paré, Z5 for Bauhin).

[5]   As Katharine Park and Lorraine Daston argue, this period sees an evolution away from Aristotelian notions of generation, toward Hippocratic views which often posited a "more equal" role for the woman in the process of generation. See their article, "The Hermaphrodite and the Orders of Nature: Sexual Ambiguity in Early Modern France," pp. 419–73.

Like Bauhin, Duval is primarily interested in the question of sexual difference, that which distinguishes the female from the male. For both authors, the hermaphrodite becomes the site for discussion of the complexities and problems inherent in this distinction. Whereas Paré's and Bauhin's discussions of hermaphrodites seem primarily focused on the various ways of knowing, and on the various discourses used to define hermaphrodites, Duval seems intent on one manifestation of sex in particular, sexuality, and its (in his view) necessary consequence, reproduction. His discussion of the hermaphrodite is therefore much narrower than Bauhin's, and his conclusions seem much more rigid in terms of designation of sexual identity. A man is revealed to be perfectly male only when he engenders life, that is, becomes a father. The accompanying definition of womanhood is effaced from the treatise, even though the work ostensibly concerns itself with childbirth, in favor of establishing unequivocal proofs of maleness. Thus, although he reiterates many of Bauhin's arguments, Duval creates a treatise that represents a backlash against Bauhin's pluralism and a return to more clearly hierarchical notions of gender.

An even more significant difference between Bauhin's treatise and that of Duval resides in their views of how knowledge is acquired and passed on. For Bauhin, working within the context of the Renaissance revival of Pyrrhonian skepticism, no sense-impressions hold any particular validity for the acquisition of knowledge; all possible perceptions are unstable, effected as they are by the various conditions of the perceiving subject, the perceived object, and the circumstances that bring the two together. In this context, poetry and myth have the same value as clinical reports and legal precedents. Unlike Bauhin, Duval clearly feels that certain forms of clinical observation have to be accepted as more accurate than others. In particular, he privileges the sense of touch as a more direct means of understanding, even "reading," the body. Appearances, when judged merely by the sense of sight, can easily deceive. The sense of touch reveals underlying forms which, precisely because they are tangible, hold greater validity for the doctor. This is particularly true in the case of childbirth, where much of the necessary information is accessible not to view, only to the touch. But it is also true in the case of Marin le Marcis, where feminine characteristics that are more easily apparent are contradicted by internal structures attainable only by means of an invasive internal examination that proceeds by means of touch. This is the other aspect of Duval's work that is striking; knowledge is obtained by penetration of the body, an invasive interference in the body's workings. Duval seems quite aware of the intrusive nature of internal medicine, and of the fact that knowledge is a sort of violation, albeit one that often prevents worse violations such as execution, imprisonment, or death in childbirth.

Also, for Duval, direct knowledge of the body is better communicated by words than by visual representations. Language is the means of mastery of knowledge that is acquired indirectly, and in its performative guise it mimics the tangible but fluid nature of the body. Language is thus invasive, and even transforming. Here, Duval elaborates a theory of the body and its representation that is in fact more complex than those fueled by skepticism. He asserts that there are underlying structures to the body which are more "real," or at least should be read as more indicative of the sex of a person, than the surface presentations. He admits that there is a gap between the surface presentations of gender, and those underlying structures; these two aspects of a person may even contradict each other. He links the surface presentations of gender to aspects of sexual difference that we might call performative, that is, behavior, dress, gesture, even environment, which can alter our understanding of a person's sex. And he argues that these performative aspects can also, to some extent, alter the underlying structures. He sketches out, somewhat tentatively, a complex relation between body and environment (mostly social context) that is based on mutual interaction. In postmodern terms, Duval recognizes neither performative nor essentialist notions of gender and sex as ideal modes of understanding the body, but describes how organic structures of the body can be altered over time by certain practices and situations, and how the body in turn can transform, even if only slightly, those practices.

Marin le Marcis

Duval is best known for his involvement in the case of Marin/Marie le Marcis, discussed at some length by Lorraine Daston and Katharine Park.[6] He opens his treatise with a brief version of this story and concludes the book with a much longer and more melodramatic version (Bb7–Ff7), claiming this case as the inspiration for this work:

> ... une fille nous a esté representé: Laquelle ayant esté baptisée, nommee, entretenue, élevee & tousiours vestue comme les autres filles de sa sorte, iusques à l'aage de vingt ans, à esté finallement recognue homme: & comme tel à plusieurs & diverses fois eu habitation charnelle avec une femme, qu'il avoit fiancee par paroles de present, avec promesse du mariage futur.
>
> Non qu'on peust appercevoir en ce subiect les marques & particules destituez aux deux sexes, telles qu'on recognoist ordinairement aux Hermaphrodits: tant en ceux qui sont entiers & parfaicts, qu'en ceux auxquels on peut noter quelque marque d'imperfection, comme il advient plus souvent. Ou bien que la nature feminine fust totalement obliteree, pour ceder à la masculine, si qu'il n'en restast vestige quelconque, comme il se voit pratiqué aux gunaneres ou filles-hommes.
>
> Mais par une merveilleuse dexterité de ce grand ouvrier, le membre viril obtenoit telle situation, qu'il se pouvoit monstrer & sortir actuellement, pour l'exercice & action qui en est requise, tant à rendre l'urine, que semence genitale: souvent aussi s'absconcer et cacher, en retrocedant à l'interieur. (*Des hermaphrodits*, A4v–A5)
>
> (... we had been told about a girl who, having been baptised, named, nourished, raised, and always clothed like the other girls of her lot, until the age of twenty, was finally recognized to be a man, and as such had carnal knowledge of a woman, many and

---

6   In "The Hermaphrodite and the Orders of Nature," cited above.

different times, to whom he had become engaged by his word before witnesses, with a promise of future marriage.

Not that one could perceive in this subject the marks and parts assigned to both sexes, such as one ordinarily finds in Hermaphrodites: as much in those who are complete and perfect, as in those in whom one can note some sign of imperfection, as occurs more often. Or that the feminine nature had been totally effaced, ceding to the masculine, so that no vestige at all remains, as one can see occurring in *gunaneres* or girl-men.

But through the marvelous skill of this great worker, the male member was so placed, that it could show itself and actually protrude, for the required exercise and action, whether to urinate or to ejaculate, but it could also often conceal and cover itself, by withdrawing into the body.)

The case is difficult, since Marie/Marin is not clearly a hermaphrodite, nor a man. Her male genitalia are hidden, yet functional. Duval is called, together with other doctors, to decide this case. The reports of the other doctors are completely opposed to his own conclusions, and the poor hermaphrodite is condemned to death for his/her apparent "sexual misconduct":

> ... ce pauvre gunanthrope qui avoit encouru condemnation de faire amende honorable, tout nud, la torche au poin, en divers endroits, de la ville de Monstiervillier, puis d'estre conduit au lieu patibulaire, pour la estre pendu estranglé, & finalement son corps reduit en cendres ... (*Des hermaphrodits*, A5v)

> (... this poor woman-man who had incurred condemnation to make honorable amends, completely naked, torch in hand, in several places, in the town of Monstiervillier, then to be led to the place of execution, to be hung, strangled, and finally his body reduced to ashes there.)

The author heroically prevents this evil fate by means of further examination of the subject in question, discovering the hidden member and its capacity to urinate and ejaculate. As Duval has suggested in other parts of his treatise, a functional penis is *the* sign of masculinity. It must be noted that this examination resembles a violation; the hermaphroditic body, in order to be recognized or categorized, must be dissected or otherwise invaded and its secrets revealed. The other doctors shrink from such an act. But Duval files a dissenting opinion and saves the life of the accused. Marin/Marie must live in limbo, dressed as a woman, for four years, until one or the other gender becomes clearly dominant (*Des hermaphrodits*, A6v). Ten years after the trial, Marin is bearded and living as a man:

> ... ce gunanthrope est de present rendu en meilleure habitude virile qu'il n'estoit auparavant, & que qualifié du nom de cadet de Marcis il exerce son estat de tailleur d'habits, entreprend, faict, execute tous exercices à homme appartenans, porte barbe au menton, & à dequoy contenter une femme, pour engendrer en elle ... (*Des hermaphrodits*, A7)

(… this womanly man is now restored to an even better manly state than he had before, and that under the name of Marcis the younger, he is practicing the profession of man's tailor, and undertakes, performs, and completes all duties pertaining to a man, he has a beard on his chin, and has that which is necessary to content a woman, and to beget children by her …)

Marin has defined himself as a man by his external attributes and actions; he has constructed himself as a man, and is apparently accepted as such by society. Duval justifies this designation by referring to Marin's sexual prowess, even claiming that the young man can beget children, but as in the case of Paré's hermaphrodites, the external attributes of sexual identity that are acquired performatively, that is, by the very exercise of those attributes, define the person as much as any physical characteristics. It is ironic that Marin is a "tailleur d'habits," creating the very signs of gender that were once so problematic for him (as he was forced to wear women's clothing) and that help to establish his identity.[7]

Duval places his paradoxical defense of Marie/Marin le Marcis, whom he designates repeatedly as a "Gunanthrope" (Dd3) and a "Gunanere" (Bb5), terms he has clearly established as describing a predominantly female being who has some male characteristics (but in whom, generally, the male reproductive organs do not function),[8] within the context of the heterosexual and reproductive imperative that he has chosen to advance. Occasionally, he has observed, such a woman is revealed to be a man. Still, Duval does not describe Marin le Marcis as unequivocally male, even though the Court demands that a clear gender designation be made, and even though Marin's life depends upon his male identity being legally established. Duval firmly believes Marin to be a hermaphrodite, who has the one important masculine characteristic: a functioning penis. He concludes that Marin's sex is ambiguous, but that he could function as a male. This refusal to assign a clear role is unusual for the period. The Court accepts this ambiguity to some degree, requiring that Marin dress as a woman until the age of twenty-five, but allowing for the possibility that Marin will choose to live as a man after that. (*Des hermaphrodits*, ch. 80, Ff4v)

The reasons for Duval's humane conduct in this case are clear throughout the narration. The sanctity of life that is attached to the reproductive imperative, which Duval emphasizes in the rest of the treatise, extends to all human beings. Duval adopts the view that the diversity of nature is a sign of divine power, rather than that

---

7   This problematic nature of apparel certainly links the tailor to homosexuality and other marginalized forms of sexuality in English Renaissance literature. See Simon Shephard, "What's so Funny about Ladies' Tailors? A Survey of some Male (Homo)sexual Types in the Renaissance," in *Textual Practice* 6 (1992): 17–30. Tailors themselves were often portrayed, most of all in the theatre, as foppish and effeminate, thus making this the appropriate profession for the ambiguous Marin.

8   This type of hermaphrodite is discussed in Chapters 53 and 54 (*Des hermaphrodits*, A3v–A4).

which sees any deviation from an established norm to be monstrous: "… nature n'a rien formé en vain, & n'a fait aucun animal ou partie d'iceluy quelque vilaine qu'elle semble estre ausquels elle n'ait inseré une grande perfection" (*Des hermaphrodits*, Ch. 68, Cc8v: "nature has formed nothing in vain, and has not made any animal or part thereof, however lowly it might seem to be, into which she has not placed great perfection"). Duval also argues that this diversity is present in all men and women, and therefore should be seen as normal in hermaphrodites: "Or d'autant que telle diversité n'est specifique en tous les autres hommes & femmes, ell n'est tant remarquable & considerable, comme en ceux du sexe desquels nous somme incertains" (*Des hermaphrodits*, Dd6: "Inasmuch as such diversity is not limited in all other men and women, it is not so remarkable or noteworthy when it is found in those about whose sex we are uncertain"). Nature continually practices these variations (Dd6), so that a model of sexual difference other than a simple male/female binary must be proposed: "… deffaillant la propre difference, nous soyons munis sinon de ce qui depend en tout de ce qui est propre à tout le moins de l'amas de beaucoup d'accidents communs …" (*Des hermaphrodits*, Dd6: "in the absence of a clear-cut difference, we might have armed ourselves if not with that which occurs or is appropriate to all, at least with an accumulation of common instances …." Thus, difference and resemblance are not clear and absolute, but cumulative impressions of similarities. For Duval, the condemnation to death of someone who does not fit neatly into the constructed categories of male and female is a violation of the sanctity of life, and a patent absurdity, since none of us fits neatly into those categories. While his fellow doctors shrink from the contamination they might endure from contact with the hermaphrodite's body, Duval condemns their deadly negligence: "… nous demeurerions chargez & contaminez du sang de ce pauvre garçon si nous ne faisons deuë visitation pour cognoistre la verité du fait" (Dd1v: "we would remain covered and contaminated with the blood of this poor boy if we do not make a proper investigation to understand the truth of this matter"). This difference of opinion and approach also marks the confrontation between empirical forms of medical investigation (including dissection and invasive internal examinations) and more traditional forms of observation based on ancient traditions. The impact of early forms of internal medicine, practiced on living beings, is hinted at in Duval's discussion of the external appearance and internal structure of Marin's body (as well as in his discussions of the pregnant body and of the body during labor):

> Auquel apres plusieurs signes exterieurs qui se sont submis à la veuë, nous tirions premierement consequence que ledit Marin estoit fille … non obstant que les signes exterieurs donnassent grande occasion de la iuger fille, si toutefois il estoit homme muni de membre viril, suffisant pour la generation & propagation de son espece …
> (*Des hermaphrodits*, Dd2v)

> (In the course of which (examination), after observing numerous external signs, we came to the preliminary conclusion that the said Marin was a girl … but notwithstanding the fact that external signs give great reason to judge her a girl, nonetheless, he was a man armed with a male member sufficient for the generation and propagation of his species.)

Marin's appearance passively "submits" (the term used of proper female sexual conduct in this period) to examination, but his male member is more defiant, a "munition" of sorts; and so the very description evokes his hermaphroditic nature. The pronouns used to designate Marie/Marin alternate between the masculine and the feminine, according to the context in which they appear. Such textual instability suggests that while Duval recognizes the public nature of gender, he does not abandon the belief in a body that may not conform absolutely to socially acceptable gender roles, even as it is shaped and molded by those very roles.

This more complex notion of gender and sex is elaborated in an exchange between Duval and a court official who wonders why Marin's penis has not been observed even once by his captors, although he has been in jail for some time (and one notes the absolute lack of privacy revealed by this question). Duval's response marks the early seventeenth century's position as the meeting-ground between medieval and modern notions of physiology. First, Duval points out that Marin's humoral "complexion" is more feminine than masculine, that is, cold and moist rather than hot and dry. But the heart of his answer is a long speech on the emasculating effect of disempowerment. He points out that Marin has had to endure several invasive, even hostile, physical examinations; and indeed, for his "hidden" penis to be located, he had to endure penetration, the stereotypically feminine role of the time. He is now no longer free, but lives in hardship and pain. He cannot exercise in fresh air, but rather languishes in a small space. He does not eat well and drink good wine, but is fed meager amounts of bread and water. He cannot enjoy the company of the beautiful widow Jeanne Le Febvre, but must pass the day alone. In short, he is leading a confined and passive existence, and thus is rendered effeminate by the conditions in which he is living (Ffv–Ff2v). For Duval, it is clear that these conditions shape the body to some extent. But Marin's penis is still there; the body cannot be entirely transformed by external influences. Nonetheless, it can appear to be radically different from what it was before. Duval underscores his recognition that the relationship between a body and the culture with which it interacts is not straightforward or easily categorized. Given this complexity, the only absolute which Duval asserts is the sanctity of life: Marin's life must be spared, precisely because his sex is indeterminate.

Sex, Gender, and Generation

The hermaphrodites in Duval's treatise are the pretext for discussion of a more widespread, immediate, and serious issue: the difficulties of childbirth and how they might be overcome. Thus, hermaphrodites are set, once again, in the context of heterosexual reproduction. Duval's treatise might be seen as far more practical, and far less about hermaphrodites, than that of Bauhin, as he prescribes methods for ensuring the survival of mother and/or child. Duval justifies his project of establishing the parameters of sexual difference by arguing that it is necessary to understand and recognize the genitalia of either sex in order to determine such complex cases (A5v). He claims that his work is a legal manual for surgeons involved in deciding cases of sex, sexuality (defloration), birth, etc. (A6). Thus, from the opening pages of this treatise, sexuality is strictly linked (even in the case of Marin) to the question of reproduction within marriage. The author particularly wishes to avoid the high infant mortality rates that have plagued France (A6v). He denies any lascivious interest in this subject (a denial that seems severely undercut by the text itself), and argues that he has many children ("heureuse lignee") and a long, happy marriage (A7). But he hopes that the gaiety of the subject will encourage midwives to read this book and learn the methods contained therein; certainly, the largest portion of the book is devoted to questions of childbirth:

> Si donc recreant & delectant la pensee des hommes, (quoi que ce ne soit mon but principal) par l'exposé des richesses viriles, & representation de utensiles reconces aux plus secrets cabinets des femmes: en l'usage desquels les uns & les autres se donnent carriere de delectation: J'eleve tellement la pensee de celles qui se disent obstetrices & matrones ... qu'elles puissent vrayement estre rendues sages femmes, dont le monde à tant de besoin ... (*Des hermaphrodits* , A8)

> (If then, in amusing and pleasing men's thoughts (although this is not my principal goal) by the description of the treasures of manhood, and the representation of the hidden utensils in the most secret chambers of woman, in the use of which each gives the other a full range of delight, I enhance the understanding of those who call themselves obstetricians and matrons ... so that they might truly be made wise women ... whom the world so greatly needs ...)

Duval thus admits his use of hermaphrodites to draw the reader into what he deems to be a more serious discussion of reproductive issues. Duval's discussion also privileges men over women as the superior sex, and places women purely in the reproductive role, accepting unquestioningly the old clichés of women as disorderly beings governed by their womb.[9] In keeping with this spirit, Duval's assertion of the need for more and more demanding training of midwives implies a desire to assert masculine control over the process of childbirth. This book can be seen as a step in the development of greater supervision over midwives by male doctors, a move which itself led eventually to the suppression of midwifery in favor of deliveries controlled at every stage by male doctors.[10] Thus, science is being called upon here to confirm

---

[9]   Some of his arguments recall to the modern reader those summarized by Natalie Zemon Davis in her piece "Women on Top," from *Society and Culture in Early Modern France*, pp. 124–51.

[10] This evolution is traced briefly by Karen Newman in her book *Fetal Positions: Individualism, Science, Visuality* (Stanford: Stanford University Press, 1996), pp. 48–51. The first stages of this evolution, contemporary with Duval's treatise, are discussed by Wendy Perkins in her study, *Midwifery and Medicine in Early Modern France*.

traditional attitudes towards the sexes, and traditionally prescribed roles. The woman is seen as almost pure physicality, upon whom the doctor works his magic.

He also, from the beginning, associates mastery of discourse with mastery over the body, constrasting his eloquence to the ineptitude of those doctors who opposed his examination of Marin le Marcis:

> Deslors ie fis curieuse recherche de plusieurs belles histoires & graves authoritez, avec ample discution de diverses causes & raisons qui pouvoyent concurrer à l'entiere cognoissance d'un si rare subiect. Lesquelles ie sceus tant bien disposer & naïvement representer, que cooperant l'ayde du tout puissant qui me daigne dessiller les yeux, & lever le bandeau d'ignorance en cette part, ie rendis ce qui en estoit, tant cler & manifeste, par l'exposé qui i'en fis à la Court, sur ce que nous fusmes faits entrer à la chambre, pour rendre & dire les raisons de la diversité de nos rapports .... (*Des hermaphrodits*, A5)

> (On this occasion I researched carefully many pleasant stories and stern authorities, with detailed discussion of diverse causes and reasons which could lead to a full understanding of such an esoteric subject. Which I knew how to put forth so well and present so earnestly, that with the help of the all-powerful one who deigned to open my eyes, and lift the band of ignorance concerning this matter, I made the case so clear and evident, by means of the report I made to the Court, that we were called into the chambers, to give and explain the reasons for this difference of opinion in our reports.)

He wishes to share this discursive mastery with his readers, among whom he includes patients, so that "those who need to consult Doctors … might respond competently to that which is proposed to them" (A6). He also wishes to aid Surgeons and midwives who might be asked to pronounce on legal matters. And he wishes to pass on his mastery of the process of childbirth to surgeons, so that they might deliver skillfully, when the midwife is not equal to the task (A6). Childbirth has been transformed in this text from a natural process to an art; this art requires knowledge of signs and forms, rather than of the body (which might nonetheless present some of those signs). Accession to knowledge of this art will save infants' lives; and thus, mastery of discourse is mastery of life itself (A6v).

This mastery is clearly linked to masculinity, as Duval makes clear in subsequent discussions of "… ce qui est en l'homme de plus plaisant & voluptueux: c'est la semence genitale, qui y est tellement copieuse & abondante, que le docte Fervel n'a fait doute de dire que *homo totus semen est*" (*Des hermaphrodits*, A7–A7v: "… that which is most pleasant and pleasurable to man, which is semen, so copious and abundant in him, that the learned Fervel did not hesitate to say that *man is entirely semen*"). Nevertheless, the mastery of language over the body is factitious at best, as Duval concedes in his discussion of the genitals:

> Mais aussi elle (nature) à par ie ne sçay quel instinct, concedé une tant voluptueuse titillation & libidineuse amorce, lors que par la nomination, ou seule signification, l'esprit est attiré à s'y encliner, que quand i'userois de lettres Hierogliphiques

empruntees des Egyptiens, ou seulement de signes expressifs repetés de l'Anglois Taumaste, pour les designer, sans autrement les nommer: encores ne pourrois-ie rescinder cette naïfve gayeté dont nature a voulu decorer & orner leur commemoration. (*Des hermaphrodits*, A7v)

(But also nature, by some instinct, has granted such pleasurable titillation and libidinous power, that by the naming or simple representation, the spirit is so drawn to this inclination, that if I were to use Hieroglyphics borrowed from the Egyptians, or merely expressive signs (hand gestures) taken from the English Thaumaste, in order to signify them, I would never be able to prevent that naïve happiness with which nature has wished to decorate and embellish their memory.)

Words or signs can prompt the body to do that to which it is already inclined, but they cannot undo this inclination or action. The performative power of words has its limits, but it is the sole form of mastery that can be conveyed by a book, so it is what Duval wishes to pass on to midwives and surgeons, so that they might save lives:

… par ce traité, estant bien entendu, ie retranche le chemin à un grand nombre de mauvais rapors, & à la perte d'une quantité d'ames presque infinie, qui sans avoir le commodité de iouyr de la lumiere de ce monde, pour rendre graces & louange à la maiesté divine, sont contraintes de rebatre promptement la mesme piste que le souverain Createur leur avoit fait tenir. Et ce à cause de l'ignorance des obstetrices, qui pour n'estre capables de lire ny entendre des livres de plus grand consequence .... (*Des hermaphrodits*, A7v)

(By means of this treatise, if it is well understood, I will block the way to a large number of bad results, and the loss of an almost infinite number of souls who, without having the capacity to enjoy the light of this world, so that they might render praise and thanks to the divine majesty, are constrained to return by the same road that the sovereign Creator made them take in the first place. And this because of the ignorance of women obstetricians, who because they cannot read or understand books of greater importance …)

The midwives are cut off from mastery of the techniques of childbirth by their illiteracy, and are replaced, even in the text, by male barbers and surgeons (A7v). These latter often do more harm than good, "(c)e qu'ils ne feront Dieu aydant pour l'advenir, s'ils se rendent dociles à l'intelligence de ce présent traicté" (A8: "which they will no longer do in the future, God willing, if they submit themselves to the wisdom of this present treatise"). Duval thus renders himself master of the entire discipline, directing his "docile" pupils.

In this context, Duval reviews various ways of knowing, for the most part linked to discourse. Both orators and philosophers use primarily discursive modes of knowing; orators cite authorities in order to confirm their assertions, and philosophers construct arguments (B–B1v). Pure discourse is fine for generalizations, "Mais quand ils descendent au particulier & individu, ils sont souvent contraints laisser arriere les arguments, pour venir à l'authorité des sens ausquels Aristote, en son second livre de l'ame, veut que pleine foy soit adioustée" (B1v: "But when they descend to the particular and the individual, they are often compelled to abandon these arguments, and turn to the authority of the senses to which Aristotle, in his second book on the soul, wishes full faith to be granted"). Faced with individual cases, empirical methods, depending heavily on the senses, are preferable. Gone from Duval's treatise are the strong skeptical doubts concerning the validity of observations or sense-perceptions, such as those expressed in Bauhin's work. Modern science depends greatly on faith in the accuracy of our perceptions; Duval already expresses this faith clearly in his accounts. It should be remembered, however, that appearances can deceive, as in the case of Marin le Marcis, and that informed observers will look beyond the obvious to find underlying truths.

Here, then, is a clearer break than is apparent in previous work, with the traditional epistemological methods (particularly as used to acquire knowledge of the body) that predominated well into the sixteenth century. Generally, in the period preceding Duval's work, medical treatises were quite dependent on citation of classical and medieval authorities, rather than on dissection or other forms of observation of the body. Duval asserts that such authorities do not recognize the existence of someone like Marin le Marcis; certainly, they discuss hermaphrodites, but do not acknowledge diversity even among hermaphrodites. Because of the boundless diversity of creatures, Nature is the sole authority to which Duval will accede. Or so he claims. He does cite Aristotle, Galen, Hippocrates, and others constantly, but reserves the right to criticize their theories and counter them with examples from nature.

Nonetheless, Duval retains traditional views of the male/female binary when he asserts that all knowledge is meaningless when divorced from masculinity/virility. In his chapter praising the genitals ("Louange des parties genitalles," ch. 2, B2v seq., and by this he means the male genitalia), Duval links them with rationality and with immortality. He claims that genitals create heat in the body, and are superior to the heart, which merely enables one to live, not to propagate. This is perhaps an extreme example of defining masculinity purely by means of the penis, and this argument seems to echo Galen's theories of heat, as well as echoing a fairly predominant view of the hierarchy of sex in which the "cooler" woman remains subservient to the "hotter" man.[11] Deprived of their reproductive organs, eunuchs show a degradation of intellect, Duval claims: "Nous y trouvons des moeurs perverses, & tres mauvaise ratiocination, & qu'à peine on peut trouver un Eunuque de bonne loy & iugment solide" (B3v: "We find in them perverse morals, and very poor reasoning, and hardly ever can one find a Eunuch of good behavior and sound judgment"). One wonders, of course, what his statistical sample was, and to what extent he really does rely on direct observation for some of the arguments he presents in the treatise. But at least in his mind, the phallus is associated with law and reason, and, further on, with the divine itself:

---

[11]   See Thomas Laqueur, *Making Sex*, p. 28.

Ie ne craindray de dire, qu'en l'usage de ces parties consiste non seulement la plus utile & necessaire action de toutes, mais aussi la plus noble & excellente: d'autant qu'au compliment d'icelle concurre manifestement la faveur du verbe Divin, qui seule s'est reservé la puissance d'engendrer, disant l'Evangeliste Saint Jean, *Omnia per ipsum facta sunt, & sine ipso factum est nihil.* (*Des hermaphrodits*, B3v)

(I will not hesitate to say, in the use of these parts consists not only the most useful and necessary action of all, but also the most noble and excellent: all the more for the fact that in support of this activity the favor of the Divine Word concurs openly, which has reserved to itself alone the power to engender, as Saint John the Evangelist says, "Everything is made by it, and without it nothing is made.")

The male role in procreation is compared to divine creation by means of the Word, and judged to be the most noble of human actions. Duval lists various terms used to designate the penis, and observes that this organ is frequently presented as life itself, or the sole source of life (B4; this contention is contradicted by his adoption of Hippocratic theories of generation later in the treatise). By means of procreation, man leaves his image (B5: "son image vif") on life. Duval repeats the divine mandate of "Be fruitful and multiply" (B5v). He makes it clear that marriage is the context of this entire discussion. Most striking, however, is the extent to which creation, and even procreation, are linked to the *Logos* ("le verbe divin"), that is, to rationality and discursive mastery. He defends language with the same ardor that fuels his praise of masculinity, attacking the hypocrisy of scandal-mongers in a manner reminiscent of Reason's discussion of words and things in the *Roman de la Rose*: "Mais laissant arriere ces hypocrites ensouffrez, qui s'efforcent de blasmer de paroles, ce qu'ils mettent en usage tant voluptueusement ..." (B4v: "But leave behind these sulphurous hypocrites, who strain to condemn those words which they use with such pleasure"). Duval even plays on the Latin term for testicles, *testes*, which also means witnesses: "ils donnent tesmoignage de la virilité" (C2: "they give proof of virility"). The parts of the body speak, act, reason, and thus represent the whole. This synecdochical dynamic of the part standing in for the whole is most picturesquely evident in Duval's description of sperm "comme pleine de petites clochettes, dans lesquelles sont enclos les esprits ouvriers, scientifiques batisseurs & edificateurs du corps humain" (D2: "as full of little bells in which the worker-spirits are enclosed, knowledgeable builders and fabricators of the human body"). This is a slightly different version of Paracelsus's *homunculus* (Duval quotes Paracelsus earlier, C4). Here, the little men are not merely tiny reproductions of the father, but in fact actively participate in the construction of those reproductions.

This proliferation of images of busy body-parts, from talking testicles to industrious sperm, might remind the reader of the passage in which the limitations of discursive and rational power are considered (A7v, cited above). The (masculine) body is not entirely subsumed into an integral self, controlled by the intellect or reason, but consists of various parts which follow their own inclinations. As has been suggested, they can be prompted by words to do that to which they are already naturally inclined; but dissuading them from these inclinations is another matter altogether. Thus, the insistence on masculine rationality and discursive power is mitigated by the depiction of automata-like body parts which follow a pre-programmed agenda.

Into this scene of turbulent activity steps yet another disruption: the "petit monde inferieur" ("little inferior world") that is woman. Obviously, man is the "petit monde superieur" (D3). Duval cites Paracelsus's argument that inferior worlds cannot influence superior ones, but counters with the observation that they can indeed, by means of "la communication des pisse-chaudes, chancres, poulains & verole ..." (D3: "by transmission of venereal diseases, cankers, sores, and pox"). Thus, woman is presented as the carrier of disease, and most significantly of those diseases which disrupt the procreative process. He has repeated several times the belief that the seed which creates a female is produced by the left testicle (B8, "l'emulgente senestre;" C2–C2v, "le senestre *thylugonon*, engendreur de femelles"). This belief confirms the notion of woman as sinister and menacing, as do the allusions to menstrual taboos in Duval's accounts of the engendering of hermaphrodites.

Rather than declaring sexuality a disorderly, messy process which defies reason, Duval reasserts the superiority and dominance of the penis, devoting a chapter to its praise. In the name of the penis, he reasserts discursive control over sexuality:

> ... Plus un instrument est cognu, remarqué, desiré & souvent mis en usage par l'un & l'autre sexe (indice de sa plus grande excellence, noblesse & dignité) tant plus grande varieté de noms luy est attribuée.
>
> Or n'y en à il en quoy cela soit plus frequent qu'en cette partie .... (*Des hermaphrodits*, D3)

> (The more a tool is known, remarked upon, desired, and often put to use by one and the other sex [an indication of its greater excellence, nobility, and dignity], the more names are attributed to it.
>
> So, there is no part more frequently in this situation than this one [the penis] ...)

A long list of names is offered, in epic fashion, to prove the importance of the penis. Again, mastery of language covers over the impossibility of mastery of the body.

Duval similarly glorifies male anatomy and male sexuality, claiming that the testicles, although themselves cold, render the body warm and robust. Therefore, a well-endowed man is a healthy man. He spends some space elaborating on the importance of ejaculation (and one remembers that this was the proof positive of Marin's masculinity), and describes the penis in some detail:

> C'est une partie de l'homme longue & prominente, souvent pendante, molle, ridee & flache, quelquesfois aussi tendue, roide, ferme, & dure, lors principalement qu'elle est preste & bien disposee à l'excretion de la semence genitale, dans le fertile & avide champ du genre humain. (*Des hermaphrodits*, D4)

> (This is a part of man which is long and protruding, often hanging, soft, wrinkled, and limp, sometimes also erect, stiff, firm, and hard, principally when it is ready and well-disposed for the excretion of semen, in the fertile and eager field of the human species.)

Thus, masculinity is not only defined in terms of the reproductive organs, but of the reproductive capacity itself. A man who does not propagate is seen by Duval as less than a man. Duval comes very close here to designating the woman as mere vessel, even though he does not fully accept this Aristotelian theory of generation.

After a long discussion of male anatomy, Duval embarks on a similar discussion of female anatomy. Proof of some adherence to a one-sex theory is the illustration offered to the chapters on the "Parties genitales de la femme" (E2v: "The Female Genitals"). The organs depicted do not seem in any way to resemble a man's organs, but the terminology used is largely derivative of male anatomy: "la veine spermatique" (E3: "the spermatic vein"); "vaisseaux spermatiques;" "rameaux spermatiques;" "les testicules feminins;" "les vaisseaux eiaculatoires" (E5v–E6: "the spermatic vessels," "the spermatic branches," "the feminine testicles," "the ejaculatory vessels"). So the female organs are being described as analogous to male ones. The vagina is simply translated from Latin into French, and becomes the "gaine du membre viril" ("the sheath of the male member"). All female reproductive organs become subject to the law of male sexuality. They are subject to the law of categorization and language as well. Duval offers a multiplicity of names used for the labia, pudendum, and clitoris, as he did for the penis (E4v, E8v). In this discussion of female genitalia, Duval cites a sermon by Anne de Joyeuse on their corrupting influence, and then cites a series of names and authoritative sources that link these genitalia to Hell. The names that he lists for the clitoris hint at the reasons for this perception of a menace: "En français elle est dite tentation, aiguillon de volupté, verge feminin, le mespris des hommes; Et les femmes qui font profession d'impudicité la nomment leur *gaude mihi*" (E8v: "In French it (the clitoris) is called temptation, the goad of pleasure, the female rod, the disdain of men. And women who make a living off of immodesty call it 'my delight'"). These names hint at the possibility of independent female sexuality, at the superfluity of the masculine member, and at contempt for men. Fear of this independent sexuality and this contempt may have driven the courts of the time to forbid one woman with an enlarged clitoris ever to use that body part (E7v–E8); this notion of the superfluity of men is also why Marin le Marcis's case caused such an uproar and why his punishment upon condemnation was so severe. This is also why Duval contends that in chaste women, the clitoris is scarcely visible, while in "indecent" women, it is more evident. It is most probably this fear of an independent, unregulated feminine sexuality which motivates Duval's lengthy and repeated discussions of the signs of virginity (ten pages in the thirteenth chapter, repeating points made earlier from E4v–E7).

Female Trouble: Feminine Sexuality and Childbirth

Thus, parts of the woman's body as well as her discourse seem to escape male domination. Duval discusses a "barre feminin" which creates a barrier to penetration, and which he claims "tribades" and "subigatrices" (two of a number of names for lesbians) use. He does not clarify whether these women use their "barre" to prevent penetration by a male, or whether they use it for their own pleasure. The clitoris seems to guarantee male access to the female body: contact with it apparently renders all women "submises à la volonté de celuy qui les touche: leur causant l'attrectation d'icelle, une si grande titillation, qu'elles en sont amorcees & ravies, voire forcees au deduit venereen" (E8: "subject to the will of him who touches them: causing the stimulation of this part, and such great titillation, that they are pushed and carried away, even forced to venereal pleasure"). Duval's use of the word *forcees* would seem to equate seduction with rape; yet he recommends this method for controlling unruly women. The clitoris can also be forbidding: "Mais en quelques unes ledit cleitoris s'est trouvé si grand, qu'il y à eu des femmes ausquelles il representoit la grandeur & grosseur d'un membre viril dressé & disposé à la culture: dont elles abusoyent les filles & femmes" (F1: "But in some the said clitoris has been found to be so large, that there have been women in whom it resembled an erect penis in length and size, one ready for cultivation: with which they abused girls and women"). Because these parts did not ejaculate, they were not male. Duval takes this opportunity to denounce lesbian practices (lesbians were called *tribades*, *subigatrices*, *frictrices*, and *ribaudes*, among other names). The fact that he returns to this topic (F2v) suggests that this independent female sexuality is obviously a source of irritation for the author.[12]

The need to control this sexuality is the author's justification for the Islamic practice of clitoridectomy:

> En Egypte cette maladie est vulgaire presque en toutes filles, ausquelles on est contraint faire couper cette barbole, quand elles sont prestes à marier, de peur que venant à dresser lors du coit, elle n'en oste le plaisir tant à elles qui les portent, qu'à leurs maris. (*Des hermaphrodits*, F2v)

> (In Egypt this illness is common to almost all girls, from whom it is necessary to cut this little rod, when they are ready to marry, for fear that if it rises up during coitus, it will prevent pleasure as much for the women who have them, as for their husbands.)

Apparently, it was believed at the time the Egyptian women were particularly "hot" in nature, and that their genitalia were consequently enlarged, sometimes to the point of resembling a male member. These phallic women, rivaling male anatomy as they do, are presented as unacceptable and monstrous. Even though Duval takes pains to defend similar characteristics in Marin le Marcis, he can only accept this conformation by designating it as male. So, when the woman's body threatens male dominance as

---

12   For more detailed consideration of this issue, see Lise Leibacher-Ouvrard, "Tribades et gynanthropes (1612–1614): Fictions et fonctions de l'anatomie travesti," *Papers on French Seventeenth Century Literature* 24 (1997): 519–36. See also Stephen Greenblatt's famous piece on *Twelfth Night*, "Fiction and Friction," in *Twelfth Night*, ed. R.S. White (New York: St Martin's Press, 1996), pp. 92–128.

well as male sexual activity, the menacing part is seen as an illness and is to be cut away, actualizing the myth of woman as castrated or lacking.

Further complicating the difficulties of controlling feminine sexuality is the belief (and Duval quotes Paracelsus on this matter) that the uterus is a separate entity, which he calls *animal*, and for the maintenance of which the rest of the female body was formed. Thus, just as the male is subsumed into his penis and testicles, rather than the reverse, the female is subordinated to her womb. For this reason, most of the rest of the treatise is devoted to the "governance" of pregnant women and of delivery. Some of these pages contain rules of conduct: women should avoid violent emotions (M4) and avoid too great an interest in visual images, which might affect the form of the child (M4v). And again Duval notes the diseased nature of woman as he discusses the signs of imminent death in the mother (O7).

The largest portion of Duval's treatise is devoted to pregnancy and childbirth, from "the formation and nourishing of the infant in its mother's womb" (K2v) to the possibility and causes of monstrous births (K6), to the appropriate behavior for an expectant mother (L7v, ch. 18). Most detailed of all is his description of childbirth in the chapter "Comment il faut accoucher une femme" (M6v seq: "How to deliver a woman"). In spite of the obvious passivity of the woman, who is supplanted by the heroic doctor in this event, much of the advice seems quite enlightened for the period. For example, Duval suggests that women should exercise during pregnancy in order to make labor easier (N4v).

Duval offers a section on natural childbirth (M6v–O6), and one on artificial or assisted births (chs 21–24, O6v–Q5: "Des accouchemens artificiels"). The techniques for assisted births include turning the infant by hand inside the womb, the use of hooks, mirrors. In such complicated cases, the loss of the mother was a real threat, and Duval lists the warning signs, so that at least the baby might be saved. But in the section on cesarean birth, he details the treatment of the mother after the procedure, to assure her better recovery. In the chapter on "How a woman should be governed after she has delivered" (ch. 25, Q5v seq.), he offers sensible dietary rules, bed rest (R6), and gives guidelines for breastfeeding. A large section is also devoted to the care of the infant (R7v–T3v: "What must be done for the newborn"). Duval is clearly concerned with the very real effects of (hetero)sexuality, and with what he sees as the necessary outcome of this sexuality. Clearly, there is a gap between his cultural biases concerning gender and the practical advice he offers on the very real bodily event of childbirth.

This portion of the treatise is really a heroic account of the virtually divine control the doctor or surgeon exercises over these unruly bodies, one that reads almost as an appropriation of the parturiant maternal role, as is clear from the comparison of the work of the doctor to a bear licking her new cub into form, an image which echoes a belief still held in the Renaissance. The doctor can even vanquish unruly nature in this divinely hermaphroditic role of mother and father:

... les anciens Payens ont attribué honneurs divins aux Medecins: veu qu'il est besoin qu'ils se monstrent avoir plus de force & energie que la nature mesme, quoy que

procedante directement de la main & toute puissance de Dieu eternel ... Voire mesme
un Dieu remplissant & parfaisant le tout par son actuelle presence. (*Des hermaphrodits*,
P1v)

(... the ancient Pagans attributed divine honors to Doctors: seeing that it is necessary
for them to demonstrate more force and energy than nature herself, even though she
proceeds directly from the hand and omnipotence of eternal God ... truly, even a God
fulfilling and perfecting everything by his effective presence.)

Once again, the Doctor assumes God-like control through his superior knowledge;
this role is to be contrasted with the deadly ignorance of midwives, due to their
unwillingness to communicate their knowledge: "Because rarely do they wish to
transmit their secret and precious experiences one to another" (E2). Again, mastery
of discourse conveys mastery of nature. One of the more brutal images of mastery
is offered in Duval's exhortation to tie the woman in labor down, so that she will
not move during an internal examination (and possible rotation of the child, P3); as
necessary as the procedure might sometimes have been, the image is striking.

But this discourse of mastery is revealed to be overcompensation, at least to some
extent, in the following chapters on cesarean sections. In his justification of this
procedure, Duval reveals that he lost his own wife and child, because the infant's head
was too large for natural delivery. His in-laws refused to allow a cesarean, so, after
his wife had been in labor for four days, Duval had to pull the dead infant out of its
mother, in pieces. Duval's wife died eight days later (P4v). This example, as Duval
himself admits, shows the extent to which nature still eludes mastery. He makes clear
that, to some degree, any cesarean is an admission of defeat as well. He asserts that
this procedure should only be used as a last resort, when the mother is dead or dying
anyway, but the child is still viable (P6v). Yet he describes the great care with which
a cesarean must be performed, each layer of tissue cut separately and carefully so
that the smallest possible amount of damage might be done, and the care with which
the mother must be treated after this procedure. He also lists and describes specific
instances of this procedure, cases in which the mother survived and even went on to
have more children (Q2v–Q5). Clearly, the goal for Duval was not merely to save
the child at the expense of the mother's life; in his experience, this choice was rarely
successful.

Singular in a midwifery manual of this period is the lack of illustrations representing
the pregnant uterus or the fetus itself.[13] Duval instead uses extremely vivid and detailed
descriptions of what physiological phenomena the doctor might encounter; he is
particularly effective in communicating what certain conditions and parts of the body
might feel like. In fact, as the illustrations Karen Newman has selected demonstrate
(although she uses them to support a slightly different argument), representations of an

---

[13]   See Newman, *Fetal Positions*, pp. 27–42, for examples and discussion of such
       illustrations.

independently active fetus, although they may serve a particular ideological agenda, are in fact useless for facilitating successful childbirth. A doctor in seventeenth-century Europe would not be able to see the fetus before birth, and would have wanted to know the meaning of what he was feeling. Duval is correct in his assertion of the importance of mastery of language; obstetrical practice of the time was only partly reliant on visual cues, and more often proceeded by touch. Duval describes with extreme care how various vital organs feel (so that a surgeon performing a cesarean might avoid damaging them), as well as how to judge the various difficult presentations of the fetus by touch. His words guide much more effectively than illustrations of the period would have; strangely, as much as he has proclaimed the mastery of language over the body, Duval's words exhort and signal a responsiveness to bodily cues that can only be read in the most direct and physical fashion. And although still normative to some extent (the surgeon is to feel for certain muscles that should be aligned in a specific way), this emphasis on verbal representations of touch allows for greater variations in physiology, in that the Doctor must locate organs and muscles for himself, rather than assuming their location based on crude visual representations. Duval's detailed descriptions of the complications of childbirth and of cesareans demonstrates an understanding of the range and variety of anatomy in pregnant women; this is in keeping with the awe he expresses at the range of physical presentations nature has concocted in hermaphrodites. This appreciation of difference, rather than a more normative approach, is crucial to the successful practice of medicine.

Thus, the sense of touch and language are described as jointly conveying mastery, just as they were in the chapters on sexuality. But, once again, touch and language must be sensitive to the natural dispositions and inclinations of the body. They convey mastery only to those who are willing to submit to the laws of the body, and understand what can, realistically, be done. The god-like qualities of the doctor, all affirmations of his mastery over nature notwithstanding, are incessantly effaced by the power and variety of nature. The doctor, as intecessor in the process of birth, plays the hermaphroditic role, acting as he submits, responding and controlling.

The Generation of Hermaphrodites

After some discussion of the proper care of the newborn and of the new mother (the word most frequently used is "gouvernance," implying the relationship of ruler and subject), Duval turns again to his discussion of female anatomy and its role in conception, in order to prepare for his tale of the hermaphrodite Marin le Marcis. He rejects the Aristotelian notion of the active male principle and the passive female receptacle, in favor of Hippocratic theories of generation:

> Ie sçai qu'en ce i'aurai repugnance des peripaticiens sectaires d'Aristote, qui ne veulent admettre deux principes actifs. L'un provenant de l'homme, & l'autre de la femme.
> (...)

> Nature n'a rien fait en vain. Elle a formé les parties seminales aux femmes. C'est donc pour engendrer la semence. S'il n'y avoit semence genitale que du masle, le seul masle seroit engendré. Or la femelle est aussi engendree par une faculté qui se trouve au sang, lequel n'est qu'excrement, comme veut l'Aristote. Et par conséquent il ne peut donner la faculté specifique de la femelle. (*Des hermaphrodits*, T7v–T8)

> (I know that I will hold in repugnance those peripatetic partisans of Aristotle, who do not wish to acknowledge two active principles; one coming from the man, and the other from the woman ...
> Nature has made nothing in vain. She has formed seminal organs in women. They are thus to form seed. If there were only male seed, only the male would be engendered. The female is also engendered by a faculty which is found in the blood, which is nothing but excrement, according to Aristotle. But logically, this cannot endow the specific conformation of the female.)

Duval rejects Aristotle's explanation of the generation of females (from *The Generation of Animals*, quoted in the introduction to this study) as irrational and self-contradictory. Nonetheless, he seems primarily concerned with reaffirming the distinctions between the sexes:

> Les sexes establis selon le commun & frequent usage de celle qui dispose de nos corps, dont tous les climats du monde sont pour le iourd'hui habitez, depuis un pole iusques à l'autre, sont l'homme, dit en Latin *Vir*, en Grec *anur*, & la femme, dicte des Latins *mulier*, des Grecs *gunu*. L'un & l'autre aussi sont nommez *homo*, en Grec *anthropos*, usurpant ces deux dictions tant au masculin, que feminin genre ...
> Ceux qui ont devié des plus frequentes & ordinaires configurations, sont l'Hermaphrodit, homme-femme, femme-homme, dictions rendues en Grec *hermaphroditoi, andraguny* & *gunanur*. Desquels il nous convient traicter separement, en faisant & constituant trois especes diverses. (*Des hermaphrodits*, V)

> (The sexes established according to common and frequent usage of she who governs our bodies [nature], which inhabit all of the zones of the world today, from one pole to another, are man, called *Vir* in Latin, *andros* in Greek, and woman, *mulier* in Latin, *gynon* in Greek. One and the other are also known as *homo*, in Greek *anthropos*, these two terms encompassing the masculine as well as the feminine sex.
> Those who have deviated from the most frequent and ordinary configurations, are the Hermaphrodite, the manly woman, and the womanly man, terms rendered in Greek *hermaphroditoi, androgyni*, and *gynanyr*. These should be discussed separately, since they form three diverse species.)

Duval's discussion seems convoluted: sexual difference is established by "common and frequent usage," but, he claims, this usage is that of nature. This sexual difference is both universal and necessary for the population of the world. Duval thus oscillates between the notion of sexual difference as a practice, and such difference as a state of being. This ambiguity is in keeping with his discussion of Marin le Marcis' sexual identity, and the way in which it is effected by his environment.

This problematic argument is further complicated by Duval's insistence on the importance of language for designating gender, and by his immediate retreat into literary and mythological examples of hermaphrodites, accompanied by an avoidance of scientific discussion of any actual cases. He begins his list of hermaphrodites with the tale of Hermaphroditus and Salmacis (V–V2v), retelling the Ovidian tale, as well as the story of the Carians and Lelegians, who were civilized by the waters of the fountain Salmacis (V2). Duval does suggest in his version of the Ovidian tale, that the hermaphrodite is a "demi-homme," and defines it as "un homme nay au vice de composition, portant nature d'homme & de femme" (V: "a man born of imperfect form, containing both male and female natures"). This suggests that Duval still perceives the male as the ideal sex, and the female as merely a defective or lesser male; and certainly the outcome of the Ovidian tale echoes this view of sex.

Nonetheless, the hermaphrodite does create confusion about sex, effacing the distinction between male and female, as Duval admits:

> ... les instruments ou particules servantes à l'un ou à l'autre sexe, sont tellement configurez, qu'on ne peut distinguer, si on doit dire du subiect qu'il soit homme ou femme, dont parlant Iean Soter d'un Hermaphrodit qui estoit dedans un baing d'eau tiede, il dict ...

> Cypris me nomme femme, Hermes homme me dit,
> Mon corps estant noté, de tous les deux ensemble.
> Ce n'est donc sans raison, qu'ils m'ont Hermaphrodit
> Mis en ce baing, dont l'eau est chaude et froide ensemble. (*Des hermaphrodits*, V3)

> (... the instruments or parts serving one or the other sex, are so configured, that one cannot distinguish whether one should say of the subject that he is man or woman, as Jean Soter said of a hermaphrodite in a tepid bath:

> Cypris calls me woman, Hermes man,
> My body was marked by both together,
> So it is not without cause that they placed me
> A hermaphrodite, in the bath of hot and cold water ...)

The image of tepid water suggests a mixing of two disparate elements that do not retain their identity, but create a third, yet again different, element. This third state is neither one nor the other, but somehow both.

Duval then reverts to stories of hermaphrodites that are more reminiscent of the "journalistic" or popular style of Boaistuau than of scientific analysis. The insistence on mastery has dissolved from these accounts. He rehearses the ancient stories of hermaphrodites told by Bauhin (ch. 33, V4–V4v); and then offers an odd chapter on "Histoires des enfans Hermaphrodits, desquels le parfait sexe n'a peu estre remarqué, à raison de leur bas aage & mort subite" (V5–V6: "Stories of hermaphroditic babies, for whom the correct sex could not be discerned, because of their young age and sudden death"). He tells of a mother who died giving birth to 364 hermaphroditic children, who also died. The boys were baptized Jean, the girls, Elisabeth; one wonders, if their sex could not be determined, how they were so baptized, but this is one of the many contradictions in Duval's arguments. He in fact repeats this error in yet another story, claiming that the sex of the child was determined by the functions (in urination) of the external genitalia:

> L'an mil six cens à sainct Sever prés cette ville de Rouen, la femme d'un nommé Roland accoucha d'un enfant qui avoit marque des deux sexes, & sur la question du baptesme, sçavoir s'il seroit presenté pour fille, ou fils: Ils observerent par laquelle des natures il rendoit l'urine, voyant qu'il l'avoit rendu par le conduit muliebre, il fut baptisé pour fille, & ne fut jouissant de longue vie. C'est enfant fut receu par Catherine Mahom obstetrice qui me l'a ainsi affermé. (*Des hermaphrodits*, V6)

> (In 1600, at Saint Sever near this town of Rouen, the wife of a man named Roland gave birth to a baby with the marks of both sexes, and on the matter of baptism, and whether he would be presented as a girl or a boy, they observed by which of the parts he urinated, and seeing that he did so by the feminine conduit, he was baptised a girl, but did not enjoy a long life. This child was delivered by Catherine Mahom the midwife who swore this was true.)

The language betrays the certainty of the conclusions drawn concerning this child. Even though she is designated a girl by the authorities, Duval insists on using the masculine pronoun when speaking of her, even when "he" is baptised as a girl. This insistence is made possible by use of the masculine noun *enfant*, but it is particularly odd given the flexibility of usage in Duval's narration of the case of Marin le Marcis. Perhaps Duval wishes to hint at some doubt about the infallibility of this method of reading the body; perhaps he is preparing the way for the dramatic story of Marin, which he will retell at the end of his treatise.

Although he has suggested that most hermaphrodites are essentially male, Duval does turn to a discussion of "perfect" hermaphrodites, "qui peuvent tirer usage de l'un & l'autre sexe" (ch. 35, V6–V8v: "who can make use of one or the other sex"). In this chapter, he repeats the accepted notion of sex roles: women submit, men act. He also reviews the notion that Adam was the first hermaphrodite, and offers the usual Neoplatonic reading of Genesis.[14] Most of the examples of perfect hermaphrodism that Duval offers are from less threatening and immediate sources, such as the distant past, distant places, and the animal kingdom. He echoes Augustine's contention that some animals are naturally hermaphroditic, and Pliny's affirmation that there is a race of Androgynes in Africa (V7v).

---

[14] For a detailed account of this myth, see Naomi Yavneh, "The Spiritual Eroticism of Leone's Hermaphrodite," pp. 86 seq.

Still, in his opinion, the existence of hermaphrodites is indisputable and this existence tests many theories of generation. So, he is particularly concerned to establish the truth of the existence of "double" hermaphrodites, that is, those who can beget and bear children:

> J'ay cogneu un Hermaphrodite ... (qui) fut marié à un homme, auquel il engendra quelque fils & fille, & ce nonobstant il avoit accoustumé monter sur les chambrieres & engendrer en icelles. (*Des hermaphrodits*, V8)

> (I knew a hermaphrodite who was married to a man, by whom he conceived a son and a daughter, and notwithstanding this, he was accustomed to mounting the chambermaids and begetting children by them.)

Although he recognizes that, for social reasons, these hermaphrodites must choose one role or another, Duval argues that such double beings do exist. Their existence is crucial for his argument against Aristotle's theories of generation; the fortieth chapter is devoted to a refutation of these theories (X6–X6v). Duval points out that these theories are incoherent and inconsistent with each other, and then he refutes them one by one. For the theory that too much material (provided by the mother) causes the generation of hermaphrodites, he argues that this excess should cause other "deformities" at the same time. Why is the location of the "deformity" so specific? Duval seems particularly offended by Aristotle's description of "the female as mutilated and imperfect." He makes the logical point that if the woman does not contribute anything but "material" to generation, then why isn't the male seed entirely to blame for malformations?

Duval also rejects theories that link hermaphrodites to pollution taboos, among them Avicenna's theory that hermaphrodites are conceived in the eighth to eleventh days after the last sign of menstrual flow, and Lemnius's theory that hermaphrodites are caused by the presence of menstrual blood (V8v–X2v). In his rejection of Democritus' theory, that when the timing of the joining of seed is off, so that it does not join perfectly, a hermaphrodite is created, Duval suggests that the hermaphrodite is not a monster, but rather some sort of super-being: "... comment pourra estre engendré l'Androgyne, ou la crase & mistion n'aura esté complete? Veu que ce n'est un corps imparfaict, mais qui à perfection d'un sexe & plus?" (X5: "how could an Androgyne be born, when the formation and mixture has not been complete? Seeing that it is not an imperfect body, but one which has one perfect sex and more?"). Here, he is returning to the Neoplatonic notion of the androgyne as the perfect being, as his vocabulary indicates. He is guiding the reader away from theories that would brand hermaphrodites as monstrous (that is, unnaturally so) towards those that reinscribe them in the orders of nature. But Duval reserves his harshest criticism for Aristotle, even if he retains some Aristotelian biases about the superiority of men. He accuses Aristotle of vagueness: the philosopher believed that monsters were the result of too much seed. Rather than resulting in multiple births, in this case some obstacle prevented normal conception; Aristotle does not explain the nature of this obstacle.[15] Duval, probably rightly, accuses Aristotle of complete lack of understanding of the function and inner workings of the uterus (X6v). He even rejects Aristotle's designation of the female as monstrous, even though he does believe in the superiority of the male.[16] He continues to refute Aristotle in the following chapter, and declares the superiority of Hippocratic theories ("Suitte de la refutation des opinions d'Aristote touchant la conception des Hermaphrodits, & comme il faut entendre Hippocrate sur le faict de la semence,"ch. 41, X7v–Z2: "Continuation of the refutation of the opinions of Aristotle concerning the conception of hermaphrodites, and how Hippocrates should be understood on the matter of seed"). Duval astutely observes that if the feminine matter were passive in conception, then it would not affect the process in any way (X8), yet Aristotle is so intent on crediting conception entirely to the male, that he begs the question:

> Mais il ayme mieux attribuer retusion en la faculté residente en ce spermeviril, comme provenant de ce sang informe, que de conceder un principe formel en la femme, par le moyen de la semence qu'elle fournit au coit. (*Des hermaphrodits*, X7v)

> (But he prefers to attribute any flaw in the faculty residing in the male sperm to this formless blood, rather than concede a formal principle to the woman, by means of the seed she provides in conception.)

Duval then argues that both male and female seed join to form any infant, and chastises Aristotle for not following the opinions of the wiser Hippocrates:

> Combien eust il esté meilleur à ce subtil Philosophe ne se departir de l'authorité des plus signalez personnages, ains suivant l'opinion du sage Hippocrate constituer les deux principes tant actif que passif à la semence genitale, qui procede tant du masle que de la femelle. (*Des hermaphrodits*, Y)[17]

---

[15] Here, Duval seems to be discussing Aristotle's *Generation of Animals*, 770b27–772b34 (pp. 1192–6).

[16] "Pourquoy il ne se trouvera en cette opinion, comme ie croy non plus de raison, qu'en l'action retuse qu'il veut estre en la semence virile, lors qu'au lieu d'un masle la femelle (dit-il) animal comme mutilé & imparfait est engendrée" (X6v).

[17] Laqueur's presentation of the Hippocratic argument, in *Making Sex*, p. 39, is clearer than Duval's and may be of some help here: "Hippocrates argues for pangenesis, the view that each part of the body of each parent renders up some aspect of itself; that the representatives of the various parts form a reproductive fluid or seed; and that conception consists of a blending, in various proportions and strengths, of these germinal substances. Hippocrates abandons any effort to attribute strong or weak seed respectively to actual males or females. Although male must originate from stronger sperm, 'the male being stronger than the female,' both are capable of producing more or less strong seed." See also Hippocrates, *On Generation* in the Iain M. Lonie edition of *The Hippocratic Treatises* (Berlin: Walter de Gruyter, 1981), 7.2.

(How much better would it have been for this subtle Philosopher not to depart from the authority of more significant figures, thus following the opinion of wise Hippocrates who establishes two principles, active and passive, to generative seed, which procedes as much from the female as the male.)

He even accuses Aristotle of stealing his best ideas from Hippocrates. Yet the final opinion which Duval expresses varies only slightly from Aristotle's theories; as he attributes conception of a male to more active and "robust" seed, that of a female to more passive seed (Y2v). Seed from the father tends to be more robust; seed from the mother tends to be weaker. Both come together, and whichever is present in greater quantity dictates the sex of the child. This model still ascribes greater perfection to the male, although Duval does add that both men and women carry stronger and weaker seed. Duval's own argument seems self-contradictory: both men and women have male and female seed, yet the seed from a man, because of its superiority, engenders a boy more often than does that from a woman. Duval, who corrected Aristotle's similar mistaken notions only a few pages earlier, falls into the same trap of presumption of male superiority (even though he does attribute some effective action to the maternal matter):

Or quand il vient plus de sperme du corps de l'homme que de la femme ce part est mieux formé, & semblable au pere, mais quand il en vient plus de la femme, ce corps est plus beau & plus semblable à la mere & nullement au pere .... (*Des hermaphrodits*, Y3)

(So when more sperm comes from the body of the man than from that of the woman, this part is better formed and resembles the father, but when more comes from the woman, this body is more beautiful, and resembles more the mother, and not at all the father ....)

This passage echoes Duval's early pronouncements on reproduction as *self*-propagation and thus immortality. But it creates a basic flaw in his argument, similar to the flaw he used to destroy Aristotle's seeming logic: if the male seed is superior, why can it not vanquish the unruly but clearly inferior female seed? If there is in fact a hierarchical relation of male to female, by which the female is merely a defective male, then the "defects" of the female seed should be effaced by the perfect male seed; in the same manner as Salmacis's identity is effaced when she is joined to Hermaphroditus. Any hierarchical explanation of generation cannot in fact account for hermaphrodites.

At the same time as he is trying to assert male superiority in his accounts of conception, Duval rejects any theory of the origin of hermaphrodites that denies the mother an equal role in the generation of the child, for example Empedocles's theory that when the father's seed predominates, a boy is conceived, when the mother's, a girl, and when both are present in equal amounts, a hermaphrodite is created. He has adopted instead a slightly more complex theory based on Hippocrates' claim that both mother and father carry strong and weak seed. As we have seen, when "robust" seed predominates, a boy is conceived; when weak seed is present in greater quantity, a girl is conceived. But if one or the other does not predominate, a hermaphrodite is born. Since the issue is one of variable quantities, a whole spectrum of "sexes" can be explained: from the manly man to more effeminate men, through a range of hermaphrodites, to vigorous women, and to very feminine women. This spectrum fits in well with the great variety in nature that Duval has remarked upon elsewhere in the treatise. While retaining the superior value of the masculine in his theories, Duval has managed to mitigate at least a bit of the misogyny and vehement prejudice against hermaphrodites present in the work of the "partisans of Aristotle" (T7v). In fact, the most coherent part of Duval's argument simply echoes Paré's explanation of hermaphrodites,[18] which did not assign higher or lower values to either sex:

> Dont resulte facilement, que s'il advient que la semence genitale soit rendue en égale quantité & qualité, tant de l'homme que de la femme ... l'une ne cede à l'autre, mais apres deue mistion agisse en patissant, patisse & endure en agissant mutuellement & esgallement l'Hermaphrodit sera engendré. (*Des hermaphrodits*, Y3v)

> (So it occurs easily, that if it happens that the generative seed is given in equal quantity and quality from the father as well as from the mother ... one does not give way to the other, but after proper mixture, acts while submitting, submits and endures while acting mutually and equally, the hermaphrodite will be conceived ....)

The concepts of *agir* and *patir*, used so often in discussions of sexual roles, are at play even at the moment of conception in this theory. But the notion of equal mixtures, equal roles, and equal power granted to each type of seed belies the constantly assumed superiority of the male which informs most of Duval's treatise.

After establishing an acceptable (to him) theory of the origin of hermaphrodites, Duval once again turns to mythological and astrological accounts. He claims that the positions of the Sun and the Moon, Venus and Mercury, are particularly important. He lingers for quite some time on the figure of Mercury, calling him a prophet, and linking him to Theuth (Y7), the Egyptian god of language, with all of the implications of mastery and loss of mastery that this form of divinity might contain.[19] Mercury, often portrayed in alchemical treatises as being of ambiguous sex, and in mythology as the father of Hermaphroditus, thus links hermaphrodites to eloquence and rhetoric. He daringly describes Mercury as the divine *Logos* (again echoing alchemical treatises):[20]

---

[18] In *Des monstres et prodiges*, ch. 6, pp. 24–5, cited above.

[19] Not only is this in keeping with discussions of language previously offered in this treatise, but this figure is analyzed as one of attempted mastery over that which remains elusive in Jacques Derrida's essays on "La pharmacie de Platon," particularly from pp. 71–133; *La dissemination* (Paris: Seuil, 1972).

[20] In particular, the *Rosarium philosophorum* compares the alchemical process to Christ's life. See the facsimile edition of the 1550 printing, ed. Joachim Telle (Weinheim: VCH, 1992), pp. 182–92.

Mais ils parlent en ces livres là d'une parole ou verbe energique & actuel, lequel ayant pour sa Venus cette masse elementaire, qui estoit lors confuse en un cahos, à creé le ciel, la terre, & tout ce qui est enclos sous la voute de ce grand temple celeste, auquel ce verbe Divin doit estre adoré avec toute humilité. (*Des hermaphrodits,* Y6v)

(But they speak in these books of an energetic and effective word, which having as its Venus this elemental mass which was previously mixed together in chaos, created the sky, the earth, and all that is encompassed under the vault of this great celestial temple, in which this Divine Word should be adored with all humility.)

Note that Mercury, often portrayed as an androgynous divinity, is here cast as the male principle which organizes and forms the chaotic female matter, represented by Venus. He is also associated with the feminine *parole* and the masculine *verbe*, both linked to Scriptural discourse and to the divine *Logos.* This cosmology echoes Aristotelian notions of generation, Platonic notions of the union of spirit and matter, and alchemical depictions of the process of conjunction (all concepts which overlap to a large degree). Mercury is then depicted as tricephalous, a representation of the trinity, but also of the pagan god's intellectual characteristics: memory, intelligence, and providence, which inform the triple-headed figure of Prudence in Renaissance iconography[21] Duval also elaborates on his nature as the serpent-killer, vanquisher of Satanic forces. But Mercury as the divine *Logos* is ineffective without the material upon which to work; bodily reality meets linguistic mastery in this image as well. So, Duval discusses Venus' qualities, and tells some mythological stories about the two (Y7v–z); but his main concern remains with Mercury as the image of salvation, propagation, and immortality. In astrological accounts of the generation of hermaphrodites, the influence of the planet Mercury is seen as key (Z1). These accounts thus place hermaphrodites in a stereotypically masculine role, one that involves mastery of discourse and control over others.

In his examples, Duval does seem primarily concerned with masculine hermaphrodites, and with establishing their social role as men, even though he has argued in theory for a continuous spectrum of sexes. For hermaphrodites with two sets of genitalia, of which only the male organs function, he uses the term *Androgyne,* arguing that "la plus excellente partie obtenant le premier lieu en la nomination" (Z2: "the most excellent part obtaining the first place in the name"). *Gynanders* are hermaphrodites in whom the female reproductive organs function, but the male do not; sometimes these people pass as men, but are eventually discovered to be women (Z2v). As was the case in Duval's opening arguments, here the primary criterion for designating a male is his reproductive capacity:

Car la perfection du sexe ne se doit iuger par l'excretion de l'urine seulement mais par l'orgasme, & emotion de nature, s'inclinant d'avantage aux particules desquelles

---

[21] Wind, *Pagan Mysteries in the Renaissance* (New York: Norton, 1968), p. 260. These triple intellectual virtues also correspond to past, present, and future.

l'Hermaphrodit peut user, en l'habitation & copule charnelle, pour le fait de la generation. (*Des hermaphrodits*, Z3)

(Because the perfection of a sex should not be judged only by urination, but by the orgasm and natural feeling, inclining more to the parts the Hermaphrodite can use, in the sexual act and in coupling for the purposes of generation.)

Neuter hermaphrodites can fulfill neither the active nor passive role (Duval's terms), neither beget nor bear children (Z5v). Thus, gender identity is linked only to reproductive capacity. This limitation of criteria is crucial to Duval's defense of Marin le Marcis, who, by all appearances, is female but for her functioning penis.

When he admits the possibility of unstable or transformed sex, the only examples he gives are mythical or animal. Duval offers the example of Tiresias, and later mentions the hyena's apparent capacity to change sex in an echo of Bauhin (Aa1v). Any "transformations" that may have occurred in recent history are explained away as misobservation in the initial determination of sex. In the reign of Louis XI, a man from Auvergne gave birth to a child (Z7). In 1575 in Paris, a young man (an altar boy) was discovered to be a girl, and allowed to live as a woman (Z7v). Duval becomes concerned that his (apparently male) audience may feel threatened, and reassures them:

... les hommes formez tels en la vulve maternelle, ne deposent iamais leur nature virile, & ne retourne arriere vers le sexe feminin, d'autant que toutes choses tendent à perfection, & n'ont regres à ce qui est moins parfaict. Or est la nature de l'homme plus parfaicte que celle de la femme. (*Des hermaphrodits*, ch. 51, Z8)

(... men formed as such in the maternal womb never lose their virile nature and do not regress towards the feminine sex, since all things tend towards perfection, and do not degenerate into that which is less perfect. So, the nature of man is more perfect than that of woman.)

The social construction of male superiority, which certainly would guarantee a strong desire to remain male, is here taken as a "natural" or biological fact. Duval seems torn between his understanding of female anatomy and biological functions and the cultural biases he has received, more from philosophical treatises than from any other source. His powers of scientific observation remain in conflict with the received attitudes towards sex that his society has trained into him. For Duval, the hermaphrodite becomes the site of his own conflicted notions of sex and gender.

It is for this reason as well that Duval emphasizes the extent to which our perceptions of external signs lead us to misjudge the sex of a person. He offers examples of men who have been discovered to be women, arguing that these men cannot have become women, but were women who merely seemed to be men. He emphasizes the social pressures that favor masculinity: "Il advint aussi qu'un Hermaphrodit estant produict sur terre, les parens plus curieux d'elever un fils, qu'une fille ..." (Z8v: "It happens as well that, a hermaphrodite appearing on earth, the parents are more eager to raise a boy than a girl"). Such social pressures bear upon the subject, causing her to maintain the masculine role she has been given, but nature will out (Aa1). Similarly, in his accounts of women who were revealed to be men, of which he gives many examples from ancient Rome (Aa6), Duval emphasizes the extent to which appearances deceive, and to which social practices may shape those appearances. He asserts repeatedly that it is the functioning of the body, not its appearance, which should be used to designate the sex of a subject.

Throughout these accounts, Duval insists that men cannot become women (Z8), and women cannot become men (Bb2v). In cases where this seems to have happened, in fact the appearance belied underlying function, the only true mark of sex for Duval. Or the subject in question was a hermaphrodite, exhibiting characteristics of both male and female, although one set of characteristics may have remained hidden for some time. As is true in his discussion of childbirth, what one sees is not to be trusted, and it is the sense of touch that reveals the truth. This view dominates the case of Marin le Marcis, and Duval's eloquent presentation of this revolutionary argument will save the young hermaphrodite's life.

For Duval, then, visual cues of gender are linked to performative presentations (dress, speech, gesture, comportment, etc.); touch is linked to the underlying body, which he considers more "essential" or more "real" than the surface presentations. Whereas Bauhin offers the various modes of presentation of sexual identity, from clinical observation or dissection to dress and behavior, as being of more or less equal value with no one more determinate than another, Duval clearly feels that the structure of the body as established by internal exam, and primarily by the sense of touch, provides a more definitive mark of sex than the surface and social presentations. To some extent, then, he is offering a view of sex that is close to essentialist theories being discussed today. But, as we have seen in the case of Marin le Marcis, Duval not only concedes but elaborately delineates a concomitant theory that environment, and what might be deemed performative practices (dress, level of activity, relative empowerment or disempowerment), can alter bodily "reality." The complex interaction between the body and the roles imposed upon it makes it difficult (although not impossible, according to Duval) to determine the sex of some subjects. While Bauhin conveys, through his contradictory uses of various ways of knowing (poetic, clinical, customary, political, etc.), that our perception of sex may be unstable, and therefore we may not be able to know what bodily "reality" underlies that perception, Duval seems to be arguing that the body itself is mutable and unstable, so that bodily reality can only be factitiously determined by given functions at a specific time. Yet he sets limits on this mutability – men can never become women – in a desperate attempt, it seems, to hold on to traditional gender roles. Like Bauhin, Duval cannot break free from the traditional misogyny so central to his profession. Yet he seems to remain at the margins of that profession, coming as close as any other author to questioning those very traditions.

The extent to which Duval differs from his colleagues in the subtlety and complexity of his understanding of sexual difference is nowhere more evident than in Jean Riolan's refutation of his work, the *Discours sur les hermaphrodits, où il est démontré contre l'opinion commune, qu'il n'y a point de vrays hermaphrodits* (*Discourse on Hermaphrodites, in Which it is Demonstrated that, Contrary to Popular Opinion, There Are No True Hermaphrodites*).[22] Riolan argues that there are only males or females, and that the distinctions between them are quite clear. His primary argument is that those who are deemed to be hermaphrodites are in fact sexually deviant women, who have enlarged clitorises due to their activities. Although he claims in his opening letter that he wishes to make hermaphrodites loved and accepted (a2), he condemns any sexual difference in the body of his text. The opening lines of his text evoke a horror at the possibility of unbridled sexuality:

> On dit que l'Afrique produit tousiours quelque monstre nouveau, c'est un pays fort sec, arrousé de peu de rivieres, & fertil en bestes sauvages, qui sont contraintes souvent d'aller boire en mesme riviere, où se rencontrans en grand nombre, ils s'accouplent pesle-mesle, & de ce meslange & copulation dissemblable naissent les monstres estranges …. (*Discours*, p. 1)

> (They say that Africa always produces some new monster. It is a very dry country, watered by few rivers, and fertile in wild beasts, which are often compelled to drink in the same river, where, encountering each other in great numbers, they couple without order, and from this mixing and diverse coupling are born strange monsters ….)

The milder climate of Paris produces no monsters; any oddities that are to be found there have gathered in Paris because of its pleasant situation (2). Again, we see the association between the animal and unbridled sexuality. This prepares the way for Riolan's condemnation of hermaphrodites as merely overly lustful women:

> Or ceste partie dicte clitoris, representant par sa figure & composition la verge de l'homme, peut croistre & grossir comme le doigt aux femmes voluptueuses & amoureuses, & en peuvent abuser pour se donner plaisir, en habitant les unes avec les autres. (*Discours*, p. 79)

> (So this part called the clitoris, mimicking by its form and its composition the male rod, can grow and thicken like a finger in libidinous and lustful women, and they can abuse it to give themselves pleasure, by living with each other.)

The threat of this form of sexuality is its exclusion of the masculine. This menace is clearly too great for the author to bear, as he displaces this form of sexuality onto distant cultures, claiming almost immediately after this discussion of female homosexuality that it is Egyptian women who are best known for this form of enlarged clitoris

---

[22]   Paris: Ramier, 1614. Riolan was a professor at the Sorbonne, and a partisan of Aristotelian medicine.

(he also adds examples of Turkish women, p. 81). The "cure" for this condition is "l'amputation des parties superflues" (p. 83: "the amputation of superfluous parts"), a suggestion which echoes the more forceful "retrancher ce qui ne leur appartient" (5: "cut away that which does not belong to them") offered earlier in the treatise. Egyptian women are more fertile, probably because their country is hotter (p. 85), and their genitalia grow overly large, and thus must be cut off (also Duval's explanation for clitoridectomy). These excesses are also linked to the myth of hypermasculinity of Egyptian men (p. 87). Riolan then devotes a chapter to the history of "the circumcision of women" (p. 89) and how they might be castrated (his term) without risking their lives. In a treatise that is otherwise a fairly conventional recasting of Duval's work (often verbatim repetition), this obsession with excessive female sexuality and its cures, and the insistence on distancing this sexuality from French culture, reveals the extent to which male dominion felt itself to be very vulnerable indeed. The precise vulnerability of this dominion is evident in Riolan's argument that "un homme sans bourses & testicules, s'il a la verge bien formee, ne lairra pas d'estre homme" (*Discours*, p. 105: "a man without scrotum or testicles, if he has a well-formed penis, does not cease to be a man"). But, if women can be castrated, and indeed if some of them must be in order to assure their femininity, then how sure is masculinity based on this one body part? The fear of castration, of sexual insufficiency, lurks below the surface of this argument, and in his insistence on clear distinctions based on examples that are hardly clear, Riolan destroys all certainty of what is masculine, what feminine. If the penis grants manhood, then the phallic woman is also a man; if the penis can be taken away, then manhood based solely upon it is easily lost.

Riolan's paranoia, along with the sinuous twists and turns of Duval's arguments, reveals the extent to which, although a biological reality, sexual ambiguity was an untenable state in French society of the time. Duval concludes his treatise with a longer narration and discussion of the case of Marin le Marcis (*Des hermaphrodits*, Bb7–Ff7), making quite clear the suffering and fear Marin and his wife Jeanne endured. Duval's melodramatic account of their lives underscores the social torment and ostracism involved for a person of indeterminate sex. Thus, he must heroically establish Marin's true nature, not only for his contemporaries, but as an uninterrupted state that already existed at birth. Even "transformation" was unacceptable; Marin had to be categorized as unequivocally male if he was to survive. Thus, although anatomical and other observations had established the fact of sexual ambiguity, a whole continuum of sexes and genders, of biological and social identities, this ambiguity was like a dirty little secret that had to be denied and repressed in order for society to function, and for individuals to function in society. Science had advanced somewhat in its understanding of anatomy, sex, and sexuality. Society, however, did not stay in step with these medical advances, and maintained rigid roles, increasingly revealed as fictional or cultural constructs, by means of capital or corporal punishment and public humiliation. The hermaphrodite, recognized at least to some degree by medicine, was repressed mostly by the legal system. But as with anything repressed, this figure resurfaced continually in the poetry, novels, and popular pamphlets of the time. Denied existence, the hermaphrodite seemed to be everywhere, invading every aspect of intellectual life. The constant ridicule or repression of such ambiguity revealed intense fear; this fear hints at the power of the hermaphroditic figure for the intellectual and the popular imagination.

Chapter 4

Hermetic Hermaphrodites

Alchemy and Sexual Difference

If medical treatises of the early modern period reflected official and cultural attitudes towards sex and gender, even as they tested the limits of those attitudes, alchemical treatises offered an alternative view. These two bodies of knowledge contain the fundamental images of the hermaphrodite that were echoed throughout sixteenth century culture; they served as sourcebooks for poets and for pamphleteers, but they were also guidelines for reading sexuality and sexual difference as natural or supernatural, as strictly regulated or infinitely varied, as debased or exalted. Also, whereas medical treatises strove more frequently at the end of the sixteenth century to naturalize intersexuality, alchemical treatises combined the monstrous and the divine hermaphrodite into one evocative figure. The monstrous hermaphrodite was sacrificed, and reborn as divine. This sequence echoed the story of Christ, but also served as a consoling narrative in times which were considered "monstrous" and disordered themselves. These treatises offered the hope that rebirth and renewal might result from destruction.

This optimistic message contained within an often violent narrative is fundamental to the practice of alchemy itself. The primary goal of alchemy is presented as the transmutation of metals, from baser to nobler ones.[1] In particular, alchemists focused on the production of gold, considered a mystical metal and associated with the sun, and silver, associated with the moon.[2] Some of the earliest origins of alchemy lie in Egyptian techniques of amalgamation and even forgery, the records of which are no longer available to us, the earliest extant sources dating from about the third century AD.[3] The development of western alchemy can be linked to that of gnosticism, described as the

---

[1] Paracelsus: "Alchemy is nothing else but the set purpose, intention, and subtle endeavour to transmute the kinds of the metals from one to another. According to this, each person, by his own mental grasp, can choose out for himself a better way and Art, and therein find truth ..." (*The Coelum Philosophorum*, in *The Hermetic and Alchemical Writings*, p. 16).

[2] Reinhard Federmann, *The Royal Art of Alchemy* (Philadelphia: Chilton, 1969), p. 3. For an excellent general introduction to alchemy, see Gareth Roberts, *The Mirror of Alchemy: Alchemical Ideas and Images in Manuscripts and Books* (Toronto: Toronto University Press, 1994). Probably the best historical account of alchemy, focusing on the Renaissance and on the seventeenth century, is Allen G. Debus' work, *The Chemical Philosophy: Paracelsian Science and Medicine in the Sixteenth and Seventeenth Centuries*, cited above.

[3] M. Berthelot, *Les Origines de l'alchimie* (Paris: Steinheil, 1885), "Les Sources égyptiennes," pp. 21–45.

result of the interaction between Greek philosophy and Judaeo-Christian theology;[4] in particular, the divisions between spirit and matter are strikingly similar.

Images of sexual difference or ambiguity, and of generation in particular, are central to much of alchemical discourse from the origins of the practice to early modern times. The sixteenth century witnessed an explosive evolution in alchemical thought, traced already in the works of Allen Debus, and a concomitant change in the depiction of the body and of gender roles in alchemical treatises. As Debus points out, from the earliest examples of alchemical thought to the publications of Paracelsus, the chemical philosopher places himself in a surrogate maternal role:

> In fact, we do find that the oldest surviving works of metal craftsmen combine an emphasis on the change in the appearance of metals with the acceptance of a vitalistic view of nature – a view that included the belief that metals live and grow within the earth in a fashion analogous to the growth of the human fetus. It was to become basic to alchemical thought that the operator might hasten the natural process of metallic growth in his laboratory and thus bring about perfection in far less time than that required by nature.[5]

Mother Earth, the feminine principle, is a slow and unreliable producer of precious metals. Thus, the male philosopher eliminates the feminine ground, and develops more efficient systems to refine matter. This appropriation of the maternal role is linked to the creation of the homunculus, that is, perfection of reproduction by separation from the maternal body. According to Paracelsus, for example, humankind could be rendered immortal if philosophers could learn to reproduce themselves from sperm only, and in a jar.[6]

But alchemical works published from the mid-sixteenth century on, although some may have been written well before Paracelsus' time, emphasize the *conjunction* of male and female, the union of spiritual and physical, as necessary for the perfection of matter. As was the case with medical treatises on the generation of animals and humans, this evolution away from an asexual ideal of reproduction towards a renewed estimation of the importance of the female in the reproductive process was based on rejection of Aristotelian notions of sexual difference, which condemned the female to the realm of the monstrous, and designated her merely as the fertile field upon which the male reproduced himself. The hermaphrodite, an increasingly important figure in alchemical works, was the symbol of this necessary but complex *conjunction* and balancing of male and female.

---

[4]   See Federmann, p. 9, and Vern L. Bullough, *Sexual Variance in Society and History* (New York: John Wiley and Sons, 1976), pp. 182–8. Bullough links gnosticism to early Christian thought.

[5]   Debus, *The Chemical Philosophy*, p. 4.

[6]   This ideal is echoed by the "transvestite" poetry of the court of Henri III, analyzed in a later chapter, in which the male poet takes on the female role, thus eliminating the female other.

Even in the later Middle Ages, alchemy and the sexed body were closely linked: a thirteenth century pseudo-Albertus wrote both on *The Secrets of Women and Men* and on *Metals and Minerals*. Roger Bacon (1214–1294) and Arnold of Villanova (b. 1235), two of the more influential adherents of the art, enlisted alchemy in the service of the natural sciences, and of medicine in particular.[7] Both philosophers insisted that the welfare of the soul depended on that of the body.

By the late Middle Ages and the Renaissance, alchemical practice evolves into recipes for medicine (*aurum potabile* and herbal remedies), embalming processes (and thus two very different forms of Egyptian lore are linked), methods of divination, and spiritual exercises. The alchemical process divides the universe into spiritual and material realms, aligning everything on a scale as it more or less approaches the spiritual ideal. Alchemy is thus perceived as a process of purification; but, at the same time, this process is dependent upon the fusion of the spiritual and material realms, for purification can express itself only in material terms for most practitioners (in the production of gold, of medicine, of incorruptible bodies). Most alchemical treatises thus revolve around an obsession with the human body as well as with metals.

These two realms are united in the hermaphroditic figure of Mercury,[8] at once the dual divinity from whom sprang the seven planets (and seven metals) and itself the metal by means of which transformations are effected (quicksilver). Mercury/ Hermes is the figure that links gnostic and alchemical systems with Christianity.[9] This conflation of pagan and Christian ideas emphasized natural as much as spiritual processes. Generally, mercury, sulphur, and salt are the three elements that form all substances.[10] From Mercury can be generated Jupiter (tin), Mars (iron), Venus (copper), Saturn (lead), Luna (silver), and Sol (gold).[11] In turn, Sol and Luna are often portrayed as a hermaphroditic brother-sister pair or *rebis*,[12] sometimes as an incestuous pair (and then as King and Queen, or Prince and Princess). Sometimes they are designated as Apollo and Diana, or Phoebus and Phoebe. Thus, the hermaphrodite becomes a recurrent image in the alchemical process. Mercury is in turn associated with the *monstrum*, the dragon or serpent, an early image of the world-creating (and

---

7   Federmann, p. 91; Debus, pp. 19–21.
8   C.G. Jung, *Psychology and Alchemy* (Princeton: Bollingen, 1980), pp. 302, 371–2.
9   Federmann, p. 25: "During the 2nd and 3rd centuries a secret Gnostic Hermes cult also flourished. Hermes was worshipped as the All-Spirit, as the Demiurge who created the material world and permeates it as Logos. He is identified with the Savior, the mediator between God and the world, which he saves from the planets' destructive influence."
10 Waite's introduction to his edition of the works of Paracelsus, xi; and Paracelsus's treatise *The Aurora of the Philosophers*, p. 65; see also Clovis Hesteau de Nuysement's *Traictez du vray sel secret des philosophes et de l'esprit général du monde*, ed. Sylvain Matton, p. 169. Debus credits Paracelsus with introduction of this new triad of elements (*The Chemical Philosophy*, p. 57).
11 See Paracelsus, *The Coelum Philosophorum*, in *The Hermetic and Alchemical Writings*, pp. 5–11.
12 Jung, *Psychology and Alchemy*, pp. 202, 243, 244; fig. 125.

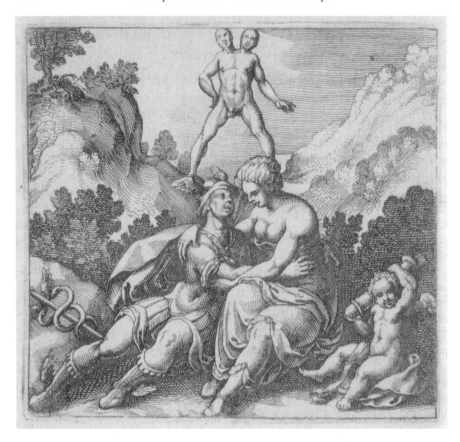

Figure 4.1   Plate 38, the hermaphroditic rebis, Hermes, and Aphrodite, from Michael Maier's *Atalanta fugiens*. Courtesy of the Division of Rare and Manuscript Collections, Cornell University Library

potentially world-destroying) spirit;[13] thus, it represents the primordial chaos, the origin and goal of the alchemist's work. It is also linked with the self-creating phoenix, representing the purified and reborn *materia*.[14]

---

[13]   Jung, *Psychology and Alchemy*, p. 292.

[14]   "This work, the Tincture of the Alchemists, need not be one of nine months; but quickly, and without any delay, you may go on by the Spagyric Art of the Alchemists, and, in the space of forty days, you can fix this alchemical substance, exalt it, putrefy it, ferment it, coagulate it into a stone, and produce the Alchemical Phoenix. But it should be noted well that the Sulphur of Cinnabar becomes the Flying Eagle, whose wings fly away without wind, and carry the body of the phoenix to the nest of the parent, where it is nourished

Many of these images link alchemical representations of the hermaphrodite to classical myths of dualistic divinity (Tiresias and the serpents, which transform him into a woman, and then back into a man; Caeneus who is transformed from a girl into a boy, and then into the phoenix). These associations are confirmed by the notion that Mercury is highly volatile and mutable.[15] This mutability, decried in its worldly form by late Renaissance moralists, is the alchemists' ideal. This dilemma suggests again the menace associated with the hermaphrodite, who takes on now one sex, now another, sometimes both.

Because of its all-encompassing nature, the mercurial hermaphrodite is most closely associated with the sixth of the seven most common steps in the alchemical work, that of *coagulatio* or *coniunctio*. After the burning of the body (of matter – *calcinatio*), its decomposition (*putrefactio*, often portrayed as a ritual dismemberment or sacrifice), evaporation (*sublimatio*), liquefaction (*solutio*), and distillation, the material is crystallized or "fixed" into a solid form. Only when this new and complete body[16] is created can the desired essence be extracted from it in the final step of the process.

Alchemy seems based on the presumption that everything can be dissolved, and that boundaries between different elements and masses can be erased and rewritten; thus, "conjunction" and "separation" are two basic concepts in this process. Even more presumptuous is the notion that this can be achieved by a mortal man. Perhaps this presumption can be seen as a conjuring away of the abject; fearing dissolution, man places it in his own control, tames it. This leads to an acceptance of the abject, but only in its own particular place. From its earliest manifestations in ancient Egypt, alchemy seems to be based on this "fear of the abject," as it oscillates between insistent classification of the natural world and dissolution of these observed or created differences.[17] Born as the fraudulent practice of minting false gold, it also has a mystical or spiritual edge to it even in the earliest manuscripts. In his discussion of ancient Greek alchemical documents, Berthelot observed a cluster of concerns and issues surrounding this proto-science:

---

by the element of fire, and the young ones dig out its eyes: from whence there emerges a whiteness, divided in its sphere, into a sphere and life out of its own heart, by the balsam of its inward parts, according to the property of the cabalists" (*The Treasure of Treasures for Alchemists*, from *The Hermetic and Alchemical Writings*, p. 40).

[15] "The spirit of Mercury, which is only subjected to the spirits above, has no determinate or certain form in itself. Hence it happens that it admits every metal, just as wax receives all seals, of whatever form" (Paracelsus, *Concerning the Spirits of the Planets*, from *The Hermetic and Alchemical Writings*, p. 79).

[16] "The fusion of the male mind and the female soul is expressed in the double-headed eagle and lion, in the Hermaphrodite, in the meeting of unicorn and hart ..." (Federmann, p. 36).

[17] M. Berthelot, *Les Origines de l'alchimie* (Paris: Georges Steinheil, 1885), p. 22.

... ces papyrus nous fournissent aujourd'hui un document sans pareil pour apprécier à la fois les procédés industriels des anciens pour fabriquer des alliages, leur état psychologique et leurs préjugés mêmes relativement à la puissance de l'homme sur la nature.[18]

(... these papyri furnish us today with a document unequalled for the appreciation at once of the technical procedures of the ancients in the fabrication of alloys, their psychological state, and their assumptions even relative to the power of man over nature.)

This statement goes beyond Jung's view of alchemy as a proto-psychology,[19] in that it suggests a "politics" of natural science, informed by that sense of control and domination over the natural world which is reflected in the social hierarchy itself. Yet the alchemical practice is at its very origins a subversion of economic authority, being as it was the art of counterfeiting gold coin.[20] Alchemy retained this double identity of fraudulent art and philosophy of man's natural authority well into the early modern period.

Of further importance is the link between alchemy and early fertility rites, by means of gnostic thought. As we shall see, early modern alchemical treatises seem fairly evenly divided between those supporting the notion of a dualistic divinity and those with a more patriarchal view of the process. The theory of an initial dualistic divinity is supported by works of hermetic philosophy, such as this fragment ascribed to Poemandres:

9. But the Mind, The God, being masculine-feminine, originating Life and Light, begat by Word another Mind Creator, Who being God of the Fire and Spirit, created some Seven Administrators, encompassing in circles the sensible world; and their administration is called Fate.
10. Immediately from the downborne elements sprung forth the Word of the God to the pure creation of all Nature, and was united to the creative Mind, for it was of the same essence, and the irrational downborne elements of Nature were left to be matter only.
11. But the Creator Mind along with the Word, that encompassing the circles, and making them revolve with force, turned about its own creations and permitted them to be turned about from an indefinite beginning to an interminable end; for they begin ever where they end.[21]

---

[18] M. Berthelot, "Introduction" in the *Collection des anciens alchimistes grecs* (Osnabruck: Otto Zeller, 1967; reimpression of the 1888 edition), vol. 1, p. 5.

[19] Most clearly stated in his two books, *Psychology and Alchemy* and *Mysterium Coniunctionis* (Princeton: Princeton University Press, 1977).

[20] Berthelot, *Collection*, vol. 1, p. 6: "Comment nous rendre compte de l'état intellectuel et mental des hommes qui pratiquaient ces recettes frauduleuses, destinées à tromper les autres par de simples apparences, et qui avaient cependant fini par se faire illusion à eux-mêmes, et par croire réaliser, à l'aide de quelque rite mystérieux, la transformation effective de ces alliages semblables à l'or et à l'argent en un or et en un argent véritables?"

[21] "Poemandres," from *The Theological and Philosophical Works of Hermes Trismegistus, Christian Neoplatonist*, trans. John David Chambers (Edinburgh: T. & T. Clark, 1882), pp. 4–6.

Even in this early medieval philosophical work, the advent of language (the Word) is equated with the dominion of the Father and with the ordering of the universe into rational and irrational. Value is not ascribed to any thing, creatures are not assigned various places in a hierarchy, until the male-female divinity creates a masculine Word. From that moment on in the text, creation itself is dominated by masculine divinities only. The male-female then remains outside of the created universe, turning it around and back to the beginning. This divinity is at once abject, in that it is excluded from creation, and embodies the recurring threat of abjection (as it turns the universe back towards Chaos, which is in fact the hermaphroditic divinity itself). This circular movement from and towards abjection, dissolution, or duality, is the very basis of alchemical thought; it is symbolized by the *euroboros*, the serpent gnawing on its own tail.[22]

There is a tension in alchemical treatises between the neopythagorean and gnostic formulation of the necessary coexistence of the female essence of the divinity as the power and the male as the act, and the simple Aristotelian and Christian hierarchized duality.[23] One half cannot function without the other in the neopythagorean scheme; in the Christianized Platonic or Aristotelian schemes, the male spirit is always trying to detach itself from the female body in order to lead a more pure existence. This tension between two very different world views is reflected in the intellectual and political life of late sixteenth-century France. That which was different was evidently not simply going to disappear; the world of the western hemisphere could not be ignored by Europe, other religions could not be eradicated by the Catholics, and even Paracelsus could not explain how to perpetuate the human race without women. For a brief time, certain intellectuals in France toyed with the notion of coexistence between that which was the same and that which was different. The alchemists in particular, soon sidelined by mainstream culture, clung to their belief in the importance of that which was different. For this reason, they were scorned by most of the academic world.[24]

In the alchemical treatises analyzed in this chapter, the hermaphrodite as *prima materia* becomes the locus for the primordial concerns hinted at in the images of

---

[22] "The examples given in the last chapter show that there is a spirit hidden in the *prima materia*, just as there was in the Nile stone of Ostanes. This spirit was eventually interpreted as the Holy Ghost in accordance with the ancient tradition of the Nous swallowed up by the darkness while in the embrace of Physis – with this difference, however, that it is not the supreme feminine principle, earth, who is the devourer, but Nous in the form of Mercurius or the tail-eating Uroboros (fig. 147). In other words, the devourer is a sort of material earth-spirit, an hermaphrodite possessing a masculine-spiritual and feminine-corporeal aspect ... The original Gnostic myth has undergone a strange transformation: Nous and Physis are indistinguishably one in the *prima materia* and have become a *natura abscondita*" (Jung, *Psychology and Alchemy*, p. 345).

[23] Delcourt, *Hermaphrodite*, pp. 116–17, citing Jamblichus.

[24] And perhaps for good reason. After all, Paracelsus did offer feces to his colleagues, declaring them unworthy if they could not accept the importance of this substance for medicine. Waite, "Preface to the English Translation," p. xiii.

monsters, incest, and cannibalism. In historical terms, late sixteenth-century France in particular must have been swept by fears of annihilation on several fronts. The country itself and its inhabitants were being torn to pieces, often literally. This fate is depicted by some authors as a form of autophagy or cannibalism.[25] This menace was further strengthened by intellectual and religious movements that questioned established authorities. Because of the Reform, there was a significant population in France that was culturally the same, and yet different in religious beliefs. This slightly shifting identity seemed most threatening to extremist Catholics, who proceeded to declare these Protestants monsters or diseases, and who attempted to annihilate these similar "others" absolutely by burning them at the stake or by hacking them to tiny pieces. The primacy of fire as a destroying and a life-giving force in the alchemical process,[26] may in part explain the fascination some French Protestants held for hermetic philosophy.[27]

This fear of religious difference couched in similarity was echoed by a strong insistence on the maintenance of sex distinctions. Given that French society was heavily dependent for its ordering on the subordination of women to men, and therefore on a clear distinction between the sexes, anything which placed this distinction in doubt, whether transvestism, homosexuality or bisexuality, or hermaphrodism, was responded to as a terrible menace. This insistence upon clear distinctions seems to spring from a fear of being subsumed by (or being) the other, a fear expressed in the many treatises on monsters. Further evidence of this fear is to be found in the recurrent images of emasculation that dominate political propaganda in the reign of Henri III. Hermaphrodites, as monstrous creatures, seem to be the ultimate expression of this menace. Thus, alchemy, with its emphasis on hermaphrodites, and on the effacement and restoration of distinction, seems to be a very threatening form of knowledge. Most alchemical treatises, and particularly those widely available in France in the late sixteenth and early seventeenth centuries, seem primarily concerned with the mutability of forms by means of the fluidity of boundaries.

Paracelsus

The "Helvetian" Theophrastus von Hohenheim (1493–1541), known as Paracelsus, was undoubtedly the most influential alchemist of the Renaissance, quoted and imitated by virtually all who were consumed by the *opus* after his time. Thus, a large portion of this chapter will be devoted to analysis of the figure of the hermaphrodite, of the definition of the natural, of methods of classification, and of the importance of language

---

25   Théodore Agrippa d'Aubigné, *Les Tragiques*, in *Oeuvres*, ed. H. Weber (Paris: Gallimard, 1969), "Misères," ll. 617–18 (for autophagy), 495–562 and 97–130 (for cannibalism).

26   See Paracelsus, "Concerning Simple Fire," in the treatise *Concerning the Spirits of the Planets* in *The Hermetic and Alchemical Writings of Paracelsus*, p. 74.

27   Bernard Palissy being the most striking example; but Béroalde de Verville and Théodore Agrippa d'Aubigné were adherents as well.

for these processes in his works. Paracelsus evidently saw alchemy as the guiding system for the workings of the universe, or at least used the process as his metaphor for these workings. Thus, the mercurial hermaphrodite is linked with the processes of generation and reproduction in the human body, and with Adam, the original man (hermaphrodite), and thus with the workings of the universe:

> We know that there are only two stones, the white and the red. There are also two matters of the Stone, Sol and Luna, formed together in a proper marriage, both natural and artificial. Now, as we see that the man or the woman, without the seed of both, cannot generate, in the same way our man, Sol, and his wife, Luna, cannot conceive, or do anything in the way of generation, without the seed and sperm of both. Hence the philosophers gathered that a third thing was necessary, namely, the animated seed of both, the man and the woman, without which they judged that the whole of their work was fruitless and in vain. Such a sperm is Mercury, which, by the natural conjunction of both bodies, Sol and Luna, receives their nature into itself in union. Then at length, and not before, the work is fit for congress, ingress, and generation, by the masculine and feminine power and virtue. Hence the philosophers have said that this same Mercury is composed of body, spirit, and soul, and that it has assumed the nature and property of all elements. Therefore, with their most powerful genius and intellect, they asserted their Stone to be animal. They even called it their Adam, who carries his own invisible Eve hidden in his body, from that moment in which they were united by the power of the Supreme God, the maker of all creatures ... Summarily, then, the matter of the Philosophers' Stone is none other than a fiery and perfect Mercury extracted by Nature and Art; that is, the artificially prepared and true hermaphrodite Adam, and the microcosm ... Our Mercury, therefore, is the same which contains in itself all the perfections, force, and virtues of the Sun, which also runs through all the streets and houses of the planets, and in its own rebirth has acquired the force of things above and things below ...[28]

In this version of the process, Mercury is the hermaphroditic offspring of the conjunction of Sol and Luna; as in Leone's philosophy, hermaphrodism becomes a code-word for marital relations (but here in the mineral realm). Paracelsus also echoes the notion of the hermaphroditic Adam, who contained Eve within himself. This concept is later repeated almost verbatim by Gerard Dorn in his *Congeries Paracelsicae chemicae* ..., published in the *Theatrum Chemicum* of 1602, which was reprinted frequently over the course of the seventeenth century.[29] The *Eva abscondita* seems to be a cross between Salmacis, lost in Hermaphroditus's transformation, and

---

[28] Paracelsus, *The Aurora of the Philosophers*, in *The Hermetic and Alchemical Writings*, pp. 65–6.

[29] Gerard Dorn, *Congeries Paracelsicae chemicae de transmutationibus metallorum*, in the *Theatrum Chemicum, praecipuos selectorum auctorum tractatus ... continens* (Ursel, 1602), cited by Jung in *Psychology and Alchemy*, 319: "This Mercurius is composed of body, spirit, and soul, and has assumed the nature and quality of all the elements. Wherefore they affirmed with most powerful genius and understanding that their stone was a living thing, which they also called their Adam, who bore his invisible Eve."

part of the Aristophanic spherical being. In this hermaphrodism, Mercury contains the four elements, and thus is linked to the universe as a whole. Finally, Mercury is expressed as self-generating in much the same manner as the Phoenix. Paracelsus has managed to bring together, with some skill, the cluster of images and theories surrounding the figure of the hermaphrodite.

The image of the *coniunctio* as the union of male and female recurs throughout Paracelsus's alchemical works: for example in the second chapter of the "Second Treatise" of *Concerning the Spirits of the Planets* ("Concerning the Conjunction of the Man with the Woman"); and the second chapter of the "Third Treatise" of the same work (also "Concerning the Conjunction of the Man with the Woman"):

> ... we now propose to describe more at length how the man and the woman meet and are joined together. This is the manner. Take Philosophers' Mercury, prepared and purified to its supreme degree. Dissolve this with its wife, that is to say, with quick mercury, so that the woman may dissolve the man, and the man may fix the woman. Then, just as the husband loves his wife and she her husband, the Philosophers' Mercury pursues the quick mercury with the most supreme love, and their nature is moved with the greatest affection towards us. So then each Mercury is blended with the other, as the woman with the man, and he with her, so far as the body is concerned, to such an extent that they have no difference, save as regards their powers and properties, seeing the man is fixed, but the woman volatile in the fire. For this reason, the woman is united to the man in such a way that she dissolves the man, and he fixes her and renders her constant in every consideration as a consequence. Conceal both in a glass vessel, thoroughly fastened, so that the woman may not escape or evaporate; otherwise the whole work will be reduced to nothing. (*Hermetic and Alchemical Writings*, p. 86)

Paracelsus seems to be trying to explain how the male and female principles may be fused, and yet remain different; this is the conceptual problem that the figure of the hermaphrodite expresses perfectly – sameness conjoined with difference. Both principles act upon each other; thus, there is no division between active and passive roles in this process. The male and female principles even exchange properties, as he dissolves and becomes volatile by her influence, and she becomes fixed and constant by his. They blend together in this exchange, and yet this fusion remains unstable. This account of alchemical conjunction is a precursor to many later descriptions of the rebis, or the alchemical hermaphrodite.

Paracelsus alternates in this treatise between a more complex and egalitarian view of conjunction, and a view which echoes Aristotelian accounts of generation:

> When you have placed the husband and the wife in the matrimonial bed, in order that he may operate upon her and impregnate her, and that the seed of the woman may be coagulated into a mass by the seed of the man, without which she can bring forth no fruit, it is necessary that the man should perform his operation on the woman.[30]

---

30   Paracelsus, ch. 3, "Concerning the Copulation of the Man with the Woman," *Concerning the Spirits of the Planets*, from *The Hermetic and Alchemical Writings*, p. 86.

The "woman" clearly designates the amorphous *prima materia*, which must be distinguished into forms by the male agent. Significantly, this "coagulation" does not at first free the feminine principle from a state of dissolution, but seems to corrupt her further, into a state of putrefaction:

> As soon as you see the woman take a black colour, know for a certainty that she has conceived and become pregnant: and when the seed of the man embraces the seed of the woman, this is the first sign and the key of this whole work and Art. Therefore preserve a continuous natural heat, and this blackness will appear and disappear through being consumed, as one worm eats another, and goes on consuming until not one is still left. (*Hermetic and Alchemical Writings*, p. 86)

The female is putrefied, then "consumed" or annihilated much in the manner of a rotting corpse; obviously, parturition even in the alchemical sense effaces the feminine. This union between male and female is also expressed as a conquest:

> But when the peacock's tail begins to appear, that is, when many and various colours shall be seen in the glass, it is a sign that the Philosophers' Mercury is acting on the common mercury, and extending its wings until it shall have conquered. (*Hermetic and Alchemical Writings*, p. 86)

The feminine thus disappears into the masculine, which, like a phoenix, produces brilliant colours along with its self-engendering. When these colours turn white and produce a flower-like mass, the King has been born: "That King has strength and power, not only for transmuting metals, but also for healing all infirmities" (*Hermetic and Alchemical Writings*, p. 87). Thus, male begets male at the expense of the female, who seems to dissolve or disappear in the process.

It is fairly apparent throughout the works of Paracelsus that this great thinker could not accept the concept of the mercurial hermaphrodite as such; much as in the Ovidian tale of Hermaphroditus, the female in these works is continually subsumed into the male. Paracelsus seems to be locked into a hierarchical, rigidly ordered, epistemological system, so that the notion of genuine coexistence of two sexes in one form is unthinkable to him. So, he rewrites the hermaphrodite in terms of a heterosexual (and married) union; in this union, the goal is for the male to beget the male. In the end, female is written out of the process along with the hermaphrodite. The intense dependence on a rigid linguistic system that expresses itself through obsessive cataloguing of every object or element observed, excludes anything which might seem confused, chaotic, or abject; anything, in short, that escapes such rigid classification. Thus, Paracelsus's notion of women and of their role in generation systematically informs his reworking of the alchemical myth of the hermaphrodite.

In turn, alchemy informs Paracelsus's reading of the world around him.[31] Particularly in his work *Concerning the Nature of Things*[32] (*De Natura rerum*),[33] the vocabulary of the alchemical process is used to represent a wide variety of natural phenomena, including monsters:

> The generation of all natural things is twofold: one which takes place by Nature without Art, the other which is brought about by Art, that is to say, by Alchemy, though, generally, it might be said that all things are generated from the earth by the help of putrefaction. (*Hermetic and Alchemical Writings*, p. 120)

Putrefaction links natural and alchemical processes with spiritual ones, as Paracelsus makes clear:

> For putrefaction brings forth great effects, as we have a good example in the sacred gospel, where Christ says, "Unless a grain of wheat be cast forth into a field and putrefy, it cannot bear fruit a hundred fold." Hence it may be known that many things are multiplied by putrefaction so that they produce excellent fruit. For putrefaction is the change and death of all things, and the destruction of the first essence of all natural objects, from whence there issues forth for us regeneration and a new birth ten thousand times better than before. (*Hermetic and Alchemical Writings*, p. 120)

One cannot help but note the consolatory nature of this belief in putrefaction, especially given the insistant fascination that Paracelsus seems to have had for this aspect of the alchemical process. He continues his treatise with a discussion of how putrefaction can lead to generation, even of men ("without natural father and mother"); this is a different, seemingly heretical notion of resurrection.

At any rate, the desire to control nature is linked to the status of women in society, who are portrayed in a long digression as menacing:

> Thus you see with regard to the basilisk, which is a monster above all others ... since a man can be killed by the very sight and appearance of it, for it possesses a poison more virulent than all others ... This poison, by some unknown means, it carries in its eyes, and it is a poison that acts on the imagination, not altogether unlike a menstruous woman, who also carries poison in her eyes .... (*Hermetic and Alchemical Writings*, pp. 122–3)

---

31   This is particularly evident in his treatise *Concerning the Generations of the Elements* (*Hermetic and Alchemical Writings*, pp. 201–34), in which his cosmography is closely linked to the three basic elements, salt, sulphur, and mercury.

32   In *The Hermetic and Alchemical Writings*, vol. 1.

33   German version published by Karl Sudhoff, *Theophrast von Hohenheim, Samtliche Werke*, vol. 2, *Medizinische, naturwissenschaftliche und philosophische Schriften* (Munich and Berlin: R. Oldenbourg, 1928).

Paracelsus explains that the basilisk is produced from the menstrual blood of a woman. Thus, "science" is put to the service of expressing and explaining a menacing and feminine nature and thereby controlling it.

As Paracelsus explains in his ninth book, *Concerning the Signature of Natural Things* (*De signatura rerum naturalium*), this science consists mainly of "signatures," that is, the naming of all natural things and their proper categorization. Man is the "signatory," or the namer, and nature is both the material on which the name is inscribed and the thing signified. This practice expresses at one and the same time the interconnected quality and the division of the universe, as each body part and each aspect of nature (plants, minerals, animals) is assigned specific but overlapping characteristics and linked to a planet. Interestingly, hermaphrodites and other such "monsters" that do not remain in one specific category are quickly dismissed:

> Many men come to the light deformed with monstrous signs. One man has a finger too many, another a finger too few; and the same may be the case with toes. Another brings with him from the womb a distorted foot, arm, back, or other member; another has a weak or hunched back. So also there are born hermaphrodites, androgyni, men, that is to say, possessing both pudenda, male as well as female, and sometimes lacking both. Of monstrous signs like this I have noted many, both in males and females, all of which are to be regarded as monstrous signs of secret sins in the parents ... These are signs of vices, and rarely denote anything good. (*Hermetic and Alchemical Writings*, p. 173)

Such monsters are a sort of "anti-signature," both in that they do not signal anything worthwhile or good (in Paracelsus's view), and in that he writes them out of his book early on:

> ... know that monstrous growths amongst animals, which are produced by other methods than propagation from those like themselves, rarely live long ... So, too, monstrous human growths seldom live long. The more wonderful and worthy of regard they are, the sooner death comes upon them ... It should be known, forsooth, that God abhors monsters of this kind. They displease Him, and not one of them can be saved when they do not bear the likeness of God. One can only conjecture that they are shapen by the Devil, and born for the service of the Devil rather than of God; since from no monster was any good work ever derived, but, on the contrary, evil and sin, and all kinds of diabolical craft. For as the executioner marks his sons when he cuts off their ears, gouges out their eyes, brands their cheeks, cuts off their fingers, hands, or head, so the Devil, too, marks his own sons, through the imagination of the mother, which they derive from her evil desires, lusts, and thoughts in conception. (*Hermetic and Alchemical Writings*, p. 123)

It should be noted that such horrible "monsters" include people who are missing fingers or have too many; as Paracelsus points out, he has encountered many examples of such "monsters" (p. 173, cited above). This work, focused so intently on language and other sign systems, and developing complex systems of the natural world, rejects the feminine, the ambiguous, the monstrous. These are designated by their own sign system, a corrupt and unstable one, linked to the Devil and the maternal imagination, both represented as deceitful and destructive, and compared here to the executioner's work.

Paracelsus's view of reproduction in this treatise is a double-edged sword for the mother. She does not contribute any seed, in his view; thus, the child should be a miniature version of the father. This is quite different from accounts of alchemical conjunction discussed later in this chapter. Yet the infant in the womb is described as being "as much in the hand and under the will of the mother as clay in the hand of the potter" (*Hermetic and Alchemical Writings*, p. 122). The mother, then, is responsible for the form of the child *if* it is born a monster: "So the pregnant mother forms the fruit in her own body according to her imagination, and as her stars are" (*Hermetic and Alchemical Writings*, p. 122). In escaping blame, the male seems also to lose a large measure of his control, and thus monsters must be condemned to an early death in order to restore this control. It is, apparently, the mother's refusal to accept the paternal inscription within her body that results in extra-linguistic (or extra-signatorial, to retain Paracelsus's own vocabulary) birth. The mother is thus associated with the monstrous; and both remain in the realm of the pre-linguistic. Both refuse paternal control, and thus are dismissed. Thus, Paracelsus marvels at the creation of the homunculus by alchemical means:

> Let the semen of a man putrefy by itself ... until it begins at last to live ... If now, after this, it be every day nourished ... it becomes, thenceforth a true and living infant ... This we call a homunculus ... Now, this is one of the greatest secrets which God has revealed to mortal and fallible man .... (*Alchemical Writings*, p. 124)

In fact, women are consistently written out of procreation in this treatise. Paracelsus argues that men can procreate with animals (which will then produce human children, *Hermetic and Alchemical Writings*, p. 121), that it is the Devil, rather than the mother, that shapes monsters (*Hermetic and Alchemical Writings*, p. 123) – thereby contradicting himself. Interestingly, however, the homunculus itself remains in a sort of extra-linguistic state: "It is a miracle and marvel of God, an arcanum above all arcana, and deserves to be kept secret until the last of times, when there shall be nothing hidden, but all things shall be made manifest" (*Hermetic and Alchemical Writings*, pp. 124–5). But this state can be seen as super-linguistic: "As by Art they acquire their life, by Art acquire their body, flesh, bones and blood, and are born by Art, therefore Art is incorporated in them and born with them, and there is no need for them to learn, but others are compelled to learn from them ..." (*Hermetic and Alchemical Writings*, p. 125). In other words, the homunculi are the embodiments of paternal control. This attempt at demystification of Nature mystifies itself, creating an obvious fiction of paternal procreation in order to bypass that which cannot be controlled. Furthermore, the monstrous, rejected as sub-linguistic or pre-linguistic and linked to the imagination, returns to haunt the fragile perfection of the supra-linguistic homunculus, who cannot be narrated, whose secret cannot be revealed, lest it be corrupted. Language is at once crucial and problematic for Paracelsus's system; it creates order, but its own instability and potential monstrosity also threatens that order.

Yet the treatise insists on man's supremacy by means of language; and this language is seen mainly as a means of classifying all the elements of the universe. Man even has the power to reclassify that which has been created, and thus recreate it. The second book of *De natura rerum* offers alchemy as the supreme example of man's control over nature (*Hermetic and Alchemical Writings*, p. 128: "The Scriptures say that God subjected all created things to man, and handed them over to him as if they were his own property ..."); thus, although this book is supposed to be "Concerning the Growth of Natural Things," it largely consists of recipes for the transmutation of metals, focusing once again on man's control over nature.

Book Three, "Concerning the Preservation of Natural Things," while again largely concerned with the transmutation of metals, establishes a dualistic system of God/ Devil, good/evil, joy/sorrow, sickness/health, preservation/corruption (putrefaction? – *Hermetic and Alchemical Writings*, p. 130). Yet this dualism is contradicted by the importance of putrefaction for the alchemical process (*Hermetic and Alchemical Writings*, p. 153). Again, the treatise belies the simple categorizations that inform Paracelsus's system. This treatise inscribes alchemy as a profoundly conservative discourse, yet one that has the potential to unravel itself over time, as it does in the subsequent works of other alchemists.

Paracelsus, in the fourth book ("Concerning the Life of Natural Things"), equates the body with that which is corruptible, and thus rejects it, expelling it to the realm of the monstrous and the feminine:

> For what is the body without the spirit? Absolutely nothing. So it is that the spirit holds concealed within itself the virtue and power of the things, and not the body. For in the body is death, and the body is subject to death, and in the body nothing but death must be looked for. For the body can be destroyed and corrupted in various ways, but not the spirit: for it always remains a living spirit, and is bound up with life. It also keeps its own body alive, but in the removal of the body from it, it leaves the body separate and dead, and returns to its own place whence it had come, that is to say, into chaos, and into the air of the higher and lower firmament. (*Hermetic and Alchemical Writings*, p. 135)

This dualistic notion of the universe and of human existence is accompanied by a fierce insistence upon classification of all things, a mode of thought present in every book of this treatise: "There are celestial and infernal spirits, human and metallic, the spirits of salts, gems, and marcasites, arsenical spirits, spirits of potables, of roots, of liquids, of flesh, blood, bones, etc." (*Hermetic and Alchemical Writings*, p. 135). These frequently repeated and amplified catalogues reveal the underlying problems with distinction and classification: odd associations are created (men are compared to minerals), and the list often ends with the open-ended, inclusive, blurring word *etc.* That is to say, something always escapes Paracelsus's mania for classification.

That something is whatever he has already rejected in order to create a coherent and comforting "science" of the natural order: women and monsters are listed in very few of these catalogues. But the hint of something beyond his own system undermines the authority of that system, creating the sense that Paracelsus cannot in fact explain all the functioning of the universe. He himself creates this impression when he refuses to offer an explanation for certain phenomena, such as the creation of *homunculi*, the recipe for which he defers to the end of time. He cannot even name or explain the human spirit, what it is or from whence it comes, except as "a certain astral balsam" (*Hermetic and Alchemical Writings*, p. 136: "I am unable to name it more clearly, although it could be put forward under many distinctive titles").

Also illuminating is the fact that Paracelsus can only describe the spirit of other things in terms of their sensory manifestations: "The life of gems and corals is mere colour" (*Hermetic and Alchemical Writings*, p. 136); "The life of sweet things, as sugar, honey ... is a subtle sweetness ..." (*Hermetic and Alchemical Writings*, p. 137). Thus, their means of classification *is* their life; a skeptic would note a certain self-defeating circularity in these definitions ("the life of a sweet thing is its sweetness"). Thus, although Paracelsus's work reflects a conservative ordering of the universe, this ordering constantly undoes itself, like the *euroboros* biting its own tail. Unable to move beyond a dualistic frame of reference, the treatise gives definitions that merely return to the initial terms defined (in a form of circular reasoning); no knowledge is gained. Thus, distinctions are impossible, and all things seem to dissolve under the intellectual gaze. Strangely, although alchemy reveals a fascination with this dissolution, in this treatise, Paracelsus consistently emphasizes the importance of division and distinction. This insistence is most obvious in the final book, on "The Signature of Natural Things."

Similarly, the fifth book, on the death of natural things (*Hermetic and Alchemical Writings*, pp. 138–45), merely defines that death as the absence of the characteristics listed in book four. Death, then, is non-being; but being has yet to be established. The reverse of the author's obsession with classification, and his consequent refusal of that which cannot be neatly classified (women, monsters, hermaphrodites, and dead bodies), is revealed in this chapter on non-being. Here again, the mineral and metallic dominates the discussion. But the "death" of these metals leads to useful compounds and formulae, and also to the following chapter, "Concerning the Resuscitation of Natural Things." Paracelsus touches upon the heretical in his section on resuscitation by distinguishing natural, predestined death from mortification, which is death inflicted by human hands. He argues that the body of a murdered man does not have its spirit, but retains a balsam which contains the potential for life. Again, this distinction underscores a basic problem in Paracelsus's approach to alchemy: while he wishes to retain a dualistic, Christian system that values soul over body, male over female, spirit over matter, the body itself is the crucial element in the alchemical process. All alchemical recipes are based on forms of matter; many based on parts of the human body. Alchemical thought remains fundamentally hostile to a philosophical or religious system that excludes matter.

Nonetheless, the alchemical process is based on the *mortification* of this matter. In the seventh book of his treatise, Paracelsus discusses the various steps involved in the "transmutation" of matter: "Calcination, sublimation, solution, putrefaction, distillation, coagulation, tincture" (*Hermetic and Alchemical Writings*, p. 151). By calcination, matter is turned into carbon and ashes (this is generally achieved by burning at a very high temperature). Next, sublimation is the separation of lower from higher elements; this is often achieved, in the case of metals, by use of a corrosive substance. Sublimated matter is then dissolved (solution), either by means of cold or heat (usually, however, it is placed in a fire). Next, the remaining substance is subjected to putrefaction (Paracelsus does not explain how this is done in this treatise); then it is distilled. Once distilled, it is again heated or cooled to coagulate it, to recreate a corporeal mass. This mass is then tinctured, that is to say, colored with extracts drawn from metals by the same processes listed above – this step may be a residual element of Egyptian forgery processes.

This book seems in many ways to be about the dissolution of differences between various metals and other forms of matter; the eighth book, then, is about the separation of these forms. Paracelsus, in rather pagan fashion, sees separation of the primordial chaos into four elements as the first step in the creation of the universe (*Hermetic and Alchemical Writings*, p. 160). He further explains the notion of separation: "I mean the segregation of three principles, as mercury, sulphur, salt, and the extraction of the pure from the impure, or of the pure and noble spirit and quintessence from the dense and elemental body ..." (*Hermetic and Alchemical Writings*, pp. 160–61). The separation of man occurs in death:

> For in death the two bodies of man separate from each other, that is to say, the Celestial and the Terrestrial, the Sacramental and the Elemental. One of these soars on high, like an eagle; the other sinks down to the earth, like lead.
>
> The elemental body decays and is consumed ... But the Sacramental body ... does not decay, is not buried, occupies no place. (*Hermetic and Alchemical Writings*, p. 161)

This second, celestial, body is the source of "spectres, visions, and supernatural apparitions" (*Hermetic and Alchemical Writings*, p. 161). Paracelsus seems to have returned at this point to a dualistic notion of the universe; still, he concentrates on matter and on the corporeal. He divides everything down to its smallest elements (or at least the smallest elements known to him): "Animals in their separation give water, blood, flesh, fat, bones, skin, body, hair, Mercury, Sulphur, Salt, etc." (*Hermetic and Alchemical Writings*, p. 162). It becomes apparent that Paracelsus's treatise, and his alchemical and philosophical systems in general, are based on such separations and classifications. However, this separation becomes cannibalistic when the human body enters into the question:

> The second separation is that of fat from flesh. This fatness being separated from human flesh, a most excellent balsam is produced, allaying the pains of gout, of contraction,

and others of a like nature, if the members affected be anointed with it while warm. (*Hermetic and Alchemical Writings*, p. 169)

Significantly, Paracelsus sees the ultimate separation as the Day of Judgment; the result of this Day will be a dissolution of distinction, yet he retains a dualistic system:

> When all these things are finished and done, all the elementary subjects shall return to the first matter of the elements, and shall be turned about for eternity, yet never consumed. On the contrary, all sacramental creatures shall return to the primal matter of the sacraments .... (*Hermetic and Alchemical Writings*, p. 170)

This notion of a dualistic universe, then separated *ad infinitum* into various categories and sub-categories, drives the final book of this treatise, "Concerning the Signature of Natural Things." As pure is divided from impure by the Archeus (*Hermetic and Alchemical Writings*, p. 160, note), man assigns names to all things within his domain, and the stars mark men with particular signs. Thus, there are three levels of language operating in Paracelsus's world: natural (Archeus – as in archetypes), human, and moral (astral). For Paracelsus, human language is primary, since the world is accessible only by means of this system:

> Now, in order that we may explain all the signs as correctly and as briefly as possible, it is above all necessary that we put forward those whereof man is the signator. When these are understood you will more rightly attain to the others, whether natural or supernatural. (*Hermetic and Alchemical Writings*, p. 172)

The examples he gives are from religion (exclusionary signs, such as the marking of Jews with yellow badges), politics (lictors and magistrates) and the military (rank), the trades (couriers marked with the sign of the municipality from which they come): "It is necessary more clearly to explain those signs which man affixes, and which lead to a knowledge, not only of rank, office, or name, but also of discrimination, intelligence, age, dignity, degree ..." (*Hermetic and Alchemical Writings*, p. 172). These signs are value-laden, and convey with them the status they indicate; therefore, they seem to operate in circular fashion, creating what they define. Paracelsus does not seem to realize the performative nature of the very examples he has chosen, linking them rather to some unnamed innate characteristic. This problematic nature of signs is also apparent in his section on "Monstrous Signs in Men" (*Hermetic and Alchemical Writings*, pp. 173–4), where deformities become the symbol of some inherent evil. This reasoning justifies the rejection of deformed children. The monstrous is the realm of the imagination, which, once aroused, can create all manner of beings outside the realm of the "natural."

Whereas the monstrous is divided off from normal manhood, even men are distinguished one from another by the signs imposed on them by the stars. Paracelsus gives a long list of physical traits that can be interpreted as a form of language; this language clearly divides the "norm," which could just as well be designated the "self," or a form of the self such as sameness of race or nationality:

> Black eyes not only denote a healthy constitution, but also, for the most part, a constant mind free from doubt and fear, healthy and hearty, truthful and loving virtue.
> Grey eyes are the sign of a crafty man, ambiguous and inconsistent ...
> ...
> A flat nose indicates a malignant man, false, lustful, untruthful, inconstant ....
> (*Hermetic and Alchemical Writings*, pp. 177–8)

Paracelsus praises long noses; a glance at his portrait explains this predilection. Every body part is classified according to value (essentially, good or bad); he classifies plants and minerals with the same thoroughness.

The signator Archeus bestows natural signs of purity and impurity, fecundity and age, upon animals (*Hermetic and Alchemical Writings*, p. 190). Finally, there are the supernatural signs, which are read by means of the arts of pyromancy, hydromancy, chaomancy, and necromancy. All of these signs are mediated by human language, although Paracelsus suggests that their meaning is constant.

It is apparent from this treatise, that although Paracelsus attempts to rationalize and put in order the alchemical process, his insistent categorizations and classifications unravel themselves as they progress into practical examples. The irrational, the monstrous, always returns in his prose, only to be rejected again as impure or unclean. Yet the vehemence with which he rejects hermaphrodites and other monsters indicates the importance of these deformed entities for his thought; just as the abjected body returns constantly as an essential element of the process.

Thus, even though Paracelsus is writing well before the rediscovery of Pyrrhonian skepticism by Renaissance intellectuals, and does not therefore reject outright rigid systems of classification of the mineral, plant, and animal realms, these systems show some strain in his exegesis. Alchemy is as much concerned with the dissolution of difference as it is with that difference itself; it lends itself well to a certain skeptical view of overly rigid philosophical systems. Although early humanists like Paracelsus tried to rewrite alchemy in a positivistic manner, and show its rational bases, the irrational nature of this pursuit became increasingly apparent as the Renaissance wore on, and particularly in France, where intellectuals such as Clovis Hesteau de Nuysement seem to have embraced the irrational and imaginative aspects of the alchemical process. Part of this difference stems, of course, from the genres used to express hermetic ideas: Paracelsus is writing in the style of scholastic scientific treatises of his day, based on rigid divisions of subject, and lists of "practical" examples; Clovis Hesteau de Nuysement is writing hermetic poetry, in which imaginative combinations of imagery, and fusion of widely varied subject matter, dominate any ordered presentation. It is undoubtedly of some significance that the late Renaissance saw the rise of alchemical emblem-books and poetic renderings of the process. The visual images of the emblem-books remain much more open to interpretation, even as they offer striking versions of the various steps in the process, and are usually accompanied by short epigrams that further obfuscate, rather than clarify, the subject-matter. The poems offer new associations and new images often not apparent in the emblems, and thus open the pseudo-scientific discipline to a variety of spiritual and philosophical uses. The evolution away from consideration of alchemy as a science, to that of alchemy as a particular philosophical or even imaginative discourse, may account for the longevity of what may seem like an absurd practice, still current well into the eighteenth century, and still fascinating to modern psychologists and philosophers.

As alchemy evolved away from the status of a scientific discipline to that of a spiritual cult of sorts, the figure of the hermaphrodite – easily dismissed by Paracelsus – takes on increasing importance. The dual-sexed being is central to Clovis Hesteau de Nuysement's "Visions hermétiques," as well as to Michael Maier's *Atalanta fugiens* (1617); it is also significant in the work of Salomon Trismosin (supposedly Paracelsus's instructor, and yet his work is published somewhat later)[34] and of Annibal Barlet (published 1653).

The predominance of the hermaphrodite in these texts seems to signal a return to the consideration of the importance of the *prima materia* and the corporeal to the alchemical process. The new significance of matter in turn signals an abandonment of the attempt to reconcile alchemical thought and Neoplatonic philosophy (an attempt apparent in the works of Paracelsus, and in a poem by Théodore Agrippa d'Aubigné which will be analyzed in another chapter). Increasingly, and somewhat in harmony with the Counter-Reformation, the spiritual is seen as immanent in the material, but indivisible from it. This fruitful union is expressed in alchemical works in the figure of the hermaphrodite.

Hermaphroditic Conjunction: The *Rosarium Philosophorum* and the *Aureum Vellus*

At the midpoint of the sixteenth century, the image of conjunction of male and female took on greater importance for alchemical expression. The *Rosarium philosophorum*, first printed in 1550,[35] bases its symbolic system on the images of marriage and parturition. This emphasis on the maternal role in the alchemical process of spiritual and physical perfecting recalls late medieval images of *Jesus as Mother* enumerated and analyzed by Caroline Walker Bynum.[36] Bynum traces a rise in the use of "explicit and elaborate maternal imagery to describe God and Christ" (*Jesus as Mother*, pp. 111–12), particularly in the twelfth and subsequent centuries. The "feminization" of

---

34 Apparently 1612.
35 See Adam McLean's introduction to Salomon Trismosin's *Splendor solis*, trans. Joscelyn Godwin (Grand Rapids: Phanes Press, 1991), p. 8.
36 Caroline Walker Bynum, *Jesus as Mother. Studies in the Spirituality of the High Middle Ages* (Berkeley: University of California Press, 1982).

Christ is widespread at this time, and reflects transformations in Christian spirituality and in notions of authority.[37]

Bynum relates the growth in use of such imagery to increased emphasis on the humanity of Christ, and on the link between man and God, of which Christ is the guarantor. This union of spiritual and physical, in complete interdependence for the work of salvation, becomes central to descriptions of the alchemical processes as well, and a justification for the materialistic approach to the perfecting of natural forms. Although sacrifice and atonement are clearly present in alchemy, in the stage of putrefaction or mortification, its creative aspect seems to echo that spirituality which Bynum locates in the twelfth century:

> Creation and incarnation are stressed more than atonement and judgment. Christ is seen as the mediator who joins our substance to divinity and as the object of a profound experiential union; God is emphasized as creating and creative; the cooperation of the Trinity in the work of creation is stressed. (*Jesus as Mother*, p. 130)

The images of the sacrificed rebis, the hermaphroditic double being, who in the *Rosarium* ascends to heaven and redescends to complete the work of the alchemical process, seem based on this notion of a dual Christ, human and divine, male and female, as mediator for the salvation of mankind.

Both the texts cited by Bynum, which describe a hermaphroditic divinity, and the *Rosarium* give new importance to the fleshly and female aspects of parturition. The result of this evolution in attitude seems to be an embracing of the natural, physical world:

> Thus, the mother was, to medieval people, especially associated with the procreation of the physicality, the flesh, of the child ... For a theology that stressed the humanity of Christ as a taking up into divinity of humankind's fleshliness, female generativity could be an important symbol. For a theology that maintained – over against Cathar dualism – the goodness of creation in all its physicality, a God who is mother and womb as well as father and animator could be a more sweeping and convincing image of creation than a father God alone. (*Jesus as Mother*, pp. 133–4)

In this context, the hermaphroditic rebis becomes a figure of the divinity achieved by the conjunction of the physical with the spiritual.

From the opening pages of the *Rosarium*, the alchemical process is described in terms of the union of male and female:

---

37 "... maternal imagery was applied in the Middle Ages to male religious authority figures, particularly abbots, bishops and the apostles, as well as to God and Christ. Moreover, the use of maternal imagery to talk about male figures was developed in the twelfth century by cloistered authors with particular reference to a cloistered setting. Thus we must locate the Cistercian devotion to mother Jesus not merely against the background of growing affective spirituality of the high Middle Ages but also in the context of a Cistercian ambivalence about authority and a Cistercian concept of community" (*Jesus as Mother*, p. 112).

... diversificatur mulier a viro, quia licet in uno genere convenient, tamen inter se habent differentiam distinctam, ut differunt materia & forma. Materia namque patitur actionem, Forma vero agit sibi assimilans materiam ... Sic liberius complectitur corpus spiritum, ut ad suma perveniat perfectionem

(... the woman differs from the man: although they come together in one type, nonetheless they have a distinct difference, just as form and matter differ from each other. For matter submits to action, and truly form acts, assimilating matter to itself ... So the body freely embraces the spirit, so that it might arrive at its own perfection).[38]

The two are united into one nature, but maintain a clear difference, which resembles that between matter and form. The matter submits (*subit*) and the form acts (*agit*); thus the body seeks out the spirit in order to achieve its own perfection. Although based on Neoplatonic or gnostic notions of matter and spirit, as well as Aristotelian assumptions of male superiority, this treatise evokes a more complex theory of sex, which asserts the necessity of union, but accompanied by ineluctable difference. The author seems to assign a higher value to the male/spirit, but as the treatise reveals, this spirit is useless without the female body. The absolute need for bodily expression of spiritual truth grants new value to the corporeal/female.

In fact, the alchemical process is compared to parturition: the necessary time to perfect the elixir should be that of the "the human foetus in its mother's womb."[39] The process is also compared to engendering: "The most natural and most perfect work is to engender a being that resembles oneself."[40] This implies absolute replication of the self; yet, paradoxically, the process is also seen as a dissolution of two bodies into one, a union within difference.[41] This paradoxical union of self and other into one being, the oscillation between difference and sameness, is the concept at the core of the entire process. The difference between the participating bodies is necessary for the success of the endeavor.[42] Venus and Mercury are the divine symbols of this conjunction; Venus as the body, Mercury as the spirit.[43]

---

[38] *Rosarium philosophorum*. Facsimile of the 1550 edition, ed. Joachim Telle (Weinheim: VCH, 1992), A3–A3v, pp. 5–6. All translations of this text are my own.

[39] "quod debet esse tempus foetus humani in utero matris" (*Rosarium*, C4, p. 23).

[40] "Naturalissimum & perfectissimum opus est generare tale quale ipsum est" (*Rosarium*, D3, p. 29).

[41] "... qualiter corpora soluuntur in argentum vivum Philosophorum, id est in aquam Mercurii nostri, et fit unum corpus novum" (*Rosarium*, D3v, p. 30: "the bodies dissolve in the quicksilver of the philosophers, that is in the tincture of our mercury, and a new body is created").

[42] "quia simile in sua simili non habet actionem" (*Rosarium*, Ev, p. 34: "the similar does not act upon its like in any way"). There is an underlying tone of condemnation of homosexuality in these passages of the *Rosarium*, echoed by other treatises.

[43] "corpus est venus et foemina, spiritus est Mercurius et masculus" (*Rosarium*, E4, p. 39).

The conjunction itself is portrayed as a heterosexual union, a marriage for the purpose of reproduction. Yet this union is incestuous, transgressive:

> Coniunge ergo filium tuum Gabricum dilectiorem tibi in omnibus filiis tuis cum sua sorore Beya quae est puella fulgida, suavis et tenera … inter se filium gignent, qui non assimilabitur parentibus. (*Rosarium*, F3v–F4, pp. 46–7)

> (Unite then your son Gabricus, who is more dear to you than your other sons, with his sister Beya, who is a radiant, pleasant, and tender girl … they will engender a son who will not be like his parents.)

The incestuous act is at once that between brother and sister, and between mother and son, for Beya takes Gabricus wholly into her womb and reconceives him as his own son (F4, p. 47; this echoes the image of the phoenix who is his own father). The boundaries established in the creation of families, the boundaries of taboo, are effaced. The result of this conjunction is in fact the hermaphroditic entity that is male on its right side, female on its left (fig., G4, p. 55). The rest of the alchemical process consists of various transformations and reconfigurations of this hermaphroditic entity, from abjection (putrefaction) to transfiguration. The embrace of male and female has created a new identity altogether, an indissoluble union (H3–H3v, pp. 61–2); but it is the maintaining of opposites within this union that gives the entity, the philosopher's stone, its power. One identity cannot simply be subsumed into the other (I4v, 72). This powerful double entity, resembling the truly hermaphroditic gods of ancient Greece, is called the rebis.[44] This hermaphroditic rebis is linked to the Virgin Mary and Christ:

> Meines Sones nam ich da wahr/
> Unnd kam mit ihm selbannder dar.
> Da ich seiner wardt schwanger/
> Unnd gebäret uff ein unfruchtbarn anger.
> Ich wardt Mutter unnd bleib doch Magt/
> Unnd wardt meinem wesen angelagt.
> Das mein Son mein Vatter wardt/
> Wie das Gott geschickt hat wesentlicher arth.
> Die Mutter die mich hat gebäret/
> Durch mich wardt sie geboren auff erdt. (*Rosarium*, M4v, p. 96)

> (I took my son and united myself with him; I became pregnant by him and gave birth on sterile land: thus I became a mother and remained still a virgin. And I received in my being this gift, that my son became my father as God wished it even in his essence. The mother who gave me life through me was born on this earth.)

---

[44] "Rebis, id est una res quae fit est duabus rebus, id est corpore & spiritu, vel ex sola et luna …" (*Rosarium*,, K, p. 73: "Rebis, that is, a unique thing made from two things, such as the body and the spirit, or the sun and the moon"). The term rebis probably evolved from the Latin *res* (thing) and *bis* (double, in two ways).

This poem invokes Christ, and links alchemical concepts to that of salvation. It again effaces the boundaries of identity that create the family, and that are enforced by the family, to move towards a spiritual unity of being that nonetheless constantly renews and regenerates individual identity. This process of conjunction and individuation seems to be endlessly repeated, in this poem, in the images of the treatise, and in the sexual language of the process, which describes the union of solar and lunar elements, as we have seen. The image of the perfect stone is the King and Queen, Sol and Luna, joined in the form of a rebis (*Rosarium*, X3v, p. 166). This union is portrayed once again as a marriage: "Quando copulate fuerimus in aequitate status ... & ego & sol cum coniuncti fuerimus, vacaturi in ventre domus clausae, recipiam à te animam adulando" (*Rosarium*, Yv, pp. 170: "When we are rightfully married according to our station ... and when the sun and I will have been united in order to remain at leisure in the womb of the closed house, I will receive your soul rejoicing"). For all the legalistic language used to express this union, this incestuous marriage rewrites the laws of society, defies social norms and recreates the notion of marriage beyond social constraints. The elixir is self-generating, independent of the laws even of nature.[45] Thus the images of marriage become almost a parody of this social construct, even as they reach beyond questions of legal status to the deeper spiritual questions of fusion and individuation, unity and separation:

> Mulier est quoddam receptaculum virili seminis, quia ipsa conservat semen in suis cellulis & matrice & ibi nutritur, & pullulate usque ad tempus maturitatis ... propinquior est sibi in simplicitate & puritate, quia nihil propinquius vir quam uxor, quae sunt homogenea. (*Rosarium*, Z3, p. 181)

> (The woman is the receptacle of the male seed. She preserves this seed in her inner chambers and in her womb, and the seed is nourished there, and grows until such time as it is fully developed ... She is close to him in simplicity and purity, for nothing is closer to a man than his spouse, since they are of the same nature.)

The conservative, Aristotelian view of generation, in which the female is merely the vessel for male self-replication, is both reinforced and confused by the identification of male and female. Yet female identity is not entirely subsumed into the male; this passage is followed by a woodcut depicting the crowning of the Virgin Mary by the Holy Trinity, itself the ultimate expression of division within unity at that time.

The *Rosarium* gathered a symbolic system of explanation for the alchemical process, based on images of marriage and of the life of Christ. This system became central to the evolution of alchemy, creating as it did a seemingly coherent, while not

---

45   "Et ipse est Draco, qui maricat seipsum, & inpregnat seipsum, & parit in die suo, et interficit ex veneno suo omnia animalia" (*Rosarium*, Y3v–Y4, pp. 174–5: "And this same is the dragon who marries itself, who impregnates itself and engenders in its own lifetime, and kills by means of its poison all animals.").

entirely self-evident, means of expression of obscure alchemical truths. Its influence is particularly to be found in the work of Salomon Trismosin, who was said to be Paracelsus' preceptor, but whose works appear towards the end of the century.[46] A French translation of the *Aureum vellus* (originally published in 1598 at Rorschach), *La Toyson d'or*, appeared in 1612.[47] This work is replete with gendered images of the alchemical process, even in the prologue, which compares science to a nurturing maternal figure:

> ... la recherche de ce soleil terrestre, rapporte autant ou plus de fruicts & de contentement aux Nourriçons doctement ellevez soubz la providente tutelle de cette Science sur-humaine & sans doute celeste, amiablement nourris de l'agreable laict de sa mammelle & amoureuse & savoureuse ... (*Toyson d'or*, A1v–A2)

> (... the search for this earthly sun brings as many rewards and as much contentment to the Nurslings, properly guided by the providential guardianship of this Superhuman science, without a doubt celestial, sweetly nourished by the pleasant milk of her breasts, both loving and delicious ...)

This maternal imagery is echoed several pages later with the mention of the *avortons* of science (*Toyson d'or*, A4v–A5). The earth is similarly portrayed as the "mere de toutes choses" (*Toyson d'or*, A6v: "mother of all things"), and the elements as conceiving each other.[48] The conjunction necessary for the process is at once sexual and nourishing: "où enfin elle se repose ayant acquis la perfection de ses pretensions, se desistant sur la iouyssance finale" (*Toyson d'or*, B8: "where at last she rests, having acquired the perfection to which she pretended, ceasing at the point of complete enjoyment").[49]

---

[46] One manuscript of his *Splendor solis* seems to be dated 1532–1535, but this is the conjecture of an archivist. The earliest printed version of the work is 1598. Again, see MacLean/Godwin, *Splendor solis*, pp. 8–9.

[47] Salomon Trismosin, *La Toyson d'or* (Paris: Charles Sevestre, 1612). All citations of Trismosin will be from this edition, and from the copy to be found in the Cornell Rare Book and Manuscript Division History of Science collection. Many copies of the book seem hastily put together, with the engravings out of proper sequence, but the Cornell copy seems reliable. All translations are my own.

[48] "... les quatre qualitez des Elemens, qui se servans de matrice l'un à l'autre ..." (*Toyson d'or*, A7: "... the four qualities of the Elements, which, serving as wombs one for the other...").

[49] "Il y a autres doctrines infinies entrelassees de mesmes ambages & figures Amphibiologique, qui doivent toutefois estre toutes ensemble, & par conionction suyvies & absolument accomplies pour recueillir enfin le fruict Nectareen de nostre moisson doree" (*Toyson d'or*, C2: "There are other infinite doctrines, interlaced with the same detours and with doubly-natured figures, which must nonetheless be all together, and perfected and finished by conjunction in order to gather that Nectar-like fruit of our golden harvest").

Thus, the hermaphroditic conjunction is portrayed as plenitude and satisfaction of all physical needs; the alchemist relates to his process as the infant relates to its mother, in dependent bliss.

Trismosin refines the Neoplatonic/gnostic division of male and female into spirit and matter by asserting that the matter is the key to the alchemical process:

> Ces deux doctrines cy dessus mentionnees signifient selon les Philosophes, cette femme noire et obscure, qui sert de clef à toute l'oeuvre, & qui doibt dominer en la force de nostre Pierre, scavoir en la noirceur, base asseuree de tout le fondement; ou bien cet homme qui est la forme de nostre matiere, laquelle nous comparons fort à propos au Soleil. (*Toyson d'or*, C2v)

> (These two doctrines discussed above signify, according to the Philosophers, that dark and shadowy woman, who serves as the key to the entire work, and who must dominate in the strength of our Stone, that is to say in the blackness, the assured basis of the entire foundation; or yet that man which is the form of our matter, whom we compare appropriately to the Sun.)

Even more than in the *Rosarium*, the feminine principle of matter has a crucial role in the process, as the basis for the work. Thus the plates which accompany the parables by which the process is expressed portray Sol and Luna as King and Queen, as in the *Rosarium* (plate 8, E).[50]

The result of this conjunction of Sol and Luna is the rebis, portrayed in the ninth figure (*Toyson d'or*, E3) as a two-headed winged creature of ambiguous sex, holding the egg which symbolizes the cosmos or universe, composed of the four elements. In an echo of gnostic dualism, the rebis/divinity is portrayed as hermaphroditic, the Sun and the Moon, Earth and Water, male and female. This dual body in turn engenders the four elements, heat and cold, which are described as masculine, and dryness and humidity, which are portrayed as feminine. The elements then produce the pure substance of white magnesium; all five of these qualities together form the Philosopher's Stone, which Trismosin names Diana.[51]

---

[50]   Plate 4, C7v in the 1627 reprint of the Sevestre edition, to be found at the Houghton (Harvard University). This concurs with the Godwin edition of the *Splendor solis*, which contains many of the same images as the *Toyson d'or*; see p. 27 of the *Splendor*.

[51]   "Les philosophes ... luy attribuent deux corps, sçavoir est le Soleil & la Lune, qu'ils disent estre la Terre & l'Eau. Ces deux corps s'appellent aussi homme & femme, lesquels engendrent quatre enfans, deux petits hommes qu'ils nomment la chaleur & froideur, & deux petites femmes signifiees par le sec & l'humide: de ces quatre qualitez, il en sort une cinquiesme substance, qui est la magnesie blanche, laquelle ne porte aucune ride de fausseté sur le front ... [Quand, dict il, les cinq sont assemblez ensemble & viennent à estre une mesme chose, la pierre naturelle se faict lors de toutes ces mixtions egales, qu'on nomme Diane]" (*Toyson d'Or*, E1–E1v). The conclusion to this quote differs somewhat from the Latin version (from the *Splendor solis*) translated by Godwin (p. 38), which does not call

The hermaphroditic philosopher's stone is thus the origin and the endpoint of the universe, the alpha and omega, self-engendering and self-destroying. This duality and self-sufficiency links the hermaphroditic stone to the phoenix, who appears in an enigmatic poem towards the end of the treatise:

Enigme

I'habite dans les mons, & parmy la planure,
Pere devant que fils i'ay ma mere engendré,
Et ma mere sans pere en ses flancs m'a porté,
Sans avoir nul besoin d'aucune nourriture.
　Hermaphrodite suis d'une & d'autre nature,
Du plus fort le vainqueur, du moindre surmonté,
Et ne se trouve rien dessous le Ciel vouté,
De si beau, de si bon, & parfaicte figure.
　En moy, dans moy, sans moy, naist un estrange Oyseau,
Qui de ses os non os bastit un tombeau,
Où sans aisles volant, mourant se revifie.
　Et de nature l'art en ensuyvant la loy,
Il se metamorphose à la fin en un Roy,
Six autres surmontant d'admirable harmonie. (*Toyson d'or*, K8v–L)

(I live in the mountains, and on the plains. Father before son, I engendered my mother, and my mother without father carried me in her flanks, without any need of food. I am a hermaphrodite, of one and the other nature, the vanquisher of the strongest, but conquered by the weakest. Nothing of such beautiful, good, and perfect form is to be found below the vaulted sky. Of me, in me, without me, a strange bird is born, which of its bones not bones builds a tomb, where flying without wings, dying it revives itself. And by this art which follows the law of nature, it transforms itself in the end into a King, conquering six others with its admirable harmony.)

This poem also links the hermaphrodite/*rebis* to the image which immediately follows it, that of a body (presumably male, since bearded, although the body itself seems strangely ambiguous in the engraving of fig. 10) being dismembered. The text which explains this act recalls ancient fertility rites based on sacrifice:

Ie t'ay meurtry & mis ton corps en pieces, afin de te beatifier & te faire revivre d'une plus longue & plus heureuse vie ... [je] brouilleray ton corps dans une vase de Terre où

---

the philosophers' Stone Diana. This would be an odd appellation anyway for the conjunction of Sol and Luna, since Diana was the goddess of the Moon. However, the name Diane is also a feminine variant of Janus (Jana), the god of beginnings and endings, thus also of double nature (looking forward and back) and so often equated with the hermaphrodite. See Wind, *Pagan Mysteries*, pp. 200–201, p. 212, p. 230. According to Macrobius, Janus predates Saturn, considered to be the original god.

ie l'enseveliray, à ce qu'y estant en peu de temps pourry, il puisse davantage multiplier
& rapporter quantité de meilleurs fruicts. (*Toyson d'or*, E4v)

(I have killed you and cut your body into pieces, in order to beatify you and to make you
live again, a longer and more fortunate life … I shall break your body into an earthen
vessel where I shall bury it, so that, having decomposed for a while, it might multiply
even more and produce a large quantity of better fruits.)

This parable undoubtedly evokes the stage of putrefaction, where the destruction of
the hermaphroditic conjoined body leads to a higher state of matter. Thus, by means
of these images, the hermaphrodite is linked to sacrifice and eternal life, to the fertile
production of new life in an endless cycle. Trismosin does not overtly link this figure
to Christ, or to any aspect of the Christian tradition, although the phoenix enigma
seems to suggest the possibility of such a link. Rather, he chooses to leave his text
more obscure, and emphasize the evocative imagery that would inform much of the
hermetic poetry of the late sixteenth century (and, in fact, much of the court poetry,
hermetic or "profane"). Trismosin also does not insist too much on the sexual imagery
of conjunction, choosing to vary his symbolism with images of child's play (*Toyson
d'or*, fig. 19), laundry (fig. 20), and pictures of the alchemists' flasks themselves,
containing various monsters such as gryphons (fig. 13), which extend the imagery of
dual nature in more complex fashion. Most of all, Trismosin emphasizes the imagery
of sacrifice (in figs 10 and 11 in particular), along with the notion of life arising from
death.

This more mystical and obscure use of the hermaphrodite, to express concepts
of self-renewal, and of the necessary union between spiritual and material realms,
contributes greatly to the evolution of this figure in alchemical lore. Certainly, Clovis
Hesteau de Nuysement's complex theories of the place of the hermaphrodite in the
alchemical process resemble those of Trismosin rather than the simple and repetitive
marriage-imagery of the *Rosarium*. The popularity of this French translation of the
Aureum vellus was assured, if only for the richness of imagery that it made available
to late Renaissance writers. The emphasis on death, destruction, and renewal in
this imagery links the hermaphrodite both to the phenomenon of religious violence
so prevalent at this time in France, and to the possibility of transcendence of that
violence. The images of fire and mutilation in the work give new meaning to traditional
alchemical representations of death, putrefaction, and rebirth, and create the potential
for connections between alchemy and the Wars of Religion in late sixteenth-century
France. In this way, the hermaphrodite becomes a symbol of hope in dark times.

Chapter 5

Gender and Power in the Alchemical Works of Clovis Hesteau de Nuysement

The Chemical Wedding in the Works of Clovis Hesteau de Nuysement

The second half of the sixteenth century witnessed the violent clashes of the French Wars of Religion (1562–1598), echoed by often vicious disputes in academic and other intellectual circles.[1] In this contested ground, alchemy split into two fairly distinct but also interconnected fields: iatrochemistry, or Paracelsian alchemy, and philosophical alchemy, which owed a great deal to Paracelsus, but had less evidently practical aims. Philosophical alchemy evolved into an alternative spirituality that presented itself as coexisting with the predominant religions, but modifying them to some degree (it should be noted that predominant religions, particularly Catholicism, condemned alchemy as heretical). Its images and ideals were spread not only by means of a large number of treatises published in the late sixteenth and early seventeenth centuries, but also through lyric poetry, which adopted many of the themes and metaphors of alchemy.

More than one writer practiced both alchemy and lyric poetry. One of these poet/alchemists was Clovis Hesteau de Nuysement (1550–16??), a court poet from 1577 until the death of his patron, Henri III of France, in 1589. Nuysement wrote a treatise on alchemy, the *Traittez de l'Harmonie et constitution generalle du vray sel, secret des philosophes & de l'Esprit universel du Monde* (*Treatise on the Harmony and General Constitution of the True Salt, Secret of the Philosophers, and on the Universal Spirit of the World* (1621),[2] a sequence of long poems on alchemy, *Les Visions hermétiques*, to which he added a defense of alchemy, the *Poème philosophic de la verité de la phisique minéralle ...* (*Philosophical Poem on the Truth concerning*

---

[1] An example of the relationship between academic and broader theological disputes is the "defenestration" of Pierre Ramus, who was attacked by his colleagues and their students on the night of the massacres of St Bartholomew's Day; see Jacques-Auguste de Thou, *Historiarum sui temporis ...* (London: Buckley, 1733) vol. 6, p. 410. This attack was the culmination of a series of disputes over the primacy of Aristotle in the university curriculum; Ramus was profoundly anti-Aristotelian as well as a Protestant.

[2] Paris: Jeremie Perier et Abdias Buisard, 1621. All citations are from this edition, and all translations are my own. A modern edition is: *Traictez du vray sel secret des philosophes et de l'esprit general du monde. Les Visions hermétiques*, ed. Sylvain Matton (Paris: Bibliotheca hermetica, 1974).

the Natural Science of Minerals),[3] and several collections of lyric (sometimes love) poetry (1578).[4] The *Traittez du vray sel* was fairly successful, reprinted and translated into German, English, and Latin. Although the *Traittez* is not entirely original, it does revise its Paracelsian model somewhat, and the *Poème philosophic* opens up a new realm for alchemy, and uses the rich alchemical imagery in imaginative and complex fashion, bringing social issues into play with spiritual and philosophical inquiries. The *Visions* offer the modern reader a clear link between alchemical lore and the baroque lyric, replete as it is with images of the phoenix, of the Sun and the Moon, of burning and drowning, of the dissolution or tearing of the body, and of hermaphrodites and androgynes. Also, in the gendered nature of the images chosen to describe the work of alchemy, and in the sexuality used to depict stages of the process, Nuysement alludes to the tradition of the *Rosarium philosophorum*, so influential in the development of philosophical alchemy.[5] After the *Rosarium*, the hermaphrodite becomes a central figure in the alchemical process, no longer as the androgynous *rebis* (a double-headed being), but as a sexually joined couple that becomes one being.

Both theological and medical anti-Aristotelianism led to a reconsideration of the status of sexual difference, and this revision of sexual norms hovered on the brink of heresy, as Aristotle's notion of woman as an imperfect man[6] both informs and is supported by St Paul's theological subordination of woman to man.[7] Among surgeon-authors such as Paré and Duval, and even professors of medicine such as Bauhin at the University of Basel (by the 1590s and 1600s, when Bauhin was writing his treatises on male and female anatomy, and on hermaphrodites, a Protestant university), Aristotelian notions of generation that privilege the male over the female were slowly replaced by observation-based accounts that credit women with an equal role in generation (more of a Hippocratic notion).[8]

In the midst of this debate, philosophical alchemy, an offshoot of medieval alchemy, diverging somewhat from the work of Paracelsus, but also indebted to it,

---

3   *Poème philosophic de la verité de la phisique minéralle ou sont refutees les objections que peuvent faire les incredules & ennemis de cet art* (Paris: Perier & Buisard, 1620).

4   Now re-edited by Roland Guillot. *Les Oeuvres poétiques, livres I et II* (Geneva: Droz, 1994).

5   As I demonstrated to some degree in my article "Salomon Trismosin and Clovis Hesteau de Nuysement: The Sexual Politics of Alchemy in Early Modern France," in *L'Esprit Créateur* 35 (1995), *Writing about Sex: The Discourses of Eroticism in Seventeenth-Century France*, ed. Abby Zanger, pp. 9–21.

6   Expressed, for example, in his treatise on the *Generation of Animals*.

7   The connections between the image of the hermaphrodite and the religious divisions scarring France in the sixteenth century have already been suggested by Catharine Randall (Coats) in her article, "A Surplus of Significance: Hermaphrodites in Early Modern France," *French Forum* 19 (1994): 17–35.

8   For more on this subject, see Lorraine Daston and Katharine Park, "The Hermaphrodite and the Orders of Nature."

offered alternatives to Aristotelian gender roles. Philosophical alchemy flourished in the mid-sixteenth century, and from 1550 on, incorporated a significant representation of gender, particularly in descriptions of the stage of conjunction, often described as a sexual encounter or even as a "marriage" (hence the Rosicrucian treatise, roughly contemporary to the works of Nuysement, called *The Chemical Wedding*). Philosophical alchemy offered a spiritual alternative to Catholicism, and thus was also particularly favored by Protestants and the moderate *politiques* in France, who supported religious toleration. It was no doubt this latter group that brought the discipline to the court of Henri III. What is quite evident in the work of this group of court alchemists is their profound questioning of the traditional distinctions on which gender roles were based. What the philosophical alchemists were doing, to some extent, can be seen as the spiritual (and potentially social) equivalent of the medical revolution of the sixteenth century: creating alternative theories of interaction and thought that break down old boundaries and hierarchies. That their theories were of no practical consequence in their time does not diminish the revolutionary nature of their thought. Philosophical alchemy continued to thrive through the eighteenth century, contributing to the Enlightenment debates that preceded the French Revolution.

In the *Traittez*, Nuysement describes the hermaphroditic nature of the universe in almost Aristophanic terms:

> Le Monde donc ayant esté creé bon par celuy qui est la bonté mesme, est non seulement corporel, mais encore participant d'intelligence (car il est plein d'idees omniformes) & comme j'ai desja dit, il n'a membre ny partie qui ne soit vitale. Pour cette cause les sages l'ont dit estre animal, par tout masle & femelle, & se conjoindre par mutuelle amour & conjonction à ses membres, tant il est convoiteux & avide du mariage & liayson de ses parties. De là, par une translation, vient la diversité des sexes aux plantes, & aux animaux qui, s'acouplant ensemble, à l'exemple du monde, engendrent leurs semblables, non autrement que le monde mesme qui de soy produit une infinité d'autres petits mondes .... (*Traittez du vray sel*, A7–A7v, pp. 13–14)

> (The world, thus having been created good by Him who is goodness itself, is not only corporeal, but even participates in the intellect [because it is full of varied ideas] and, as I have already said, there is not a limb or part that is not alive. For this reason, wise men have called it an animal, male and female throughout, and joined by mutual love and union of its limbs, so great and eager is its desire for the marriage and joining of its parts. From this, by means of transmission, comes the diversity of sexes in plants and in animals, which, coupling together, like the world itself, engender those like them, not in any manner different from the world, which from itself produces an infinity of other little worlds ....)

Although the image of heterosexual marriage enters into the treatise, its inscription within a hermaphroditic model of self-generation destabilizes the Aristotelian model on which western European theories of sexuality were based. Even the rhetoric of the passage is mutable and suggests the coexistence of active and passive roles in one being. This representation of conjunction effaces the assigned gender roles of active and passive, which in turn structure the marriage-contract. The Aristotelian echo that all plants and animals generate those just like them (from the *Generation of Animals*, pp. 1187–8, mentioned above) is already skewed by the suggestion of difference inherent within the same. This difference is "translated" into sexual diversity in plants and animals, suggesting that sexual difference is not the ideal, but rather that diversity within the same being is. The treatise implies that sexual difference is only necessary in an imperfect world. But the figure of perfection, which opens and closes the treatise, is the amorphous, all-engendering Demogorgon/Saturn, a chaotic figure of asexual reproduction out of whom all material and spiritual being springs (*Traittez du vray sel*, A2, p. 3; E, p. 65; G6v, p. 108).[9]

Nuysement also revises the Aristotelian/Paracelsian model of generation to some degree, when he leaves some doubt as to which partner has the significant role in the process:

> Quand donc nous disons que la Lune est mere de l'esprit & matiere universelle, nous ne parlons pas sans raison apparente, & n'y a rien d'absurde: Mais il nous fault faire voir d'où vient cette maternité. Chaleur & humeur sont les deux clefs de toute generation: la chaleur faisant l'office de masle, & l'humeur celuy de femelle. Par l'action du chault sur l'humide se fait premierement la corruption, qui est suivie par la generation … le mesme arrive en la generation de l'homme, qui est amene à un corps accomply de toutes ses parties, par l'assemblement de deux spermes, l'un masculin & l'autre feminin, dedans la matrice, à l'aide de la chaleur naturelle de la femme. (*Traittez du vray sel*, C3v–C4, pp. 38–9)

> (When we say that the Moon is the mother of the spirit and universal material, we are not speaking without obvious reason, and there is nothing absurd in it. But we must show from whence comes this maternity. Heat and humidity are the two keys of all generation: heat does the work of the male, and humidity that of the female. By the action of that which is hot on that which is humid, corruption is first made, which is followed by generation … The same thing happens with the generation of man, who is made into a body perfected in all its parts, by the joining of two seeds, one masculine and the other feminine, in the womb, with the help of the natural warmth of the female.)

To a large extent, this account may seem typically Aristotelian; the male is equated with dry and hot, the female with cold and moist elements. Yet Nuysement contradicts himself here, and attributes heat to the female as well. He also leaves unclear what the difference between male and female "sperm" might be. Following Hippocratic and Galenic models, he suggests that both partners contribute this seed to the process of generation, rather than the male sperm acting on inert female matter. This represents a rejection of the Aristotelian model which essentially writes women out of a process

---

[9]   Also interesting is Nuysement's portrayal of Medea as the first alchemist, since she taught Jason how to pursue the Golden Fleece (which Nuysement reads as the art of alchemy) and how to restore sickly bodies (*Traittez du vray sel*, S2–S5, pp. 295–301).

for which they are crucial, and thus encapsulates the debate occurring in early modern academic circles over the relative value of Aristotelian and Hippocratic notions of generation. Nuysement goes even further when he invokes Luna, often represented in the alchemical process as female, as the "universal mother of spirit and matter," thus eliminating the binary associations established by Aristotle between the male and spirit, and the female and matter.

Another significant element of Nuysement's argument, one linked closely to his complexly gendered representation of the process of generation, is the belief that corruption, or putrefaction, is essential for creation. There must be some dissolution of the two separate forms of seed, some fusion between microscopic versions of the "Self" and the "Other" in order to create another self, yet one which is somehow different. Thus, dissolution can be seen as the very basis for generation: "J'appelle icy corruption le changement & passage de forme en forme, qui ne peult arriver sans le moyen de putrefaction, qui est le vray chemin de generation ..." (*Traittez du vray sel*, C4, p. 39: "Here I call corruption the mutation and passage from form to form, which cannot occur without the aid of putrefaction, which is the true way to generation"). One can only sense the subversive potential of such a dynamic model of generation. The Aristotelian model essentially calls for cloning of the father; the ideal offspring resembles the father exactly (this is taken to an extreme in the image of the homunculus). The very foundation of this model is the notion of stasis as an ideal; change is invariably perceived as corruption, and corruption is only perceived as a negative force. Aristotle's model of generation hints at an ideal Golden Age, when men were perfect, and from which the world has since declined; the goal then becomes a backwards movement towards the original father. In contrast to this tradition, Nuysement suggests that the transformation resulting from dissolution of boundaries, from the movement away from the "same" towards the "different" is an evolution towards a more perfect form. Since Nuysement universalizes this evolutionary model, one can hypothesize a social model of evolution as well as a biological one; the words "vray chemin" at least suggest a theological context in which this process can be worked through.

Nuysement struggles with the notion of distinction, and with the reasons for differences between species; unlike Paracelsus, he does not take these distinctions for granted. He tries to explain difference as the effect of the Universal Spirit on diverse sorts of matter, made up of the elements in various proportions:

L'ame de l'univers se feinct donc & imagine diverses formes d'especes, que l'esprit recevant dans les entrailles des Elements corporifie, & produit en lumiere. C'est pourquoy les animaux engendrent seulement des animaux; les plantes des plantes & les mineraux des mineraux ... Non que je veuille dire qu'il [l'Esprit] n'ait en luy l'action des autres vertus; Mais il ne les desmontre que selon les especes où il est accommodé. Autrement il faudroit que chacune chose en produist une dissemblable; Assavoir, que l'homme engendrast un arbre: la plante feist un boeuf, & le metal une herbe. Ce que je dy seulement à l'esgard de la specification des choses .... (*Traittez du vray sel*, D7–D7v, pp. 61–2)

(The soul of the universe enters into reverie and imagines diverse forms of species, which the spirit, receiving in the entrails of the elements, renders corporeal, and brings to light. This is why animals engender only animals, plants plants, and minerals minerals. Not that I wish to say that the Spirit does not contain in itself the power of other qualities. But he only reveals them according to the species [or type] in which he resides. Otherwise, each thing would have to produce something unlike itself. That is to say, a man would engender a tree, a plant would create a bull, and metal grass. What I say is only in regard to speciation of things.)

The material world proceeds from a simulachrum or even counterfeit of the soul of the universe (*anima mundi*), which through its imagination begets the various species on the spirit. Not only is this the reversal of biological roles (the female begetting on the male); in a disruption of Neoplatonic ideals, which value reason and intellect over the imagination, itself portrayed as too corporeal a faculty to be of real worth, the imagination is seen as the means by which the species receive their form and diversity. While reason is the faculty that fosters categorization by resemblances, it is the imagination that creates the diversity that is life. Nor is the action of the spirit on material forms a unilateral movement; it can only reveal diverse species according to the species in which it is lodged. The matter itself thus acts upon the vivifying spirit, to effect the creation of specific forms. The significance of this reversal of the Aristotelian perspective is still playing itself out in biomedical studies of conception and fetal development. Indeed, quite logically, if outside forces such as the spirit had full control of form, then there would be nothing to prevent a man from fathering a tree, as Nuysement absurdly points out. There is a certain force within the material form itself that dictates resemblance within a species, itself inscribed in the diversity of all things.

Nuysement seems to shuttle back and forth between the Paracelsian notion of rigid distinction, that everything can be categorized and then subcategorized until each individual stands completely apart from the rest of creation, and the belief that all of creation shares in one essential being. The two systems work well in tension with each other: emphasis on individual identity counteracts the conformist aspects of belief in one essential being; the more unified view of sameness in identity counteracts the rigid hierarchies of value that seem to result from over-emphasis upon individualism. Taken separately, each system leads to a sort of conformism of ideal being. First, individualism is a system that can only be established by distinction; but the bases for distinction are not clear, and often seem circular in nature ("man is not woman; woman is not man"). Then, difference is established through relative "value;" but this value in fact establishes itself rather than being based on some essential distinction ("men are superior to women"). Yet similarity also rises from the starting-point of difference; how can one even say that "women are just like men," if some distance has not been established which makes comparison possible? If women *were* just like men, then they would *be* men; so the phrase destroys itself. In creating difference, in the act of separation, difference is destroyed, as the *Traittez du vray sel* suggests: "Cette medecine opere comme le feu en consommant l'impur qu'elle separe du pur, par un banissement perpetuel des parties Etherogenes, et une adoption des Homogenes" (H6v, p. 124: "This medicine operates like fire by consuming the impure, which she separates from the pure, by means of perpetual banishment of the heterogeneous parts, and adoption of the homogeneous ones"). The punitive language, of fire and banishment, once again suggests the religious context of this discussion. The enforcement of resemblance or sameness requires a destruction of that which is different, seen as impure. But this destruction is also potentially self-destructive, putting at risk that which is the same as well (since, as Nuysement has hinted, there is difference inherent in the same).

The only solution is an uneasy balance between the two forms of identification, similarity and difference, taken with the understanding that neither is sufficient: "either/or; neither/both." It is at this juncture between similarity and difference that the figure of the hermaphrodite is to be found; expressing in its form the epistemological trap that any attempt at cosmology (as the discipline which purports to explain the universe as an orderly system) creates:

> Et comme l'enfant qui est naturellement participant des humeurs de ses pere & mere, par la commixion de leurs semences, ayt esté des sages anciens appellé d'un nom proprement composé des noms de ses deux geniteurs, assavoir Androgine: que les poetes ont dit Hermaphrodite; par ce qu'il ne pouvoit encore estre appellé homme ny femme, estant incapable de produire les effects de l'un n'y de l'autre: aussi est il convenable d'attribuer à cette vierge le nom d'Uragonee, ou Ciel terrifié, puis qu'estant terre elle a neantmoins en soy, par leurs vertus, tous les Cieux enclos & joints d'un lien indissoluble: desquels elle fait voir les operations admirables. (*Traittez du vray sel*, H6v–H7, pp. 124–5)

> (And as the child who naturally partakes of the humours of both his father and his mother by the mixture of their seed, was called by the ancient wise men a name properly composed of those of his two parents, that is to say, Androgyne, which the poets call Hermaphrodite, because he could not yet be called man or woman, being incapable of producing the effects of one or of the other, so it is appropriate to attribute the name Uragonée to this virgin, that is, earthly sky, since even though she is earth, she has in her, through their powers, all the heavens contained and indissolubly joined, from which she can do admirable things.)

The hermaphrodite is at once both man and woman, and neither. Strangely, Nuysement declares the hermaphrodite sterile, but then compares it to the powerful earthly and celestial virgin medicine engendered at the center of the earth (by which he means salt in the sense of an essential mineral that forms the basis for all other things). Thus, the dual entity is at once sterile and fecund, moribund and life-giving, abject and triumphant.

These paradoxes are echoed in Nuysement's characterization of the active and the passive (often seen as male and female roles in generation): "... ce qui patit inseparablement coexiste avec ce qui agit" (*Traittez du vray sel*, E2, p. 67: "... that which is acted upon coexists inseparably with that which acts upon it"). Here, he seems to remain within the Aristotelian system; describing fire or heat as the active element which directs generation and development of living beings (E2–E2v, pp. 67–8). Yet, it cannot function without the "passive" water, an observation which calls into question the already value-laden terms, active and passive. If fire cannot act without air or water, then one could argue that air or water are acting upon the fire (which Nuysement in fact has suggested, Ev, p. 66).

Nuysement has a similar problem with what he calls *excrement*, the impure waste that results from creation of anything. He states "rien ne se corporifie sans l'excrement" (*Traittez du vray sel*, , Hv, p. 114: "nothing can become corporeal without excrement") and that "le but auquel tend Nature est de vivifier en separant, afin d'eviter la mort qui ne vient d'ailleurs que de l'abondance des excremens qui suffocquent la pure et naturelle substance" (*Traittez du vray sel*, H2, p. 115: "the goal which Nature seeks to attain is to give life by separating, in order to avoid the death which comes only from the abundance of excrement which suffocates the pure and natural substance").[10] The undefined impure is perceived as a constant menace: "Car la chose impure qui enveloppe le pur de la substance & se mesle parmy, ne cesse de la quereller et combatre jusqu'à ce qu'elle l'aye surmontee & suffoquee ..." (*Traittez du vray sel*, I5v–I6, p. 138–9: "Because the impure thing which surrounds the pure aspect of the substance, and mixes with it, never ceases to quarrel with it and fight it until she has conquered and suffocated it ..."). Nuysement clearly equates the physical with the moral in this passage, when he compares man's lot on earth with the general degradation of the celestial purity of matter: "Car nostre aage plus vicieux et desbordé que celuy de nos ayeuls, a fait de nous pire portée que celle de nos peres ..." (*Traittez du vray sel*, I7v, p. 142: "Because our age, more vicious and debauched than that of our ancestors, has done worse by us than that of our fathers ..."). The process of mixture or mortification effects this degradation. He seems insistently concerned with decrying corruption in the second book, even as he praised it as the basis of generation in the first. Like Paracelsus, Nuysement applies his theories of separation of the pure from the impure to medical treatments; and purging is one method he calls for.

Here, as in the work of Paracelsus, separation is the basis of life: "Car si elle [Nature] ne separe, il est necessaire qu'elle mortifie" (*Traittez du vray sel*, H3v, p. 118: "For, if Nature does not distinguish or separate elements, she will necessarily mortify

---

10 Nuysement returns to the question of pure and impure when he discusses the creation of the World: "Or separation en general n'est autre chose que division & distinction des choses dissemblables; comme du ciel d'avec la terre, du Soleil d'avec la Lune; & autres choses que j'ay desja dittes. Comme aussi du pur d'avec l'impur ..." (*Traittez du vray sel*, Iv, p. 130: "So, separation in general is nothing other than the division and distinction between unlike things; as the sky from the earth, the Sun from the Moon, and other things I have already mentioned, such as the pure from the impure ..."). Note the use of the term *d'avec*, which links conjunction and distinction into one process.

them [or die]" 203).[11] Nuysement even distinguishes two forms of separation: the first is between things that are different, but not contrary (and he gives the example of leaves and branches on trees); the second is between opposites (and here he gives the example of the pure and the impure). One could well question the second category by positing more detailed examples (one being food and excrement), as even seeming opposites are often connected to each other.

Alchemy seems based on confusion of this second distinction; mortification is a crucial step in the alchemical process, leading to renewed life. Since Nuysement previously praised corruption as the source of all life, in his view existence as we know it depends upon the abjection, and subsequent expulsion, of certain elements. So, although the "pure" substance seems to be the ideal, it is defined by that which has been designated "impure," which in turn creates another circular trap. One cannot escape that which is expelled, even as one sets it aside in the ordering of the universe. Without the oscillation between distinction and abjection, between separation and union, the world would be static and empty of life:

> Et qui plus est, aucune generation ne pourroit estre faite au monde inferieur, ny ayant point d'alteration ny mutation des formes, qui n'auroient toutes qu'une mesme face: sans distinction de haut ny de bas ... Ce fut donc chose necessaire d'entremesler ces feces grossieres à la substance subtile: Car où il ny a que pureté il n'y peut avoir d'action, parce que rien ne peut agir sans patient .... (*Traittez du vray sel*, L3, p. 165)

> (And what is more, no generation could occur in the inferior world, as there was no alteration or mutation of forms, which would all have the same appearance, without distinction between higher and lower ... So it was necessary to mix this crude excrement with the refined substance. Because where there is only purity, there can be no action, because nothing can act without something to act upon.)

Perfect uniformity equals stasis; difference is essential to the process, which itself is the basis of philosophical alchemy (as opposed to the product). Furthermore, just as in the case of fire and water, male and female, the pure is a non-functional category without its opposite, the impure. Nuysement wrestles with the question of the nexus between body and spirit, the answer to which he perceives in excrement itself. If the body or the corporeal is of such importance, then why do we expel the same mass we take in (whether food or water)? He concludes that it is the spirit trapped in the bodily mass that we ingest (*Traittez du vray sel*, L3–L3v, pp. 165–6). Yet he is troubled by this

---

[11] This sentiment is echoed later in the treatise: "Car separation est le commencement de toutes choses, et la premiere operation qui distingue les membres confus du corps universel" (*Traittez du vray sel*, H8v, p. 128: "This separation is the beginning of all things, and the first operation which distinguishes the confused members of the universal body"). This is a fairly traditional view of the creation of the universe, which Nuysement inevitably problematizes by blurring the very distinctions he deems necessary for existence.

observation, because the spirit does not seem to exist outside of the body; they both live only in conjunction, and only the body is clearly observable. Thus, the importance of the body cannot be denied, if only as a vehicle for the spirit (*Traittez du vray sel*, L3v–L4, pp. 166–7); and division between body and spirit seems impossible.

The treatise continues with elaborate analogies between Christianity and alchemy (*Traittez du vray sel*, N6–Qv, pp. 203–42), the processes of spiritual and physical purification. Invariably, the introduction of Christian doctrine into the discussion has confused Nuysement's arguments, as a rigid system of hierarchical values that privileges what we cannot observe over the corporeal world we can observe displaces a system that cannot free itself of the physical nature that seems so basic to life. The body must be mortified – but not destroyed. Nuysement denigrates the body (*Traittez du vray sel*, N6v, p. 204), but then points out that God himself appeared in corporeal form to save man (O7v, p. 222). Thus, even in the case of the Christian religion, the distinction between spiritual and corporeal is effaced in order to produce action. Even here, the treatise oscillates between the duality of spiritual-pure/corporeal-impure and the recognition of the necessary conjunction of this duality. The purpose of life is death, but the purpose of death is life:

> Et de vray cette acquisition de vie par la mort se prattique naturellement en toutes creatures vitalles: Car il faut que tout sperme ou semence aux animaux se mortifie en la matrice, & aux vegetaux dans la terre, avant qu'aucune croissance vegetable, ou specification se puisse faire. (*Traittez du vray sel*, Pv, p. 226)

> (And truly, this acquisition of life by means of death takes place in all living creatures. Because all sperm or seed in animals must die in the womb, and for plants in the earth, before any plant growth or development into a particular species can take place.)

Nuysement cites "la similitude du grain qu'il a dit ne pouvoir fructifier s'il ne meurt premierement" (P2, p. 227: "the metaphor of the grain which cannot bear fruit unless it first dies"). Ordering thus becomes an effacement of death itself, an expulsion of omnipresent nothingness to the periphery of human experience. Death becomes merely the prelude to renewed life (and here the treatise joins Christian and Pythagorean thought neatly). But the insistence with which death returns, with which Nuysement must displace it and all that is corporeal, reveals the weakness of this system of ordering that supposedly grants life.

Nuysement's rigid categories have already collapsed as he tries to explain numerous exceptions to the various clear oppositions he has established, such as the plant that can kill under some circumstances, and heal under others (*Traittez du vray sel*, I4v, p. 136). Nuysement seems to inhabit a Paracelsian universe in disarray. The categories and theories remain, but they do not function as they did at the dawn of the sixteenth century. Philosophical alchemy no longer even carries the veneer of functioning as a practical system; it has evolved into a self-consciously impossible struggle to systematize the universe, to subject the world to human control. By the end of the sixteenth century, this failure to define and control has become as important to the intellectual and spiritual process of alchemy as the control itself. It is as if the whole intellectual process of alchemy mirrors the physical one of putrefaction and dissolution; alchemy is in the process of placing categorization and rational discourse alongside the imaginative and irrational.

This unusual intellectual experiment is most evident in the alchemical poetry and emblem-books, which defy explanation even as they themselves over-explain the process. Alchemy becomes a process of intellectual abjection that suggests a hope of creating new scientific methods from the rubble of the old. At the same time, it calls into question social roles and beliefs that have been supported by "old science": most notably the hierarchy of man over woman, and the belief in the primacy of the spirit over the body. Although philosophical alchemy may not succeed in defining itself, it survives for centuries as an alternative system of thought that perpetually calls Christianity and feudal/aristocratic social hierarchies into question by taking the very terms and images of these conceptual/social structures, and twisting them to mean something other than what they are accepted as representing by the authorities (the Sorbonne and other Catholic institutions, the monarchy and its institutions and apologists). In this, alchemy can been seen as a subversive, almost parodic, cultural form, enacting monarchy, marriage, and other institutions in a way that puts the institutions themselves into question. Instead of ruling over his wife, the husband loses himself in her, and she in him, thus effacing the hierarchy within which the stage of conjunction, often represented as a marriage, is enacted. This is even more clear in the *Poème philosophic*:

> Mercure est le mary, & Venus est la femme.
> L'Art en a fait deux corps, mais ces corps n'ont qu'une ame.
> L'un et l'autre patit, puis agit à son tour,
> Sous les effects divers d'un mutuel amour.[12]

> (Mercury is the husband, and Venus the wife. / The Art made them in two bodies, but these bodies have but one soul. / One and the other is acted upon, and then acts in its turn, / Under the varying effects of mutual love.)

It should be noted that, the sexual behavior described here would have been seen in the sixteenth century as bisexual, and therefore forbidden. This is clear from Ambroise Paré's reiteration of Claude de Tesserant's injunction against hermaphroditic bisexuality in *Des monstres et prodiges*, cited in the first chapter of this study.

Nuysement is positing a mixture of the active and passive roles as the ideal for each partner in the stage of conjunction. This blurring of legally hierarchized sexual roles transforms identity in some fundamental way: "Sa femelle l'embrasse, il l'embrasse à son tour, / Et vivement épris d'un amour mutuelle, / Elle se glisse en luy, & luy se

---

12   *Poeme philosophic de la verité de la phisique mineralle* (Paris: Jeremie Perier & Abdias Buisard, 1620), D5, p. 57. Again, all translations are my own.

fond en elle" (*Poeme philosophic*, C3v, p. 38: "His female embraces him, he embraces her in turn / And strongly taken with mutual love, She slips into him, and he melts into her"). Thus, the husband not only loses his hierarchical domination over his wife, he loses himself in the conjunction and cannot be distinguished from her. This is clearly a revision of the Ovidian myth of Hermaphroditus, in which the girl/nymph Salmacis disappears into the boy's identity.

This problematizing of marital roles extends into the larger social context as well. Instead of ruling over his subjects, the King in alchemy is shown sacrificing himself for the process, succumbing to illness, being torn by wolves, or drowning.[13] These are the transformations that Nuysement enacts in the *Poème philosophic* as does his contemporary, Michael Maier, in his *Atalanta fugiens*. It is this transformative thought that explains the close ties between alchemy and secret societies such as the Freemasons,[14] themselves linked almost two centuries later to Revolutionary movements in Europe and America. Perhaps seemingly unworldly theories can lead to social change.

The Hermaphroditic Origins of the World: Problems of Distinction

In his *Poème philosophic*, Nuysement also designates the *prima materia* as a hermaphroditic entity. In this passage, as at every point in this poem, gender and power are linked as crucial elements of the alchemical process; gender, because the problems of distinction and dissolutions of boundaries are basic to alchemy, and power, because distinction tends, at least in the social context of sixteenth-century monarchy, towards hierarchization. Nuysement's alchemical works oscillate between a presentation of gender as a distinction within the same that puts the lie to hierarchizing binaries, and gender as informing the binary value system (spiritual over material, male over female, for example) that structures power relations.

---

[13] For example, in Michael Maier's *Atalanta fugiens*, emblem 24 depicts the wolf devouring the King; emblem 28 depicts the King being purged of illness; emblem 31 depicts the King drowning; emblem 44 depicts the burial and rebirth of the King; and emblem 48 depicts the King suffering another illness. For an English version of the epigrams, see the translation by Joscelyn Godwin (Grand Rapids, MI: Phanes Press, 1989); this edition also contains the emblems and the fugues, but not the lengthy prose commentaries. A facsimile editon of an earlier version (Oppenheim: Galleri, 1618) contains the full text (Kassel: Bärenreiter, 1964).

[14] The connection between alchemy, secret societies, and religious dissent has already been suggested by Frances Yates in her book, *The Rosicrucian Enlightenment* (London: Routledge and Kegan Paul, 1972). The political aspect of links between alchemy and secret societies was traced in a paper written for my seminar on "Alchemy and Abjection in Early Modern France" in the spring of 1996 by Todd Stevens, on "Alchemy and Secret Societies."

Nature a composé de feu, d'air, d'eau, & terre,
Un principe à cet Art qui est Pierre & non Pierre.

...

Grand Roy, qui sans autre ayde a pris son origine
De cet Hermaphroditte, ou de cette Androgine.
De ce Cahos Phisic en qui vivent cachez
Sept esprits mineraux, par Art sont arrachez
Leurs quatre geniteurs, en la double semence
Dont l'Embrion Chimic doit tirer sa naissance.
Les deux sont au Mercure, & les deux autres sont
Au souphre; et tous ensemble en mourant se parfont.
Mercure est le mary, & Venus est la femme.
L'Art en a fait deux corps, mais ces corps n'ont qu'une ame.
L'un et l'autre patit, puis agit à sont tour,[15]
Sous les effects divers d'un mutuel amour;
Amour qui les rassemble, & des deux morts fait naistre
Un tiers tout dissemblable à ceux dont il prend l'estre.
Voila cet un mystique, & cette trinité,
Qui comprend tout mystere en sa triple unité. (*Poeme philosophic*, D4v–D5, pp. 56–7)

(Nature has composed of fire, air, water, and earth, / A principal for this Art which is stone but not stone. / ... Great King, who without other help was born / Of that Hermaphrodite, or of that Androgyne, / Of that Physical Chaos in which seven minerals / live hidden, by the Art / their four progenitors are torn out, in the double seed / From which the Chemical Embryo must take its birth. / Two are of Mercury, and the two others are of sulphur; / And all together perfect themselves by dying. / Mercury is the husband, and Venus is the wife. / The Art has made two bodies of them, but these bodies have but one soul. / One and the other submits, and then acts in its turn. / Under the influence of the different effects of a mutual love; / Love which brings them together, and from two dead beings gives birth / To a third completely unlike those from whom he takes his being. / Behold this mystical one, and this Trinity, / Which enfolds every mystery in its triple unity.)

The hermaphrodite is the chaotic material from which the world is created by means of distinction (first of the four elements, then of individual creatures). It is a state in which subject and object are (con)fused ("One and the other submits, and then acts in its turn"). The highest state of this material, the perfected version of this "dead" double being, is the King of Metals, scarcely distinguished from, and later overtly compared to, Christ. The message of this text seems to be at one and the same time

---

[15] This line recalls Agrippa d'Aubigné's accusation that Henri III had turned his pleasures to those of "patir au lieu d'agir," that is, of passivity as opposed to action, taking on the stereotypically feminine role, according to French Renaissance norms; see the *Histoire universelle*, ed. André Thierry (Geneva: Droz, 1980–99), vol. 6, bk 10, ch. 12, p. 208.

politically conservative and theologically heretical. That is to say, the ideal is still posited as some form of categorization and distinction. Furthermore, this distinction is consistently described in the terms of monarchy.

Yet the instability of sexual roles, as each partner in the alchemical process takes the active and then the passive role in turn, runs counter to the social norms of the time, according to which this behavior is bisexual, and thus extremely threatening. This recalls Claude de Tesserant's injunction against hermaphroditic bisexuality, echoed by Ambroise Paré in his treatise on monsters:

> Hermafrodites masles et femelles, ce sont ceux qui ont les deux sexes bien formez et s'en peuvent aider et servir à la generation: et à ceux cy les loix anciennes et modernes ont fait et font encore eslire duquel sexe ils veulent user, avec defense, sur peine de perdre la vie, de ne se servir que de celuy duquel ils auront fait election, pour les inconvenients qui en pourroyent advenir. Car aucuns en ont abusé de telle sorte, que par un usage mutuel et reciproque paillardoyent de l'un et de l'autre sexe, tantost d'homme, tantost de femme ....

> (Male and female hermaphrodites are those who have both sets of sexual organs well formed, and can use either for begetting or conceiving children. These ancient and modern laws made and still make choose which sex they wish to use, with the prohibition, upon the pain of death, against using any but that which they have chosen, because of the inconveniences that might arise. For some have abused in such a way, that both mutual and reciprocal use, they have debauched one and the other sex, sometimes a man, sometimes a woman ...)[16]

As has been stated before, *agir* was the term used to describe the male, or active, role in the sexual act; *patir*, linked to our *passive*, was used to describe the acceptable female role. When he ascribes both roles to each partner in the stage of conjunction, Nuysement is contravening clearly stated sexual norms, and describing an act prohibited by law. He inscribes bisexuality, clearly a vehemently prohibited act, within the model of heterosexual marriage, which provides the dominant images of the stage of conjunction.

Throughout the *Poème philosophic*, religion is also implicated in the discussions of power, and it is also skewed by the alchemical context. The comparison of occult processes to the Trinity cannot be seen as anything but heretical; all the more so because the alchemical trinity more closely resembles pagan triads of father, mother, son. Furthermore, at certain points, Nuysement's theories, as well as those of other alchemists, seem to indicate a Manichean belief in the essential duality of the universe. Matter is frequently described as essentially evil, entrapping the good spirit within; matter must be dissolved or destroyed in order to free this spirit. The alchemical

---

[16] Ambroise Paré, *Des Monstres et prodiges*, pp. 24–5. The passage he expands upon is from Claude de Tesserant's continuation of Pierre Boaistuau's *Histoires prodigieuses*, p. 223.

process is thus described as one of mastery, although this mastery is also frequently overturned or frustrated by that which is to be mastered. As Jung points out, alchemy is heavily dependent on dualisms for its exposition:

> The factors which come together in the coniunctio are conceived as opposites, either confronting one another in enmity or attracting one another in love. To begin with they form a dualism; for instance the opposites are *humidum* (moist)/*siccum* (dry), *frigidum* (cold)/*calidum* (warm), *superiora* (upper, higher)/*inferiora* (lower), *spiritus-anima* (spirit-soul)/*corpus* (body), *coelum* (heaven)/*terra* (earth), *ignis* (fire)/*aqua* (water), bright/dark, *agens* (active)/*patiens* (passive), *volatile* (volatile, gaseous)/*fixum* (solid), *pretiosum* (precious, costly; also *carum*, dear)/*vile* (cheap, common), *bonum* (good)/*malum* (evil), *manifestum* (open)/*occultum* (occult; also *celatum*, hidden), *oriens* (East)/*occidens* (West), *vivum* (living)/*mortuum* (dead, inert), *masculus* (masculine)/*foemina* (feminine), Sol/Luna.[17]

That these binaries involve hierarchization, or categorizations involving value judgments, becomes apparent as Jung's list progresses. Yet, given the nature of the conjunction itself, and the necessity of the presence of the "lower" elements in order for the process to succeed, alchemy seems at once to confirm and erase such categorization. Its emphasis on the importance of dissolution or of the abject for the process would indicate some questioning of the fundamental unities of French culture (expressed as "One King, one law, one faith" – but one could also add "one sex").[18] Furthermore, alchemy's emphasis (as expressed by Nuysement) on the importance of dissolution and destruction of the body for resurrection in a higher form counters Catholic belief, so dearly held, in the need for an integral body in order to effect resurrection. This belief is expressed in the extreme attempts made by Catholic persecutors to annihilate the bodies of Protestants (attempts that extended from burning them at the stake to grinding their bones and skulls into dust or cutting the bodies into tiny pieces).[19] Given how many Huguenots dabbled in alchemy, including Béroalde de Verville,[20] Bernard Palissy,[21]

---

[17] Carl Jung, *Mysterium Coniunctionis*, p. 3.

[18] Here, I am thinking of Thomas Laqueur's book, *Making Sex*, particularly the chapter "New Science, One Flesh," pp. 63–113. Although some scientists were questioning the one sex theory by the end of the sixteenth century, in academic circles this model still predominated.

[19] See Catharine Randall Coats, "The Sundered Body and Its Return," in *(Em)bodying the Word: Textual Ressurections in the Martyrological Narratives of Foxe, Crespin, de Bèze and d'Aubigné* (New York: Peter Lang, 1992), p. 76. This view is confirmed by d'Aubigné's account of the treatment of Gaspard de Coligny's body: "Le peuple resveillé par l'orloge du palais court au logis du mort, en coupe toutes les parties qui se pouvoyent couper: sur tout la teste, qui alla jusques à Rome ..." (*HU*, ed. Thierry, vol. 3, bk 6, ch. 4, p. 332).

[20] Author of *Les Recherches de la pierre philosophale* (Paris: T. Jouan, 1584) and of *Le Moyen de Parvenir* (one edition by C. Royer, Geneva: Droz, 1970).

[21] See for example the *Recepte véritable*, ed. Keith Cameron (Geneva: Droz, 1988).

and Agrippa d'Aubigné,[22] it may well be that this alternative belief in the importance of corporeal dissolution for final resurrection was a seductive one.

Thus, Nuysement's work seems to establish and dissolve the contemporary norms of gender difference (for example when he presents heterosexual marriage as a bisexual relationship), of monarchy (by presenting the King as the sacrifice made to ensure the process), and of religious orthodoxy (by presenting the Trinity as Father, Mother, and Son). The work of alchemy could be compared to that of Donna Haraway's cyborgs, problematizing the dualisms cited above, effacing and creating boundaries in order to extend the self beyond that which is designated as "natural":

> To recapitulate, certain dualisms have been persistent in Western traditions; they have all been systemic to the logics and practices of domination of women, people of colour, nature, workers, animals – in short, domination of all constituted as others, whose task is to mirror the self. Chief among these troubling dualisms are self/other, mind/body, culture/nature, male/female, civilized/primitive, reality/appearance, whole/part, agent/resource, maker/made, active/passive, right/wrong, truth/illusion, total/partial, God/man. The self is the One who is not dominated, who knows that by the service of the other, the other is the one who holds the future, who knows that by the experience of domination, which gives the lie to the autonomy of the self ...
>
> High-tech culture challenges these dualisms in intriguing ways. It is not clear who makes and who is made in the relation between human and machine. It is not clear what is mind and what body in machines that resolve into coding practices.[23]

The alchemists themselves played with these dualisms, and extended boundaries, often using themselves as the ground of this work. Paracelsus hoped, in his *homunculus*, to create artificial life that was immortal and that would replace mankind. Other alchemists as well united their "natural" world with "artificial" devices and recipes in order to extend the body (in the homunculus or automaton) and redefine the self. They dissolved the presumed boundaries of organic and metallic substances in order to create new substances. Even as they "worked" the process, they were worked by it, and transformed. And although they described this process as the perfecting of the self and the surrounding world, the infinitely cyclical nature of the work renders any teleology problematic.

This cyclical nature of the process is evident in the passage previously cited from the *Poeme philosophic* (D4v–D5, pp. 56–7). Nature is described as the chaotic hermaphrodite who produces the King, or the "chemical embryo." This occurs by the division of Nature into masculine and feminine, Mercury and Venus, who then combine in more gender-ambiguous, that is to say, alternating between

---

22 See his autobiography, *Sa Vie à ses enfants*, ed. Gilbert Schrenck (Paris: Nizet, 1986), pp. 63–4.

23 Donna Haraway, "A Cyborg Manifesto," *Simians, Cyborgs, and Women* (New York: Routledge, 1991), p. 177.

active and passive, roles. This ambiguity suggests that Mercury and Venus are also hermaphroditic in some way. What is born of this union is a third being who resembles neither parent, both contains both of them within himself, in a multi-gendered trinity. This being is called the King. But the process as described by Nuysement begins and ends with the Hermaphrodite, with the intervening stages also participating in this duality.

In political terms, the alchemical process seems conservative in that it calls for a restoration of hierarchical order under some all-powerful King. The process is radical in its acceptance of dissolution and chaos as crucial to the restoration of this order (or the establishment of a higher order). This oscillation between abjection and an order based on rigid categorization must have been a reassuring image for a country ravaged by the Wars of Religion. The spiritual or psychological need for such reassurance would explain the increasingly widespread practice of alchemy and publication of alchemical treatises in the face of Church censorship.

The Transgressive King

That alchemy is primarily concerned with boundaries and transgression is confirmed by Nuysement's association of hermaphrodism with incest and cannibalism. The taboo practices of incest and cannibalism, generally seen as threatening to society, are portrayed in the *Poème philosophic* as foundational to it:

> Mais ce Roy des Metaux, unique en sa nature,
> Se produict à peu pres comme la creature.
> Il a une femelle où gist tout son amour;
> Sa femelle l'embrasse, il l'embrasse à son tour,
> Et vivement épris d'une amour mutuelle,
> Elle se glisse en luy, & luy se fond en elle.
> Dans la claire matrice en tel accouplement
> Des deux spermes conjoints se fait premierement
> Une matiere informe, & comparable à celle
> Qu'entre les animaux Embrion l'on appelle.
> Cet Embrion s'anime, & s'en forme un enfant,
> Qui naist Roy, puis devient Monarque triomphant;
> ...
> Quoy qu'il ait merité que ce feu le moleste
> Comme insigne pecheur, qui comet double inceste,
> Abusant de sa mere & de sa propre soeur
> Quand il se perpetue, & cree un successeur.
> Vray est que de ce crime il fait bien penitence,
> Alors que de son sang expiant toute offence,
> Il substante & nourrit, comme les Pelicans,
> Ses freres, ses neveux, sa mere, & ses enfans. (C3–C4, pp. 37–9)

(But the King of Metals, unique in his nature, / Produces himself almost like a creature. / He has a female in whom he places all of his love, / His female embraces him, he embraces her in turn, / And strongly overtaken by mutual love, / She slips into him, and he dissolves into her. / In the bright womb, in such a coupling / Of two joined seeds an unformed material creates itself first, / And it is comparable to that which is called Embryo among the animals. / This Embryo brings itself to life, and forms an infant of itself, / Who is born King, and then becomes a triumphant Monarch; / ... Although he deserves to be ravaged by the fire / As an infamous sinner who commits double incest, / Abusing his mother and his own sister / When he perpetuates himself, and creates a successor. / It is true that he does penance for this crime, / So that with his blood, expiating any crime, / He sustains and nourishes, like Pelicans, / His brothers, his nephews, his mother, and his children.)

Here, human sacrifice and incest are related causally – the dissolution of familial identity leads to a dissolution of the self; both are the result of an absolute sexual union, recalling that of Salmacis and Hermaphroditus (Ovid, *Metamorphoses*, bk 4, lines 285–388), one that eliminates all distinction between self and other, and that reduces the self to an abject state. The King is torn to pieces, a further abjection of the body, in order to recreate distinction, that is, to extract that which is good (that is, desired). The incest and the resulting sacrifice are mentioned again, thus confirming the importance of these stages for the process (C8v, p. 48: "Phoebus l'a engendree, et Phoebé enfantee"):

> Car c'est nostre Arsenic, qui d'Art emerveillable
> Est arraché des reins du frere, et de la soeur,
> Par les ongles poignants de l'Aigle ravisseur. (*Poeme philosophic*, Dv, p. 50)

(For this is our Arsenic, which, with marvelous Art, / Is torn from the body of the brother and of the sister / By the sharp talons of the ravaging Eagle.)

In this insistence on the forbidden and sacrificial nature of the process, Nuysement echoes a vast alchemical tradition, one which draws on pagan rituals.

Master Dedalus: The Role of the Alchemist

He refines this tradition, however, by playing out the sacrificial images within a larger mythological context, drawing an analogy between Dedalus and the ideal hermaphrodite.[24] This passage also raises the issue of what is natural, in its depiction of the relationship between the alchemist and nature:

---

[24]   This analogy apparently is a caution to moderate the use of water and heat in the sublimation and fixation of Mercury.

Ces esprits transcendants ailleurs sont à priser,
Mais c'est vice en cet art de trop subtiliser;
Se voulant peindre en l'air maints succès impossibles,
Et frayer des sentiers en lieux inaccessibles.
Il faut par les raisons, & d'un jugement sain,
Considerant Nature imiter son dessain.
Fuyr les lieux ruyneux, & les voyes obliques
Où nous vont esgarant les labeurs sophistiques
Il faut marcher sans crainte au chemin naturel,
Aysé, commun, certain, droict, & continuel.
Enfin quittant Icare, il faut suivre Dedalle;
Vollant entre deux airs d'aelle toujours egalle.
Quoy qu'on puisse au labeur pere et fils appliquer,
Si l'on sçait bien leur fable au vray sens expliquer.
Dedalle est le corps double en son premier meslange,
Lors que la terre lourde en se dissolvant change
Sa nature grossiere, & monte en s'eslevant
Sur les aelles de l'eau, non de l'air ny du vent. (*Poeme philosophic*, D2, p. 51)

(These transcendent spirits should furthermore be cherished, / But it is a vice in this art to make things too subtle [to refine too much]; / Wishing to paint too many impossible successes in the air / And create paths to inaccessible places. / We must by means of reason, and a healthy judgment, / Contemplating Nature, imitate her design. / Flee ruinous places and indirect paths / Where sophistic labors go leading us astray / We must walk without fear on the path of Nature, / Calm, unremarkable, sure, straight, and unflagging. / Finally, leaving Icarus behind, we must follow Dedalus, / Flying between the two atmospheres with our wings always level. / Although one can use both father and son for the work, / If one knows how to explain the real meaning of their fable. / Dedalus is the double body in its first mixture, / As the heavy earth by dissolving itself changes / Its lowly Nature, and climbs by raising itself / On wings of water, not of air or wind.)

Icarus is portrayed as abandoning his body to the water, in his desire to rise too high above the corporeal (D2, p. 51); Dedalus represents the correct combination of body and spirit. One cannot be transformed without the other. Nuysement thus does not privilege one half of the *coniunctio* over the other, but creates a balance between the two opposites; this is the perfect hermaphroditic form, the "corps double." Dedalus also becomes the image of the alchemist himself at work, mediating between the physical and the spiritual realms; thus, with Jung, one must wonder whether (at least in this poem), the alchemist is not the matter of his own work, the hermaphroditic entity itself. Alchemy thus becomes a means for man to reconcile his corporeal and spiritual natures rather than abandoning the physical world for another life. Nuysement's alchemy does not deny the importance of the body, but makes it a necessary component of any transcendence.

A striking aspect of the rhetoric of the *Poeme philosophic*, is the insistent use of reflexive (pronominal) verbs, most frequently linked to the hermaphrodites and related figures or stages. These verbs suggest the self-contained nature of the process, and a freedom from external forces. Paradoxically, this freedom is punctuated by menacing, even violent, interventions such as burning or tearing, but after these periods of annihilation, the process begins again, like a phoenix rising from the ashes.

It should further be noted that Dedalus, in essence the servant of the King Minos in many mythological sources, is the master of the alchemical process, the one who creates the King. As is also suggested by the sacrificial role of the King in this process, power relations do not form a solid hierarchy in which control is wielded from the top. The King depends on his craftsman to make him, and in turn the craftsman's importance is validated by the creation of the King.

The Limits of Acceptable Transgression

In spite of the hermeticism of alchemical rhetoric, it must be admitted that even Nuysement's conjunction of opposites exudes contemporary cultural views of gender in its insistence on heterosexual union. Although some hierarchies may be effaced, others are maintained, particularly those linked to the condemnation of male homosexuality. In this, Nuysement work does not reflect attitudes at the court of Henri III, but rather those instilled by Catholic doctrine against homosexuality, attitudes that were "in the air" in that this doctrine was being used to ruin Henri's reputation in a large volume of scurrilous political propaganda published from his coronation in 1574 until his death, and particularly vehement in the late 1570s and early 1580s.

> Car j'ay mis Sol & Lune en liqueurs diaphanes,
> Et cuits avec Mercure à tres lente chaleur:
> Mais cet ingrat travail fut de mesme valeur;
> Nature veut Nature, & l'espece l'espece,
> Aborrant au congrez la semence diverse.
> Celuy ne peut pas rendre un pays bien peuplé
> Qui a masle avec masle au coït accouplé:
> Crime contre Nature, & faute abominable,
> Que tout le feu d'enfer d'expier n'est capable. (*Poeme philosophic*, D3, p. 53)

(For I have placed Sol and Luna in diaphanous liquors, / And cooked them with Mercury over very slow heat. / But this thankless work was of the same value; / Nature calls for Nature, and each species, its own species, / Abhorring the joining of diverse seed. / He cannot people a country well / Who joins male with male in sexual union; / A crime against Nature, and abominable error, / Which all the fire of hell is not capable of expiating.)

Apparently, Sol and Luna, brother and sister, are considered to be of the same "species," but it is the conjunction of the two "males," Mercury and Sol, that is considered criminal. Nuysement suggests that conjunction between representatives of the same sex is harmful, but incest is fruitful. Thus, alchemy excludes itself from the realm of some social taboos, but is governed by others. This is only explicable if Nuysement is focusing the work of alchemy on reproduction in accordance with the Aristotelian theory of generation, which was also accepted to some degree by Paracelsus. If the female contributes no seed, but does contribute the vessel necessary for that seed to grow, then one can see where the conjunction of two males might prove unproductive. The female, then, is seen as an extension of the male (his incubator, so to speak), rather than a separate being. So, in fact, Nuysement seems to revert to a rather conservative duality of male/female, spirit/body that belies his earlier discussion of Dedalus. Alchemy, as potentially subversive as it might seem in its privileging of the abject, nonetheless continues to inscribe itself in the traditional discourses of sexual difference. Perhaps in the context of Nuysement's own work, the crime of male homosexuality is that it does not offer a widely accepted code of behavior – as do heterosexual marriage, monarchy, and Catholic doctrine – that he can overturn. Homosexuality, itself already seen as subverting established order, cannot itself be subverted.

This continued oscillation between Aristotelian theories of generation and the more egalitarian Hippocratic view occurs with a fair degree of frequency in alchemical texts. The frequency with which these two opposing views meet would suggest that the tension between them is itself productive for understanding the alchemical process. Thus, the condemnation of homosexuality can be read in the context of Church teachings and state repression of homosexual practices,[25] but it can also be read as a warning against uniformity, in favor of difference. Alchemical texts were frequently coded in the terminology of acceptable Catholic doctrine, so that the author might avoid the charge of heresy. But this doctrine was almost always skewed, so that a straightforward reading is frustrated. This technique was also used by more mainstream authors such as Montaigne, and by surgeons such as Paré, particularly in his discussion of the existence of demons and sorcerers, which he infuses with skepticism, even as he cites Catholic doctrine. In a culture where practices of censorship sometimes included burning an author with his books, such "coding" or ambiguous writing, which seemed both to criticize and support Church doctrine, may have been a wise survival mechanism. But it must be noted that moderate Catholic humanists also developed highly complex forms of writing that allowed them to criticize Church practices even while accepting doctrine, in the mode of Erasmus.

The All-Engendering Hermaphrodite

Alchemical writing, then, is "hermaphroditic" in nature, often calling for two very different, even opposing, readings. In turn, the hermaphrodite becomes the archetypal

---

[25] Of which an account is given by Guy Poirier in his book, *L'homosexualité dans l'imaginaire de la Renaissance* (Paris: Champion, 1996), particularly in the chapters on "Les discours de la condamnation," pp. 23–73.

figure of the process, embodying the ambiguities and paradoxes that fuel the work. It should not be surprising, then – and this is most obvious in the works of Clovis Hesteau de Nuysement – that the hermaphrodite is linked to most of the other major figures of the alchemical process, such as the King, the self-devouring Euroboros, the crucial Mercury, and the Philosopher's Stone.

In confirming the hermaphroditic nature of Mercury, Nuysement links it once more to that primordial incest that creates the transcendent entity:

> Il faut trouver conjoincts d'un naturel lien
> Dans nostre vif argent le Soleil & la Lune.
> Non argent vif commun, Sol ny Lune commune,
> Mais ce couple jumeau que Jupin enflamé
> Au ventre virginal de Latone a formé. (*Poeme philosophic*, D4, p. 55)

> (One must find joined in a natural bond / In our quicksilver the Sun and the Moon. / Not common quicksilver, nor common sun nor moon, / But that twin couple that passionate Jove / Formed in the virginal womb of Latona ...)

Thus, it is redundant to unite Sol and Luna with Mercury, which already contains both natures. Nuysement's account of the hermaphrodite as that primordial Chaos from which all of creation was formed follows this discussion of difference and sameness. Confusion of different elements is the productive basis upon which all creation occurs; but the act of creation itself is a division, a clarification of these differences. This is reminiscent once more of the Gnostic belief that the feminine is the power, the masculine is the act; or the Lacanian belief that the woman is the phallus, the man has (or controls) the phallus; and further, that the man acts by means of language. This language is used to create difference through its expression (a notion especially evident in the works of Paracelsus); thus it seems that the concept of creation as purely an imposition of order is a masculine one (and also merely a rhetorical one). The value of this act is belied to some extent by the necessity of the feminine *materia* with which to work; a necessity belied in turn by the privileging of the act of division, of distinction by means of language in most cultures. This privileging is most evident in the vehement defense of laws, doctrines, and traditions that may not seem to have any evident basis in nature (for example, the Salic law prohibiting women from governing France; the tradition that women do not contribute anything significant to the generation of children; the doctrine of transubstantiation) but are so longstanding as to take on the appearance of "natural" laws. These laws are held to tenaciously in order to push back the chaos of nature, that which is uncontrolled by man, which seems to menace constantly.

But Nuysement, in his rewriting of Ovid's myth of the Hermaphrodite, seems to embrace this productive chaos even more than he praises orderly division. He commences this myth with an echo of the hermaphroditic, or even masculine, Venus (*Venus genitrix*):

Deesse engendre-amours, germeuse Citheree ...

...

Ta vertu genitrice espands egallement
Dans les reins amoureux de chacun element.
Comme au grand univers ta feconde influence
Par l'esprit general à tout donne naissance,

...

C'est pourquoy de ton nom nostre terre on appelle,
Car nostre Hermaphrodit est conceu & nay d'elle,
Apres qu'estant recuitte au bouillon de son eau,
De sa tombe funeste elle a fait son berceau.
Gentille Salmacis, que tu vis glorieuse
D'embrasser le subject de ta flame amoureuse,
Baignant un corps si noble & des membres si beaux,
Dans le flot cristallin de tes larmeuses eaux!
Honteux adolescent, ton heureuse infortune
Te rend en t'offençant cette gloire commune:
Soit que ton double sexe à ses flots s'unissant
Tu sois fait pour produire Agent ou Patissant!
Mais qui est le docteur tant subtil & tant sage
Qui prouvant par exemple ou monstrast par usage,
Qu'on puisse unir deux corps, de centres si divers
Que l'un aspire au Ciel, l'autre aspire aux enfers,
Qu'en muant leur Nature, & changeant leur substance? (*Poeme philosophic*, D5v–D6,
pp. 58–9)

(Goddess who begets love, seed-filled Cythera ... / Your generating power spreads
equally / In the amorous bodies of each element. / Just as, in the great universe, your
fecund influence / Gives birth through the spirit which is in everything, ... / That is why
we call our earth by your name, / Because our Hermaphrodite is conceived and born of
her, / After having been cooked in the broth of her own water, / Of her funereal tomb
she has made a cradle. / Gentle Salmacis, that you might live triumphant / To embrace
the cause of your amorous flame, / Bathing such a noble body and such beautiful limbs
/ In the crystal flood of your tearlike waters! / Shameful youth, your happy misfortune
/ In compromising you, restores you to this conjoined glory, / May your double sex in
being united to these waters, / Allow you to create either by acting or submitting [in
the male or female role] / But who is the expert so subtle and so wise / Who, proving
by example or demonstrating by custom, / That one might unite two bodies, of such
different origins, / That one aspires to the Heavens, while the other aspires to Hell, /
Only by transforming their nature, and changing their substance?)

From the all-engendering Venus comes the independently engendering Hermaphrodite,
a self-sufficient entity that is empowered by its dissolution. According to the *Traittez
du vray sel*, Hermaphroditus is the Philosophers' Mercury which purifies all that with
which it comes into contact; and he and Salmacis are none other than Sol and Luna
conjoined. In this version of the Ovidian myth, Nuysement wrestles with the problem

of difference: how can these two bodies be joined without dissolving into each other? How can they remain different, and yet in harmony? At this point, he does not seem to accept the Ovidian version, which calls for the disappearance of Salmacis and the diminution of Hermaphroditus. Yet he has not returned to the ancient fertility gods or the Aristophanic androgyne, which maintained two natures in one being, both of which created a supernaturally powerful entity.

Alchemy: Dissidence Triumphant

Nuysement still speaks of the union of "l'esprit agille au corps lourd & stupide" (D6, p. 59: "the agile spirit with the heavy and stupid body"), of cold with hot, of dry with humid. The discord in these conjunctions must be minimized. The potential political subtext of this treatise seems to come into evidence here:

> Et tous vivent en paix en se faisant la guerre.
> Voyla comme ces corps miraculeusement
> Se changeant changent tout, & vont tout reformant. (*Poeme philosophic*, D6v, p. 60)

> (And all live in peace, while warring with each other. / Behold how this body miraculously / Changes everything by changing itself, and reforms everything.)

The notion of *reformation* is particularly charged in the late sixteenth and early seventeenth centuries; one wonders if Nuysement is trying to create an alternative alchemical world, a utopia in which differences rest in suspension, neither resolved nor eradicated. He evidently has trouble conceptualizing such an unknown realm, since he returns repeatedly to images of hierarchy, of male or spiritual superiority over the female/body. Nonetheless, the fact that he has already modified Paracelsian hierarchies and formulae, even in confused or inconsistent fashion, suggests the potentially subversive nature of the alchemical process. This subversion, it must be recognized, is not actualized on the level of gender roles, but on the level of religious controversy, and only in a subdued fashion. The images of fire suggest Protestant sympathies, above all in Nuysement's Apocalyptic visions:

> Lors que des bienheureux les glorieuses ames
> Prendront leurs corps purgez par le Ciment des flames. (*Poeme philosophic*, D7, p. 61)

> (As the glorious souls of the blessed / Take up their bodies, purged by the mortar of flames.)

Only in alchemy, or in Huguenot lore, could burnt bodies be resuscitated gloriously. The once destructive flames now bind the bodies back together. And in fact, the concluding pages of the *Poeme philosophic*, overtly inscribe alchemy in the domain of Christianity (Paracelsus frequently does so, as well, although in a more mechanical, and less visionary, fashion), first comparing the "twin couple," Sol and Luna, with the males and females paired on the Ark (D7, p. 61); then comparing the conjunction of Sol and Luna with the descent of Christ into the body of the Virgin Mary and his ascent to Heaven (D8v, pp. 64 seq.). The alchemist daringly compares himself to Christ, but notes that he will be divided when his soul rises and his body remains on earth. In the end, the spirit will again unite body and soul. As Jung suggests, alchemy is an allegory of sorts for spiritual and psychological processes of growth. This is abundantly clear in Nuysement's poem, which seems to read alchemy backwards, using the processes to mirror and explain humanity's struggle for self-definition (which he also compares to Theseus's combat with the Minotaur (Ev–E2, pp. 66–7). The battle is with the chaotic, bodily self, which resists control, which defies definition; which must be tamed but not destroyed. Similarly, Nuysement inscribes the tales of Hercules's labors within the alchemical system. His treatise/poem ends on a menacing note, threatening all those who doubt with torments and destruction. Yet it is difficult to know what one is expected to believe, since Nuysement shuttles back and forth, from one system to another, trying to express a concept which he is too rooted in his own culture to comprehend. One senses the presence of a mind trying to reach beyond the limitations of its own culture, into the past, into the distance, into the other. Nuysement's success is limited, since he is restricted by the images his own culture has granted him; but the struggle itself is instructive, as it demonstrates how untenable that limited culture had become in the presence of those who were radically other (Huguenots, women, natives of the Western Hemisphere). Nuysement is trying to make the struggle against the other (Theseus's battle against the Minotaur) into a harmonic conjunction which does not threaten the self. He does not seem to succeed, but the struggle itself is significant.

Clearly for Nuysement, the interaction between the individual and the process is the fundamental aspect of alchemical thought; unlike Paracelsus, he offers no workable recipes, no clear formulae. The conclusion of the *Poeme philosophic* is almost a spell to ward off evil thinkers and doubters, to silence and petrify them:

Empruntez de Pallas l'effroyable bouclier,
D'où l'horrible Gorgonne eslançant maint esclair
De ses gros yeux fataux empierre l'ignorance,
Qui d'un dart espointé combat cette science.
Et conseillez à ceux qui blasment tel secrets,
D'estre un peu plus sçavants, ou beaucoup plus discrets. (*Poeme philosophic*, E4, p. 71)

(Borrow her terrifying breastplate [the aegis] from Pallas, / From which the horrible Gorgon, throwing many a lightning-bolt, / With her huge, fatal eyes turns ignorance into stone, / Which battles this science with pointed darts, / And counsel those who criticize such secrets / To be a little more knowledgeable, or much more discreet.)

The alchemist thus excludes, repulses, expels those who mock his science; that is, those who would expel him. He thus reverses the usual role of abjection, which is to enforce cultural norms disguised as natural laws. That which is supernatural, unnatural, or monstrous chases away the "natural," and establishes its own transcendence. Nuysement thus creates a bizarre mirror world of Western culture (as is evident in his frequent use of Greek and Roman mythology), one that seems to call that culture into question, and at times to offer a different version that reflects critically on Western norms. The reader may sense already in this text the subversive potential of the hermaphroditic figure, which if triumphant, would redefine the "normal" in its own terms.

Chapter 6

Lyric Hermaphrodites

Sexual Politics

Poets of the court of Henri III of France were surrounded by alchemists, and often practiced alchemy themselves. They then adopted the images of alchemy, the evocative and obscure metaphors of the Art, to their more worldly verses. These verses seem primarily concerned with the mutable sexuality of the alchemical process, and with the sacrificial nature of the hermaphrodite. Such interests are reflected in both of the poetic traditions that dominate the Court: the Petrarchan lyric, in which gender roles are frequently reversed and in which the poet sacrifices himself or is brutally sacrificed for his love; and political poetry, in which the unstable nature of power and the violent clashes of the Wars of Religion are depicted. Needless to say, these two traditions often overlapped, and were supplemented by many others, such as the Neoplatonic tradition, in which the image of the hermaphrodite links sexuality with power.

In many of these poems, difference, particularly sexual difference (and most of all intersexuality in the forms of hermaphrodism and transvestism) is at once celebrated and violently repressed. This combination of destruction and creation of new forms is typical of alchemical processes; but in court poetry, this combination takes on a more negative aspect, perhaps in response to the chaos dominating France at this time. In alchemy, destruction inevitably leads to renewal; in the lyric poetry, this renewal is viewed with skepticism. This new twist on an old tradition prepares the way for extremely negative uses of the figure of the hermaphrodite in political propaganda, a move which signals a return to more conservative attitudes towards sexual difference, and a rejection of many of the medical discoveries and innovations of the time.

Thus, the interests of courtiers and intellectuals in late sixteenth-century France led away from the Platonic and Neoplatonic models of ideal hermaphrodism to a more skeptical view of the problems of gender, and the confusion that can arise from cases of ambiguous sex. Rather than attempting to explain the fusion of two sexes as an allegory of spiritual perfection, as earlier poets such as Barthélémy Aneau, Pierre de Ronsard, and Louise Labé did, poets of the court of Henri III (and later) were fascinated with this confusion for its own sake, as a sort of intellectual puzzle which did not necessarily point to God's wisdom.

The Problematic Body: D'Aubigné's Androgyne

Théodore Agrippa d'Aubigné, sometimes on the margins of court society, sometimes at the center, but never fully accepting of court mentalities, fuses Neoplatonic and alchemical thought in much of his work. This mixture creates an unusual oscillation between portrayals of sexual difference which conform to the predominant social standards, and occasional subversions of those very same standards. This problematic dualism echoes that of the hermaphrodite, which is forced to conform to the social norms of male *or* female, but which also calls those norms into question. But it also echoes d'Aubigné's own relationship to the society in which he lived, and in which he was expected to be *either* Catholic *or* Calvinist, even if he could not perfectly conform to either role (the Genevan Calvanists asked him to leave the city because of his literary salons). His intersection with both cultures may have facilitated his ability to combine disparate philosophies in his own work.

The most complete expression of the conflation of spiritual and heterosexual union, one that initially confirms the traditional binaries of male/female, spiritual/corporeal, superior/inferior, and therefore the hierarchized notions of gender that operated in sixteenth-century French society, is to be found in his *Printemps*, a collection of love poetry. The seventeenth *Stance* ("Mesurent des haultz Cieux tant de bizarres courses") elaborates at some length upon the Aristophanic/Platonic myth of the Androgyne:

> Ceste perfection fut la mesme Androgene
> Qui surpassa l'humain par ses divins effortz,
> Quant le cors avecq' l'ame et l'ame avecq' son cors
> Vit l'essence divine unie avecq' l'humaine.
> Le terrestre pesant n'engageoit de son pois
> Le feu de son esprit à sa rude nature,
> Mais ces deux unions en mesme creature
> Souffroient de l'un' à l'autre et l'amour et les loix. (*Stances*, 17, ll. 21–8)[1]

> (This perfection was the same Androgyne / Which surpassed the human by his divine efforts, / when the body with the soul and the soul with the body / Saw divine essence united with the human. The heavenly, earthly one did not weigh down / The fire of his spirit by his rough nature. / But these two united in the same creature / Bore one another's love and laws.)

In his version of the Aristophanic myth, d'Aubigné portrays the divinity as cutting the spirit off from the body. When the two are perfectly joined by means of the soul, then man is a demigod:

> L'ame est l'esprit uni avecq le cors femelle,
> Dont l'homme le premier esprouvant l'union

---

[1]   From *Le Printemps: Stances et Odes*, ed. Eugénie Droz (Geneva: Droz, 1973), pp. 44–53.

Estoit homme plus qu'homme et sa perfection
Par l'acord de ses deux fut supernaturelle. (*Stances*, 17, ll. 41–4)

(The soul is the spirit joined with the female body, / Thus the first man, experiencing this union / Was more than a man and his perfection / Surpassed nature by the joining of these two.)

Divided, living in discord with himself, man is powerless and pitiful (ll. 51–3).

In this *Stance*, d'Aubigné conflates Diotima's story of the origins of love with the myth of the Androgyne by comparing Penia with the body, Poros with the spirit, as well as by calling Eros "l'autre Androgene" (l. 80). Although the body is given a somewhat subordinate role in this tale, d'Aubigné also emphasizes the spirit's critical need of the body in order to function, thus echoing the alchemical notions circulating in the French court at the time (most likely the 1580s). The spirit gives its intellectual gifts to the body, and in return the body offers the medium of the five senses to aid the intellectual processes:

Elle ne peut gouster ny les os, ny les restes
Du nectar de l'esprit ...

...

L'esprit fait tout divin est emeu à pitié,
Se couple avecq' le cors, et en ce mariage
Donne prevoir, juger, et souvenir pour gage
De l'union du cors et de son amitié;
Le cors loge les trois ...

L'esprit apprend au cors les ars et les sciences
De nature et d'acquis, et fidelle amoureux
Preserve sa femelle et des fers et des feuz,
Par l'aigu jugment et les experiences.
Commant pourroit ainsi ce mari sans son cors
Exercer sa vertu, car sans sa bien aimée,
Les effetz ne seroient qu'une ombre, une fumée,
Sans execution, sans oeuvres, sans effortz?
L'esprit, peintre parfait, emprunte la painture,
Les tableaux, les pinceaux des cinq sens de nature. (*Stances*, 17, ll. 91–110)

(She cannot taste the bones, nor the remains / Of the nectar of the spirit ... / The completely divine spirit is moved to pity, / He couples with the body, and in this marriage / Gives foresight, judgment, and memory as a token / Of the union with the body and of his friendship; The body holds all three ... / The spirit teaches the body the arts and sciences / Of nature and of culture, and faithful lover / He protects his female from swords and from fire, / By his keen judgment and his experience. / How could this husband practice his virtue (power) without / His body, for without his beloved, / The effects would only be shadow and smoke, / Without completion, without works, without effort? / The spirit, perfect artist, borrows the paint, / The canvas, and the brushes from the five senses of nature.)

D'Aubigné seems to remain within the traditional Neoplatonic hierarchy that privileges the spirit over the body; nonetheless, he also gives evidence of a sort of skeptical crisis reminiscent of Sextus Empiricus's rejection of indicative signs. Sextus denies that the existence of the soul can be deduced from the movements of the body: "An indicative sign, they say, is that which is not clearly associated with the thing signified, but signifies that whereof it is a sign by its own particular nature and constitution, just as, for instance, the bodily motions are signs of the soul."[2] Sextus continues by suggesting that the indicative sign does not exist as such, and that which is non-evident, for example the soul, cannot be represented by that which is apparent, the body.[3] Being a Pyrrhonian skeptic, he presents this argument mostly as a series of questions. This questioning of the possibility of representing and perceiving non-evident or invisible things by means of visible signs has profound implications for Christian culture in the sixteenth century, and is linked to the rise of atheism in early seventeenth-century France.

D'Aubigné does not go quite as far as Sextus in his argument, but points out that the spirit would be ineffectual and invisible without the body as the canvas, paint, and brush to render it. One wonders if the spirit in fact exists without the body through which it manifests itself. This conflict between the perception of the necessity of representation for existence itself, and the apparent imperfection of this representation, destabilizes at least to some extent the Neoplatonic hierarchy of spirit over body. Thus, d'Aubigné is turning away from the notion of gender as an accepted hierarchical norm, to that of gender as an identity created at once by and upon the body.

D'Aubigné devotes the rest of this poetic treatise to the question of sexual union: "nostre amour naturelle," which he portrays as indistinguishable from spiritual union:

... l'amour des cors endure
Mesme cause que l'autre et mesme liaison:
Il brusle l'un et l'autre et de pareilles flammes
Unit l'amour des cors et celuy de noz ames. (*Stances*, 17, ll. 117–20)

(Bodily love suffers / The same cause as the other and the same ties: / Both burn, and similar flames / Unite corporeal love with that of our souls.)

D'Aubigné echoes at this point the alchemical belief in putrefaction as both degradation and apotheosis of the body, in a manner that may well have inspired Baudelaire:

---

2   Sextus Empiricus, "Concerning Sign," *Outlines of Pyrrhonism*, trans. R.G. Bury (Cambridge, MA: Harvard University Press, Loeb Classical Library, 1976), bk 2, ch. 10, pp. 213–17.

3   Chapter 11, "Does an Indicative Sign Exist?," pp. 217–37.

Comme le soleil chaud r'engrege les odeurs
D'une charogne infecte et en forme la peste,
Et de mesme raion le mesme nous apreste
En sa bonté le much et le baume et les fleurs:
L'amour allume ainsi en nos espritz les flammes,
Certains eschantillons et mirouers de nos ames. (*Stances*, 17, ll. 125–30)

(As the hot sun increases the odors / Of a putrid corpse and makes a plague of it, / And from the same ray the sun gives us / In its goodness moss, sweet-smelling plants, and flowers: / Love lights thus in our spirits the flames, / Sure signs and mirrors of our souls.)

For all the hints of the more revolutionary alchemical process, however, d'Aubigné remains within the bounds of a very traditional discourse of love. It may be a measure of the degree of late sixteenth-century misogyny that he reverses the usual lyric roles of superior woman and inferior man, to impose a more Aristotelian view of gender roles in love:

Tout ainsi que l'amour unist la difference
De cors et de l'esprit, c'est luy tout seul qui peult
Unir deux autres cors en un seul, quant il veult,
Lors que des deux espritz il tire sa naissance.
Par l'homme et son esprit Pore est representé
Où l'amour a premier sa naissance et sa vie,
Puis l'ame de la femme est la pauvre Penie
Qui surprend nostre esprit yvre d'une beauté:
C'est le troisieme sens, et l'amour corporelle
En cela suit les loix de la spirituelle. (*Stances*, 17, ll. 131–40)

(Just as love unites the difference / Of body and soul, it is he alone who can / Unite two other bodies in one, when he wishes, / When from two spirits he is born. / Plenty (Poros) is represented by man and his spirit / Where love first was born and brought to life. / Then the soul of the woman is poor Poverty (Penia) / Who surprises our spirit, drunk with beauty: / This is the third sense, and corporeal love / Follows the laws of spiritual love in this.)

The body/spirit analogy is used to define the relationship between men and women; but here, the importance of women for the relationship is suppressed, whereas previously in this poetic treatise, d'Aubigné recognized the impossibility of expression of spiritual love without the mediation of the body. Man is Poros, spiritually complete; woman is Penia, destitute of the very qualities that illuminate Poros. Nevertheless, sympathy must exist for love to be born, and this sympathy must exist in the body as well as the soul. The following stanzas suggest a complicity between body and spirit in the creation of love (ll. 151–70); this would seem to imply a similar complicity or agreement between the woman (/body) and the man (/spirit). Yet the spirit is designated as "plus parfait," not deigning to enter into union with the body except when it is unconscious. Thus it is the woman who lulls the man into love:

> La femme ...
> Endort l'esprit de l'homme aux raions de son oeil.
>
> ...
>
> L'homme est fait amoureux et par l'oysiveté
> Il s'acommode aux meurs de la femelle aymée.
> Comme l'ame se voit par le cors transformée
> Espouser son humeur, voulloir sa volunté ... (*Stances*, 17, ll. 181–8)

> (The woman ... / Lulls the spirit of man to sleep with the rays of her eye. / The man falls in love and by idleness / He changes to suit the habits of the woman he loves. / So the soul sees itself transformed by the body / Marrying her moods, wishing what she wishes ...)

Ironically, the "perfect" male/spirit is entirely dominated by the female/body, which has somehow become the active principle; and thus, the misogynistic argument confounds itself by arguing too much. The inferior feminine principle is solely "responsible" for love; the superior male principle remains passive.

In his discussion of the "humours" of love, d'Aubigné reverses his earlier insistence on the importance of the body, to insist that perfection lies in that which is the least corporeal:

> L'esprit qui a un cors vif, subtil et ignée,
> Qui sent moins la terre et qui est moins pesant,
> Sent cest organe beau, agreable et plaisant,
> Et jamais de ses deux l'amour n'est terminée.
> Mais l'esprit qui se loge en un cors froid et lent
> N'aime qu'avec long temps sa nature perverse. (*Stances*, 17, ll. 191–6)

> (The spirit which has a lively, refined, and fiery body, / Which seems less earthly and is less heavy, / Feels this instrument to be beautiful, agreeable, and pleasant, / And the love of these two never ends. / But the spirit which is housed in a cold and slow body / Loves only after a long time this perverse nature.)

Cold, earthly humours are not conducive to love; that which is least material is most loving. This seems to contradict the previous assertion that it is primarily the corporeal female who is responsible for love. The spirit, then, is responsible for creating the proper environment for love:

> Il faut ainsi souvent que l'esprit du feu face
> Avant bien posseder son cors sortir la glace. (*Stances*, 17, ll. 219–20)

> (So the spirit must often use its fire to make the ice / Depart, before it can truly possess the body.)

Just so, the man must court the woman, and induce her into love; after, of course, she has lulled him into love:

> Ainsi l'homme amoureux, vrai esprit de la femme
>
> …
>
> Comme souvent les cors mesprisent les espritz,
> Les hommes sont ainsi reffusé par les dames … (*Stances*, 17, ll. 221; 235–6)

> (So the loving man, the true spirit of the woman / … As often the body disdains the spirit, / Men are often refused by ladies.)

As in much of Petrarchan poetry, the relationship between male and female seems to be a struggle for power. When this struggle is presented as being between spirit and body, a certain Manichean element arises. But d'Aubigné seems to want to reconcile this struggle, and presents the importance of this union as a matter of life or death. This could be a matter of simple seduction, or a reflection of the murderous divisions present in France at the time:

> … le corps sans esprit, la dame sans amy
> N'ont ne plaisir ne vie ou vivent à demy.
> Pas un d'eux separé n'a ne forme, ne estre. (*Stances*, 17, ll. 232–4)

> (The body without spirit, the lady without a lover, / Have no pleasure or life, or only half live. Neither one of them has form or being when separated from the other.)

The Petrarchan male lover's suffering and loss from lack of love is projected onto the female object of love. Yet it is also implied that neither half can even exist without the other. D'Aubigné seems to imply that the body without spirit, the woman without man, is lifeless and empty:

> Que l'ame vit encor quant le cors s'en delogne,
> Et que le corps n'est rien sans ame que charogne. (*Stances*, 17, ll. 239–40)

> (That the soul still lives when the body is taken away, / And the body without the soul is nothing but a carcass.)

In fact, the image is one of a decaying corpse "charogne," thus linking the female/ body to alchemical notions of putrefaction and impurity. Whereas putrefaction is a productive and important part of the alchemical process, here, the *Stance* portrays it as leading nowhere, as death without rebirth, even though previously the decaying corpse was seen as giving life.

D'Aubigné betrays his championing of the spirit towards the close of his poetic treatise, as he again hints at the significance of the corporeal:

> Sans la conjonction leur amour est donc vaine,
> Leurs effectz separez sont songes impuissans,
> Mais eux unis, de l'un et l'autre joïssans,
> Font germer en s'aymant leur amour et leur peine. (*Stances*, 17, ll. 241–4)

> (Without conjunction their love is thus empty, / Their strengths when separated are
> powerless dreams, / But when they are united, enjoying each other, / They make their
> love and trouble grow, loving each other.)

The use of the word "conjonction," which designates the crucial union of male and
female principles in the alchemical process, returns the argument to a more hermetic
context. In this process, the male element is useless without the female. D'Aubigné
ends the poem on this note of interdependence, even if he still attempts to champion
the superiority of the spirit:

> Si noz espritz qui ont prins au Ciel leur naissance
> Sont rien sans leur moitié, faitz mortz et impuissans,
> Que sera il des cors mortelz et perissans
> Sans amour, qui ont prins de l'autre amour substance … (*Stances*, 17, ll. 251–4)

> (If our spirits, which were born in Heaven / Are nothing without their other half, dead
> and powerless, / What will be the fate of mortal bodies, dying / Without love, which
> had taken sustenance from the other love.)

The poet repeats the word "conjonction," thus affirming his return to alchemical
vocabulary. He also asserts that love without this union is an "avorton," an aborted
thing. Thus, as in alchemy, the purpose of this conjunction is the creation of a third
element. The obsessive point of the poem is the union of male and female, particularly
of the lover with his "Belle." The inordinate desire for this union underscores the often
denied importance of the corporeal, at the expense of the spiritual, which apparently
seems insufficient to the poet:

> L'inutille regard d'une vaine beauté
> N'est qu'une pure mort, sans unir l'androgene.
> Imitons les secretz de Nature et ses loix
> …
> Car la desunion est la mort de Penie,
> L'acord la ressucite et luy donne la vie. (*Stances*, 17, ll. 263–70)

> (The useless gaze of empty beauty / Is only pure death, without uniting the Androgyne
> / Let us imitate the secrets of Nature and her laws. / … Because separation is the death
> of Penia, / Union revives her and gives her life.)

The poet has placed himself in the rather awkward role of suppliant to a woman
whose own neediness he uses as the excuse for his supplication. He is clearly the one

demanding physical union, which grants a certain degree of power to her; but he claims that she needs this union as well. The orderly hierarchy of male over female, spirit over body is somewhat destabilized by this obviously factitious argument. As in alchemy, power becomes an unstable element in the process, as it shifts from male to female, and back again. This fluidity, which creates the possibility of movement and change in the alchemical process, seems less productive in the context of this *Stance*.

Spurious argumentation notwithstanding, by means of the insistence on physical plenitude and conjunction, d'Aubigné makes his supposedly spiritual Androgyne approach the realm of the very corporeal hermaphrodite. In this melding of spiritual and corporeal, he approaches the spirit of the Aristophanic original, although not with quite the same understanding of the comic possibilities that the original evinced. D'Aubigné also brings the sensual nature of his Androgyne into the domain of alchemy; where, too, the corporeal and the spiritual are closely and problematically linked. His work is clearly of a transitional nature, in that he cannot free himself of the traditional hierarchies that inform French thought about sexuality, yet he cannot entirely abandon his sense of the importance of the physical, the female. Like many of the alchemists and medical researchers of his time, d'Aubigné cannot free himself completely from the system within which he lives, yet he cannot simply accept that system, either. This *Stance* is also significant as one of the earliest examples of the incorporation of alchemical imagery and philosophy into the Petrarchan tradition of love poetry. Many other examples of the alchemical lyric will appear in the court of Henri III of France.

Gender Blending: The Work of Philippe Desportes

This court, with which d'Aubigné was familiar, was the site of poetic explorations into the ambiguities of gender, either subtle or overt in nature. Philippe Desportes, eventually Henri's official court poet, wrote a collection entitled "Les Amours d'Hippolyte," containing numerous allusions to the Amazon warrior; for example, sonnet 40 ("Quand premier Hippolyte eut sur moy la victoire," "When first Hippolyta had her victory over me") and sonnet 50 ("Bien souvent Hippolyte à grand tort courroucée / Arme son coeur de glace ... Elle qui fait trophée et d'Amour et de Mars, / Dedaigne une despouille à ses pieds renversée," "Often Hippolyta, wrongly angered / Arms her heart with ice ... She who took Love and Mars as her trophies, / Disdains the spoils thrown at her feet.").[4] Most open, however, is his comparison of Henri, then Duke of Anjou, to the transvestite Achilles:

> Lors que le preux Achille estoit entre les dames,
> D'un habit feminin deguisé finement,

---

4   Philippe Desportes, *Les Amours d'Hippolyte*, ed. Victor Graham (Geneva: Droz, 1960), pp. 85 and 99.

Sa douceur agreable en cêt accoustrement
Allumoit dans les coeurs mille amoureuses flames,
En voyant ses attraits, sa façon naturelle,
Les beaux lys de son teint, son parler gracieux,
Les roses de sa joue, et l'esclair de ses yeux,
On ne l'estimoit pas autre qu'une pucelle.
Mais, bien qu'il surpassast la plus parfait image,
Qu'il eust la grace douce et le visage beau,
Le teint frais et douillet, delicate la peau,
Il cachoit au dedans un genereux courage,
Dont il rendit depuis mille preuves certaines,
Faisant sur les Troyens les siens victorieux,
Et s'acquist tel renom par ses faits glorieux,
Qu'il offusqua l'honneur des plus vieux capitaines.
Ainsi ceste beauté qu'on voit en vous reluire
Vous faict comme celeste à bon droict admirer;
Amour dedans vos yeux s'est venu retirer,
Et de là droit aux coeurs mille fleches il tire.
Mais, bien que vous ayez une douceur naisve,
Et que rien de si beau n'apparoisse que vous,
Que vos yeux soyent rians, vostre visage doux,
Vous avez au dedans une ame ardente et vive.
Et serez comme Achille au milieu des allarmes,
Foudroyant les plus forts, tuant et renversant;
Et, tout ainsi qu'un ours se fait voye en passant,
Vous passerez par tout par la force des armes.
Heureux en qui le ciel ces deux thresors assemble,
Qu'il ait la face belle, et le coeur genereux!
Vous, l'honneur plus parfait des guerriers amoureux,
Nous faites voir encor Mars et Venus ensemble.[5]

(When the brave Achilles was among the ladies, / Cleverly disguised in women's clothes, / His agreeable sweetness in this dress / Lit a thousand amorous flames in hearts. / Seeing his attractive features, his natural manner, / The beautiful lilies of his skin, his gracious speech, / The roses of his cheek, and the light of his eyes, / They thought him only a maiden. / But, although he surpassed the most perfect image, / Although he had sweet grace and a beautiful face, / A fresh, soft complexion, delicate skin, / He hid within himself a magnanimous courage, / Of which he offered a thousand certain proofs since then, / Making his men victorious over the Trojans, / And acquired such fame by his glorious deeds, / That he obscured the honor of the oldest captains. / So this beauty that we see glow in you / Makes you rightly admired as divine; / Love has come to hide in your eyes, / And from there he shoots a thousand arrows at others' hearts. / But, although you have an innocent sweetness, / And nothing seems as beautiful as

---

5   Philippe Desportes, "Pour Monseigneur le Duc d'Anjou," *Cartels et masquarades. Epitaphes*, ed. Victor Graham (Geneva: Droz, 1958), pp. 30–31.

you, / Although your eyes are laughing, your face kind, / You have inside a burning and lively soul. / And you will be like Achilles in the midst of battle, / Striking down the strongest, killing them and throwing them down; / And just as a bear clears a path wherever he is passing, / You will go everywhere by the strength of your weapons. / Happy is he in whom Heaven joins these two treasures, / May he have a handsome face, and a magnanimous heart! / You, the most perfect honor of warriors in love, / You make us see Mars and Venus together again.)

Desportes plays with ambiguity of gender on three levels: that of dress, of disguising the male as female; that of sexuality, whether heterosexuality, homosexuality, or bisexuality; that of the body, which seems at once male and female. He begins astutely with the most outward signs of gender, that of dress. Achilles's youth allows him to pass as female, when in feminine attire. Rather than condemning such ambiguity, as the rigid gender roles operating in late sixteenth-century law and philosophy might demand, Desportes describes this disguise as "fine" ("deguisé finement"). He emphasizes the feminine physical traits with sensuous detail ("Les beaux lys de son teint," "Les roses de sa joue," "Le teint frais et douillet, delicate la peau"), and lingers over this description of the seeming "pucelle." He also underscores the seemingly gratifying response to this ambiguity, that is, the love that this beautiful "girl" inspires. Desportes does not make clear the nature of that love. Disguised as a girl, Achilles did father Pyrrhus by Deidameia.[6] But the "mille amoureuses flames" might well include the male gaze, given the circumstances. Desportes' refusal to specify the nature of the love elicited by the boy's girlish good looks leaves open either or both possibilities of male and female admirers.

The "image" of feminine traits covers that which is portrayed as a stereotypically masculine personality, "un genereux courage." Achilles' honor is emphasized, and the Duke's violent bravery is described: "tuant et renversant … Vous passerez par tout par la force des armes." Yet "Amour" has also retreated to some space within the Prince, and "de là droit aux coeurs mille fleches il tire." The destructive force of the feminine principle of love is conjoined with that of war; thus, Venus and Mars cohabit in the Duke's person, with some confusion between the two, as if they are neither entirely the same nor distinct.

Perhaps in order to make the comparison with Achilles even more favorable to Henri in the context of French militarism, Desportes makes the contrast between Henri's "innocent sweetness" ("douceur naisve"), even repeating the word "doux" later in the poem, and his aggressive qualities as clear and striking as possible. Although the first seven lines of his description of Henri do contain some violence, as Love shoots a thousand arrows out of his eyes, they convey a lulling sense of beauty and sweetness that is shattered by the force of the next five lines. The image of Henri as lightning striking down his enemies grants him the divine power hinted at earlier. This power makes him superior to Achilles, in that his lightning-like force links him

---

6   Robert Graves, *The Greek Myths*, vol. 2 (Harmondsworth: Penguin, 1957), p. 160j.

to Jupiter. The comparison to a bear clearing its own way is a less refined, but more vivid and menacing image of brutish violence. The problem with the poem is that the conceit of Venus and Mars combined in one person undermines the masculinizing force of these vivid images, and destroys the otherwise effective contrast between Henri's loving nature and his capacity for powerful action. It is as if Desportes has enacted poetically the emasculation of Hermaphroditus by means of his union with Salmacis, and the poem, once powerful, becomes precious.

This conjunction of Venus and Mars creates a new version of the hermaphrodite, one that becomes significant in later representations of Henri III and his followers, the *mignons*. Although this poem is couched in the most servile terms of praise ("l'honneur plus parfait des guerriers amoureux"), these terms are used in later political doggerel (see chapter seven, below) to hint at or openly mock Henri's perceived homosexuality or bisexuality. It is clear from this satirical response to the Venus/Mars conjunction, that Desportes was working with concepts and imagery that many found offensive or deviant. His poem was not merely read as overly effusive praise, but as something more problematic still, as a declaration of the beauty of ambiguity. It is fairly easy to see from this poem why Henri's own program of mythological propaganda might have failed. His court poets seem to have a sensibility that is completely out of touch with popular demands for clear distinctions between men and women, Protestants and Catholics, foreigners and Frenchmen. Ambiguity does not play well in times of war, except as the target of harsh criticism.

The phoenix, used by Desportes as the symbol of poetic creation and linked in alchemical treatises to the hermaphrodite, may be another figuration of this ambiguity or duality. Like the hermaphrodite (particularly the hermaphroditic Venus), the phoenix is portrayed as self-engendering:

> ...
> Naist l'oyseau merveilleux, dont nous sommes nommez,
> Miracle de nature, et son plus bel ouvrage.
> L'or, le pourpre et l'azur s'eclate en son pennage;
> Il s'engendre soy-mesme, et presque en un moment
> Se sent vivre au berceau qui fut son monument;
> Car lors qu'il a passé dix siècles de sa vie,
> ...
> Et couché sur le haut d'un palmier odorant
> S'offre, heureuse victime, à la flame celeste,
> Pour renaistre plus beau de sa cendre qui reste. (ll. 4–14)[7]

(The marvelous bird is born, for which we are named, / Miracle of nature, and her most beautiful work. / Gold, purple, and azure burst forth in its wings; / He gives birth to himself, and in almost a moment / Feels himself come to life in the cradle that was

---

7   Philippe Desportes, *Cartels et masquarades*, "Pour les Chevaliers du Phenix."

his tombstone; / For, once he has lived for ten centuries, / ... Lying at the summit of a sweet-smelling palm tree / He offers himself, happy victim, to the divine flame, / To be born again, more beautiful, from the ashes which remain.)

Like the alchemical hermaphrodite, Desportes' phoenix is refined and reborn through the process of burning, and thus becomes the charged image of life after death achieved through martyrdom: "je renais de ma cendre" (*Les Amours de Diane*, vol. 2, sonnet 15, p. 217).[8] This self-generating process of triumph over death is also circular: "je retourne en ma forme premiere" (*Les Amours de Diane*, vol. 1, sonnet 37, p. 78). This self-sufficiency, this power of self-engendering, while admirable in the phoenix, is most often considered a threatening quality in the hermaphrodite. Self-sufficiency potentially excludes the hermaphrodite from the social structures of marriage and family considered necessary for reproduction. Given that these structures were considered basic to both society more generally and to political structures, self-sufficiency thus becomes menacing. The phoenix, on the other hand, evolves into a consolatory figure, more like the alchemical hermaphrodite, symbolizing life after death and rebirth out of destruction.

Love is compared to the phoenix in its self-regenerating nature: "L'Amour ... ressemble au Phenix." The burning flame of love merely perpetuates itself. This confusion between love and the phoenix is cleverly exploited by Jacques Davy du Perron in his praise of Desportes:

Voicy le beau Phénix ...
Car les ailes d'Amour font qu'il est un oiseau;
Mais ce qu'il est si rare en ce temps, le fait estre
Un Phenix, dont la tombe est l'unique berceau,
...
Amour, nouveau Phenix, pour chercher nouvelle ame
Sur un lict de senteurs ses ailes agitant,
S'oppose à ce soleil ardamment bluettant,
Tout flammeux de rayons, tout rayonneux de flame,
Voila ses os brulez dessus un lict d'encens,
Voila soudain que l'ame en a esté ravie,
Ces beaux vers animez heureusement naissans
De la cendre d'Amour, où l'Amour reprend vie.
Or estant le Phenix ...
... unique comme il est,
Rien qu'un ver seulement de ses cendres ne naist
Et, petit Phenisseau, d'autres ailettes pousse:
Mais ces beaux vers éclos pour faire des Amours,
Sortent en si grand nombre à la fois de leur cendre,

---

8   Philippe Desportes, *Les Amours de Diane*, vol. 2, ed. Victor Graham (Geneva: Droz, 1959).

Et prennent en naissant tant d'ailes tous les jours
Que les nommant Phenix h'ay crainte de mesprendre.
Soyent Amours ou Phenix, leurs ailes sont bien fortes,
Mais si tant de beaux vers aux Amours destinez,
Portent autant d'Amours amoureusement nez,
Que d'Amours porteront les Amours de Des-Portes?
Et si c'est un Phenix que chacun de ces vers,
Que de rares beautez …? (ll. 17–46)[9]

(Here is the beautiful Phoenix … / For the wings of Love make him a bird; / But the fact that He is so rare these days, makes him / A Phoenix, for whom the tomb is his only cradle, / … Love, a new Phoenix, to find a new soul / Fluttering his wings on a sweet-smelling bed, / Stands against this sun so ardently blue, / All flaming with rays, all radiant with flame, / Here are his bones, burned on a bed of incense, / Here suddenly the soul is taken away, / These beautiful lively verses being happily born / From the ashes of Love, where Love takes on new life. / So, being the Phoenix … / … unique as he is, / Nothing but a worm is born from his ashes / And, little Phoenix, it grows new wings: / But these beautiful worms [verses] hatched to make Love, / Come out from their ashes so many at a time, / And grow, when they are born, so many wings every day / That in naming them Phoenix, I'm afraid I am mistaken. / Whether they are Loves or Phoenix, their wings are quite strong / But if so many beautiful verses [worms] destined for Loves / Carry so many Loves born from Love, / Which Loves will carry the Loves of Des-Portes? / And if each of his verses is a Phoenix, / How many rare beauties …?)

The Phoenix is equated with Love, with the poet, with the poet's loves, with the poet's verses. All are self-generating, multiple identities in one unique being. The poet in particular forms an image of self-sufficiency in these lines: from the ashes of lost love, he recreates himself as immortal in the form of his poetry. The presence of the beloved is not even necessary for this generation; we seem to have returned to Paracelsus's *homunculus*, created by the alchemist as both father and mother, without the benefit of a woman. This desire to occlude or usurp the female's role in reproduction, either actually or in literary form, creates the alchemist/poet as a sort of hermaphroditic being that contains both sexes in himself. To some extent, this is the logical end of Petrarchan lyric, in which the feminine becomes more and more a part of the male poet's perspective, less and less of a separate identity. The feminine body, like the monstrous hermaphroditic body, becomes merely a blank page on which the poet inscribes his own reading of what is no longer there, and thus creates his own body anew. The effaced presence of the female is covered over by a monstrous or miraculous poetic body which ascribes to itself all feminine functions.

The language of this poem itself enacts the ambiguity it seeks to evoke, particularly by means of wordplay. The most insistent wordplay is that on "vers," which alternates

---

[9]   Jacques Davy, Sieur du Perron, "Stanses sur les Amours de Monsieur Desportes," reprinted in *Les Amours d'Hippolyte*, pp. 164–5.

between meaning "worms" and "verse," a popular pun in baroque poetry. Poetry is thus born out of death, out of the ashes: *cendres* was also the term used for decomposed human remains in the sixteenth century. The worms/verses signify at once death and life.

Another wordplay is that on *porter* and Desportes. Desportes's poetry carries and is carried by itself. It creates itself and disappears into itself, like the alchemical euroboros, the snake eating its own tail, the symbol of death and eternity. It is self-creating and self-consuming, like the Phoenix. We have seen this self-sufficient, self-contained, but also self-destructive, nature in the alchemical hermaphrodite. The pun, playing on multiple meanings of a word, becomes an important aspect of "hermaphroditic:" language, as well as of baroque writing in general. The ambiguity of wordplay lends itself well to expression of hermaphroditic subversion of social norms and linguistic ordering.

Intersexuality in Baroque Poetry

This tendency towards "transvestite" (or hermaphroditic) writing is apparent in the works of other poets present at the court of Henri III. Clovis Hesteau de Nuysement, champion of the hermaphrodite in his alchemical works, also creates ambiguous personae in his love poetry. His poetic persona often confuses feminine and masculine roles, and even, like d'Aubigné, conflates these ambiguous roles with those of animals:

Je tordrai mes cheveux et ferai de mes pleurs
Accroitre des Tritons l'impétueux empire ...

Amour sous un plaisir m'a tramé mille maux,
Il m'a rendu captif, comme les animaux,
Au joug d'un désespoir, le désespoir me donne
La fureur, le regret, le dépit, le courroux,
La pâleur et la peur, qui me conduisent tous
Sous le fatal pouvoir de la Parque félonne.

De mille et mille traits il m'entrouve le flanc,
Il se baigne cruel dedans mon tiède sang,
Il me suit en tous lieux amoindrissant ma force,
Jamais je ne le vois apparent à mes yeux,
Mais, hélas, je le sens dedans moi furieux,
Et mon corps ne lui sert que d'une vaine écorce ....[10]

(I will twist my hair and increase the Tritons' / Impetuous empire with my tears ... /
Love, hidden in pleasure, wove my evil fate, / He made me captive, like an animal, /

---

[10] "Or que le grand flambeau qui redore les Cieux," reprinted in part in *Eros baroque: Anthologie thématique de la poésie amoureuse*, ed. Gisèle Mathieu-Castellani (Paris: Nizet, 1986), p. 227.

To a yoke of despair, and despair leads me to / Fury, regret, spite, anger / Paleness and fear, which all drive me / Into the hands of murderous Fate. / With a thousand and a thousand arrows he cuts my side, / He bathes cruelly in my warm blood, / He follows me everywhere, diminishing my strength, / I never see him before my eyes, / But I feel him, alas, mad within me, / And my body serves only as an empty shell for him.)

The manner of mourning resembles more traditionally that of a woman than a man. The "violation" of the persona's body is at once sexual and murderous, as if the victim is at once trapped in the role of a "woman" and an animal, hunted and penetrated. The victim "incorporates" the persecutor, internalizes him (the use of *Amour* permits Hesteau de Nuysement to portray the violator simply as "il" throughout the poem), and the distinction between persecutor and victim vanishes. Self and other become one, and this gesture, at least fantasmatically, shifts the power to the victim. This appropriation of an ambiguously passive role is apparent in the work of Desportes as well (and is fairly typical of Petrarchan poetry):

[je] sens de mille traits ma poitrine entamer,
Je n'oze seulement vostre serf me nommer,
Et mourant par vos mains je crains de vous le dire. (*Les Amours de Diane*, vol. 2, p. 291)

(I feel my breast cut by a thousand arrows, / I only dare to call myself your slave, / And dying at your hands, I fear to tell you.)

This use of role reversals borrowed from the troubadours becomes extreme in the poem by Clovis Hesteau de Nuysement, in which one senses the absolute invasion of the lover's body by at best a possessing spirit. Similarly, Jean Godard equates feminine cruelty with masculine impotence, but celebrates both:

Je voudrais être ainsi comme un Penthée,
Nouveau toureau pour me voir déchiré
De la dent croche et de l'ongle acérée
D'une panthère à la peau tachetée.

Je voudrais voir Diane une nuitée
Baigner à nu, pour être dévoré
Comme Actéon, le trépas assuré
Aurait bientôt ma douleur limitée.
…
Ce m'est assez de perdre seulement l'oeil
Qui mon coeur brule au rais d'un beau Soleil,
Il n'est plus d'eau quand la source est tarie ....[11]

---

[11]　Cited in *Eros baroque*, p. 263.

(I would like to be like a Pentheus, / A new bull, to see myself torn / By the fang and the sharpened nail / Of a panther with spotted skin. / I would like to see Diane one night / Bathing nude, so that I might be devoured / Like Actaeon, my death assured, / Would soon have ended my pain. / … It is enough for me to lose my sight / Which burns my heart in the rays of a beautiful sun, / There is no more water when the spring is dry.)

Godard is indulging in a favorite pastime of poets at the court of Henri III: imitating, even parodying, the poetry of Pierre de Ronsard, in this case one of his most famous sonnets:

> Je vouldroy bien richement jaunissant
> En pluye d'or goute à goute descendre
> Dans le beau sein de ma belle Cassandre,
> Lors qu'en ses yeulx le somme va glissant.
> Je vouldroy bien en toreau blandissant
> Me transformer pour finement la prendre,
> Quand elle va par l'herbe la plus tendre
> Seule à l'escart mille fleurs ravissant.
> Je vouldroy bien afin d'aiser ma peine
> Estre un Narcisse, & elle une fontaine
> Pour m'y plonger une nuict à sejour:
> Et vouldroy bien que ceste nuict encore
> Durast toujours sans que jamais l'Aurore
> D'un front nouveau nous r'allumast le jour.[12]

(I would like to richly descend, drop by drop in yellowing showers of gold, into the beautiful lap of my beautiful Cassandre, as sleep slips into her eyes. / I would like to transform myself into a gleaming white bull, to take her cleverly when she goes over the most tender grass, alone and apart ravishing a thousand flowers. / I would like, in order to ease my troubles, to be a Narcissus, and she a fountain into which I could dive for a night. / And I would like that night to last forever, without Aurora lighting up the day with a new face.)

While this sonnet enacts a number of scenes of male power, as Ronsard imagines himself as Jupiter raping Danaë and Europa, the imagery he uses is already ambiguous. Jupiter/Ronsard dissolves into a shower of gold. Later, Ronsard as Narcissus plunges into the fountain, joining self with other. But Godard takes this notion of the dissolution of the self even farther, echoing Jupiter's disguise as a bull, but linking the bull to the victim Pentheus, torn apart by the Bacchantes for having desecrated their rituals with his presence. Similarly, his transgressive gaze brings on his own destruction in the second stanza, as he wishes to be Actaeon gazing upon Diana, so that he might be devoured by her. Finally, he speaks of being burned by the eye of

---

[12] Pierre de Ronsard, *Les Amours (1552)* in *Oeuvres complètes*, ed. Paul Laumonier (Paris: Nizet, 1982), pp. 23–4.

the Sun. Godard desires his own violent destruction at the hands of another, so that he might become one with this other. His eye, and the eye of the other – goddess or Bacchante – upon which he gazes, become one, and he disappears into this union. As in alchemical texts, this conjunction arises from dissolution, and also leads back to it.

This poetic self-portrayal of the man as victim also echoes the apparent threat that women posed to male power at the end of the century. In political pamphlets, all Frenchmen were described as castrated by the domineering Catherine de Medicis.[13] Desportes' warrior-like, controlling Hippolyte was apparently inspired by Marguerite de Valois, wife of Henri de Navarre and mistress of Bussy d'Amboise.[14] The *perception* of feminine "usurpation" of power created a sense of emasculation, which in turn rendered the male poet (or political propagandist) effeminate.[15] Thus, the presentation of gender roles as potentially unstable could be as much for the conservative effect of defending "traditional" roles as for the revolutionary effect of questioning those roles.

Nonetheless, there was a certain aesthetic or intellectual interest and pleasure expressed in relation to destabilized roles:

> A l'heure que Madame en homme se déguise,
> Une toque portant sur ses cheveux dorés,
> Elle semble un Adon aux yeux noirs admirés,
> Ou un nouveau Pâris ou quelque jeune Anchise,
>
> Soit qu'elle ait un habit en dame de Venise,
> A demi découvrant ses tétons empourprés,
> Ou soit qu'en habit plein elle se vête après,
> Ou soit qu'elle se vête à la nouvelle guise,
> …
> Toujours très belle elle est, et voit on clairement
> Que tout sied toujours bien à la belle personne.[16]

---

13   Pierre de l'Estoile, *Registre-journal du regne de Henri III*, eds Madeleine Lazard and Gilbert Schrenck (Geneva: Droz, 1996–2003), vol. 1, p. 172, p. 184, and pp. 189–90.

14   See Victor Graham's introduction to *Les Amours d'Hippolyte*, p. 8.

15   This is reminiscent of the process described by Susan Faludi in her book, *Backlash: The Undeclared War Against American Women* (New York: Crown Publishers, 1991), in relation to historical cycles in American history. Particularly interesting parallels can be found in Faludi's third chapter, "Backlashes Then and Now," pp. 46–72. Faludi cites a Victorian tract that accuses women of "losing their femininity to 'hermaphrodism'" (p. 49). Invariably, women's *perceived* accession to power is accompanied by an almost pathological fear of loss of "traditional" gender roles (roles which often only exist in the most theoretical aspects of culture); this is certainly true of late sixteenth-century France.

16   Jean Godard, from *Eros baroque*, p. 158.

(When Madame disguises herself as a man, / Wearing a cap on her golden hair, / She seems like an Adonis with admired dark eyes, / Or a new Paris or some young Anchises, / Or she wears the dress of a Venetian woman, / Her red nipples half uncovered, / Or she dresses herself in full clothing, / Or she dresses in the latest fashion, / ... She is always very beautiful, and one can see clearly, / That everything looks good on a beautiful person.)

The variety of the woman's disguises seems to contribute to her beauty; even though it is true that the poet emphasizes the woman's beauty as an underlying constant. Her true identity is that of "la belle personne," that is, her appearance. Yet her appearance is repeatedly reinvented and recreated, so that the "essential" person is covered over. Even her masculine guise is unstable, she resembles either "un Adon" or "un nouveau Pâris" or "quelque jeune Anchise." She herself is only *Madame, elle,* or *la belle personne,* which makes her at once everywoman (and man) and no one, freed from any individual identity that she may have had. Clearly, the costume has replaced the person, and it is the aesthetic quality of the costume, and particularly of its mutability and its destabilizing effect on the person, which is being appreciated. Appearances are valued above underlying essences, which may not be available to the perception at any rate; the sign in its own right takes on a life independent of that which it is purported to signify; in this case, masculinity or femininity. The very real concerns about the nature of power and the possibility of immortality and transcendence, expressed in the lyric poetry oriented towards alchemical thought, are balanced by a skepticism concerning the external signs of gender, which are aesthetically pleasing but potentially misleading.

The Mysterious Hermaphrodite

In this atmosphere of mysticism mixed with skepticism and the freeplay of gender roles that Pierre le Loyer wrote his sonnet on the hermaphrodite (a translation of the Latin poem of dubious origin discussed above in the introduction):

Ma mere de moy grosse un jour voulut apprendre
Des Dieux quel ie serois: Un fils, dist Apollon,
Une fille, dist Mars, nul des deux, dist Iunon:
l'estois hermaphrodite alors qu'elle m'engendre.
Demandant quelle fin ma vie devoit prendre,
Par fer, dist la Deesse: au gibet, Mars felon:
Dedans l'onde, Phebus: & tout cela Clothon
Et ses severes soeurs ferme voulurent rendre.
Grimpant d'une arbre un iour les rameaux bien feuillus,
Mon espee coula & ie tombé dessus,
Mon pied, par cas fortuit, dans un rameau se lie,
Ma teste se noya dedans un fleuve creux:

Ainsi moy femme, homme, & nul de tous les deux
L'eau, le gibet, le fer, fut le bout de ma vie. (Pierre Le Loyer, *Sonnets politiques ou meslanges*)[17]

(My mother, pregnant with me, one day wanted to learn / From the gods what I would be: A son, said Apollo, / A daughter, said Mars, neither, said Juno: / I was a hermaphrodite when she gave birth to me. / When she asked how my life would end, / By the sword, said the Goddess, on the gallows, said villainous Mars: / In the water, said Phoebus: and all of this Clotho / And her severe sisters wanted to make certain. / I was climbing a tree with leafy branches one day, / My sword slipped, and I fell upon it, / My foot, by chance, became stuck in a branch, / My head was drowned in a deep river: / And so woman, man, and neither of the two / Water, gallows, and the sword brought my life to an end.)

The entry of this originally Latin poem of dubious origin[18] into the realm of French lyric signals the evolution away from idealized Neoplatonic versions of hermaphrodism towards more skeptical and alchemical forms of thought. The poem reads like a riddle, a secret code – an intellectual game of some sort. At first, the effacement of individual identity through loss of specific gender is underscored, and this effacement seems closely linked to the insistence on fate, the individual's utter lack of free will. Apollo, Mars, and Juno seem to be amusing themselves at the expense of the child to be born. The cruelty of this game is made clear by their insistence on a triple, repetitive, death by sword, gallows, and water. Clotho and her sisters, that is, the three Fates, seal this pact. The child seems to have no life; what is important is the triple death, which occurs in "clever" fashion as he slips from a tree and falls on his sword, hanging head-first into the river. The dead hermaphrodite, who seems to be the narrator of this poem, designates himself as both man and woman, and neither.

This sonnet revises somewhat the problematic attitudes towards gender expressed in the previously cited "hermaphrodite" or "transvestite" poems. While the ambiguously gendered being is doomed to destruction (and a destruction resembling annihilation in its threefold nature), it also has some supernatural status, which allows it to speak from beyond the grave. Its plenitude of sexual identities makes it threatening, and therefore it is cut (in two, perhaps, as were Aristophanes' hermaphrodites), drowned (as were hermaphrodites in ancient Rome), and hanged (like a common criminal, but also upside-down, like the hanged man of tarot).[19] The triple death argues for a triple identity: male, female, neuter.

---

17 From *Les Oeuvres et meslanges poetiques de Pierre Le Loyer, Angevin* (Paris: Jean Poupy, 1579). My thanks to Catharine Randall Coats for calling my attention to this and two similar poems collected in the anthology edited by André Blanchard, *La Poésie baroque et precieuse* (Paris: Seghers, 1985); see her article, "A Surplus of Significance," cited above. This poem is to be found on p. 38 of that anthology.

18 Cited by Caspar Bauhin in his treatise *De hermaphroditorum*, and attributed by him to a Latin poet "Pulicis" and to Angelo Politiano. See the introduction to this study.

19 For the hanged man of tarot, see Grillot de Givry, *Witchcraft, Magic, and Alchemy*, trans. J. Courtenay Locke (New York: Dover, 1971) pp. 284–8.

The popularity of this mysterious reading of the hermaphrodite is evident from later incarnations of this poem. Jean Loys, whose *Oeuvres poétiques* were published posthumously in 1612, wrote another version of this piece. In the title, he tries to render the narration of the poem somewhat more realistic: this is "L'Epitaphe d'un Hermaphrodite, prins du latin":

Lorsque ma mère en son ventre me porte
Pour s'aviser vers les Dieux se transporte:
Phoebus lui dit, qu'un mâle enfanterait,
Mars répondit que femelle serait,
Et Junon dit ni mâle, ni femelle;
Ainsi naquis-je avec forme jumelle
Et s'enquérant de mon dernier destin,
Junon par fer vient arrêter ma fin,
Mars par la croix, et Phoebus dedans l'onde,
Et leur oracle en vérité se fonde.
Un arbre était ombrageant un ruisseau,
Auquel monté tombe de mon fourreau
Par un hasard mon épée toute nue
Dessus laquelle en tombant je me rue,
Mon pied soudain s'accroche à un rameau,
Et contre bas ma tête penche en l'eau,
Ainsi par eau, par fer, et croix je meure,
Mâle femelle, et tous deux à même heure.[20]

(When my mother was carrying me in her womb / She went to the gods for advice: / Phoebus told her that she would give birth to a male, / Mars answered that it would be a female, / And Juno said, neither male nor female: / And so I was born with a double form. / When she asked about my final fate, / Juno said the sword would bring my end, / Mars the cross, and Phoebus the wave, / And their oracle was founded in the truth. / A tree shaded a brook, / In which I climbed, when by chance / My naked sword fell out of its scabbard, / Falling, I dashed upon the sword, / My foot suddenly was trapped in a branch, / And downwards my head plunged into the water, / And so by water, by the sword, and by the cross I died, / Male, female, and both at the same time.)

Loys, perhaps influenced by the resurgence of interest in alchemy, emphasizes the "double form" (*forme jumelle*) of the hermaphrodite, rather than its neutral status. This revision is repeated at the end of the poem with the insistent "Mâle femelle, et tous deux ..." Whereas le Loyer's hermaphrodite was already self-annihilating in that the male aspects of that being seemed to cancel out the female, and vice versa, Loys offers a creature that is "too much," undone by divine forces because it reaches beyond nature.

---

[20]   From André Blanchard's anthology, *La poésie baroque et precieuse* (Paris: Seghers, 1969), pp. 52–3.

Most significant of all, however, are the revisions made on this tale by Tristan L'Hermite, in *La Lyre du Sieur Tristan*, published in 1641:

Les dieux me faisaient naître, et l'on s'informa d'eux
Quelle sorte de fruit accroîtrait la famille.
Jupiter dit: un fils, Vénus dit: une fille,
Mercure: l'un et l'autre, et je fus tous les deux.

On leur demande encore quel serait mon trépas:
Saturne d'un lacet, Mars d'un fer me menace,
Diane d'une eau trouble: et l'on ne croyait pas
Qu'un divers pronostic marquât même disgrâce.

Je suis tombé d'un saule à côté d'un étang,
Mon poignard dégainé m'a traversé le flanc,
J'ai le pied pris dans l'arbre, et la tête dans l'onde.

O sort dont mon esprit est encore effrayé!
Un poignard, une branche, une eau noire et profonde,
M'ont en un même temps meurtri, pendu, noyé.[21]

(The gods brought about my birth, and someone asked them / What sort of fruit would increase the family. / Jupiter said: a son, Venus said, a daughter, / Mercury: one and the other, and I was both. / Someone asked them again what would be my death: / Saturn said a noose, Mars menaced me with the sword, / Diana with turbulent water: and they could not believe / That such varied predictions indicated the same shameful fate. / I fell from a willow beside a pond, / My unsheathed sword pierced my side, / My foot was stuck in the tree, and my head in the water. / O fate which horrifies my spirit still! / A dagger, a branch, water black and deep, / At the same time stabbed, hung, and drowned me.)

To some extent, Tristan has made the intervention of the gods, somewhat obscure in the previous versions, seem more logical here. Jupiter represents masculine sexuality; Venus, feminine. In depicting Mercury as the arbiter of the hermaphrodite, Tristan is following a long tradition in alchemical lore. Melancholy Saturn imposes the hangman's rope; warlike Mars, the sword. Diane, who used water as her weapon, to transform Acteon into a wild beast,[22] calls for drowning. Tristan labels death by hanging and drowning a "disgrâce;" and indeed, hanging was for common criminals, and murder by drowning was practiced on those rejected by society (hermaphrodites themselves in ancient Rome, but also unwanted children, political enemies under the

---

21   "La Fortune de l'Hermaphrodite," again from Blanchard's anthology, *La poésie baroque et precieuse*, p. 203.

22   Ovid, *Metamorphoses*, bk 3, ll. 186–98.

Catholic League, and Huguenots in late sixteenth-century France).[23] The poem seems to suggest that the hermaphrodite is castrated by his sword, which pierces his "flanc." In fact, the emphasis on execution-like death ("meurtri, pendu, noyé") in Tristan's version suggests the context of the earlier pieces. The death of the hermaphrodite resembles ritual executions such as that practiced on the body of Gaspard de Coligny:

> Le peuple resveillé par l'orloge du palais court au logis du mort, en coupe toutes les parties qui se pouvoyent couper: sur tout la teste, qui alla jusques à Rome: il le trainent par les rues (selon ce qu'il avoit predit sans y penser) le jettent en l'eau, l'en retirent pour le pendre par les pieds à Montfaucon, et allument quelques flammes dessous, pour employer à leur vengeance tous les elements.[24]

> (The people, awakened by the bell in the palace, ran to the home of the dead man, cut off all the parts that could be cut: first of all the head, which was sent to Rome: they dragged him through the streets (which act he had predicted without knowing) threw him into the water, pulled him out so that they could hang him by the feet at Montfaucon, and lit some flames under him, so that they would have used all of the elements for their vengeance.)

This sacrificial aspect connects the hermaphrodite of the Loyer, Loys, and l'Hermite poems to the alchemical *rebis*, which is burned, dissolved, or otherwise annihilated in order to be recreated. These poems appear during the period of intense publication of books on spiritual alchemy, from the first printing of the *Rosarium* in 1550, through the works of Salomon Trismosin (ca. 1612) and Michael Maier (for example the *Atalanta fugiens*, 1617). Other authors such as Annibal Barlet are working well into the 1650s. These works are reprinted repeatedly until the end of the seventeenth century. Alchemical emblem-books, such as the *Atalanta*, offer striking images of the rebis and of its destruction. This sacrifice is echoed by that of the King, who is also destroyed in a variety of ways. In the *Atalanta fugiens*, he is devoured by a wolf (emblem 24, p. 105; then the wolf is burned and the King escapes); he drowns (emblem 31, p. 133); he is hacked to pieces and reborn whole (emblem 64, p. 185). Annihilation of the rebis or the King is thus balanced by rebirth or renewal on a higher plane of existence.

These images could thus be seen, in the alchemical context, as a working through of the traumas of the Wars of Religion, an attempt at least on the level of the imagination to move beyond violence. Yet the violence remains, for example in most of the images of the *Atalanta fugiens*. It is constantly re-enacted, as if the author is trapped in that

---

[23] See Elie Barnavi, *Le Parti de Dieu: Etude sociale et politique des chefs de la Ligue parisienne, 1585–1594* (Brussels: Nauwelaerts, 1980), p. 183. Note also Théodore Agrippa d'Aubigné's description of the rivers of France, choked with bodies, in "Les Fers," *Les Tragiques*, from *Oeuvres*, ed. Henri Weber (Paris: Gallimard, 1969), ll. 1447–96.

[24] Théodore Agrippa d'Aubigné, *Histoire universelle*, ed. André Thierry (Geneva: Droz, 1985), vol. 3, pp. 332–3.

moment, and cannot in fact transcend it. There is a message of hope even in all of these images of violence, but this hope is in constant conflict with pain and death.

The political discourse of this period adopts this more negative version of the hermaphrodite as an image of conflict and dissolution. That which is uncomfortably close to those who dominate culture (either masses or the elite, depending upon the situation), but is not enough *like* them, must be ritually destroyed in order to dissolve its power. Those who are seen as destabilizing the social order in any way must be eliminated; for this reason, ritual execution was most often performed on regicides who were also described as parricides, Ravaillac being the best-known case. The Huguenots were French, but not Catholic. They were, or were increasingly perceived as, members of the ruling classes, and seemed to gain many concessions from the government, in the period prior to the massacre of Saint Bartholomew's Day. The Edict of Saint Germain (1570), coming as it did after the resounding Catholic victories at Jarnac and Montcontour, seemed to concede too much to the Huguenots.[25] Yet the Huguenots had hardly gained anything: they were allowed to remain in four towns they controlled already. They were supposedly allowed to attend services wherever they had been able to previous to the Third War of Religion. It was the *perception* of their new-found power which drove French Catholics to massacre them.

Like women who were perceived as too powerful, the Huguenots seemed to threaten the social order, and had to be eliminated not merely by massacre or execution, but in ritualistic fashion, to purge society of the potential contagion. The threat was heightened by the proximity of the victim to the perpetrator; Huguenots were not so obviously different, so clearly monstrous. Under these circumstances, the hermaphrodite becomes an iconic representation of that which is alike but different, that which threatens the integrity of male, Catholic identity. Acceptance of that which is not the same, but not entirely different, menaces the boundaries that were drawn in the creation of social order.

Thus, the hermaphrodite is ritually destroyed in order to reassure the denizens of France that their society remains whole, untouched, unchanged. Yet the voice of the hermaphrodite, speaking from beyond the grave, hints at the supernatural power of that which is alike but different (the abject), which perpetually threatens our self-image (particularly on the social level of groups of sex, race, nationality, or species). The images borrowed from alchemy and the tarot hint at the cyclical nature of this battle for purity of caste or category; this is a war which has not been one by either combatant, and which will be renewed in each successive age.

Thus, hermaphroditic poetry of the Renaissance clearly aligns itself with the political issues of the time, more so even than the scientific treatises or alchemical discourses on the subject. While scientists and alchemists find themselves resisting to some degree the culture that surrounds them, torn between the empirical evidence before their eyes and the cultural assumptions that informed their training, poets enter

---

[25]   Pierre Miquel, *Les Guerres de Religion* (Paris: Fayard, 1980), pp. 268–70.

right into the fray and become entangled in the misogyny and the cultural conservatism of their time. Although their work hints at displacements and instability of gender, these poets do not question gender roles to the same extent as their scientific counterparts. In fact, some of these poets, Clovis Hesteau de Nuysement and Théodore Agrippa d'Aubigné in particular, seem more revolutionary in their non-lyric work (alchemical treatises, histories, epic) than in their love poetry. This disparity suggests either that their work was largely controlled by political factors (court patronage, censorship, polemics) or that revolutions occur last of all on the personal level. Perhaps that which appears problematic to the rational mind is hard to shake from the collective or even personal unconscious. At any rate, this peculiar strain of conservatism in the late sixteenth-century lyric links such poetry to the political propaganda of its time.

Chapter 7

The Royal Hermaphrodite:
Henri III of France

Transgressive Rulers

After the death of Charles IX in May of 1574, and before the return of Henri (III) from Poland in September, Catherine de Medicis ruled France as Regent. During this period, a number of satirical pamphlets circulated, as well as an infamous pseudo-biography, the *Discours merveilleux de la vie, actions, et deportements de Catherine de Médicis, Royne-mère* (*Marvelous Discourse on the Life, Acts, and Behavior of Catherine de Medici, the Queen Mother*, originally published as the *Legenda S. Catharinae*, the *Legend of Saint Catherine*).[1] Upon Henri's return, however, his apparent lack of interest in ruling and Catherine's continued involvement in matters of state led to a proliferation of pamphlets that linked her virility with his effeminacy. Eventually, they became a masculine-feminine "couple infernal," linked in the popular imagination to Nero and Agrippina or Heliogabalus and Soaemias. Catherine is frequently depicted in this material as a castrating Cybele who has rendered the heroes of France effeminate (see L'Estoile, vol. 1, pp. 172, 184, 189–90, for example); in several leaflets, her virago-like behavior is directly linked to Henri's sexual ambiguity, so that one cannot tell who is the Queen and who is the King (L'Estoile, 1.219, for example, where there is a play on the term "Sa Majesté"). Eventually, the popular propaganda against Catherine is overshadowed by the vehemence of that against Henri, who seems to have forfeited the right to rule by transforming himself into a woman.[2]

This political propaganda found abundant sources of material in popular literature of preceding decades, which often linked sexuality with politics. Pierre Boaistuau's *Histoires prodigieuses* (1560) and Claude Tesserant's continuation of this collection

---

[1]   Edited under the direction of Nicole Cazauran (Geneva: Droz, 1995).

[2]   For a thorough analysis of the propaganda campaign against Henri, as well as a more detailed presentation of the historical context as regards homosexuality, see Guy Poirier's important study, *L'homosexualité dans l'imaginaire de la Renaissance*, particularly the fourth part, pp. 109–61. This is probably the most complete assessment of the literature written against Henri, particularly in relation to his sexuality (or the public hypotheses concerning his sexuality). I find Poirier's approach from the perspective of the *imaginaire* of the period to be particularly convincing, since all we have are polemical texts concerning this question.

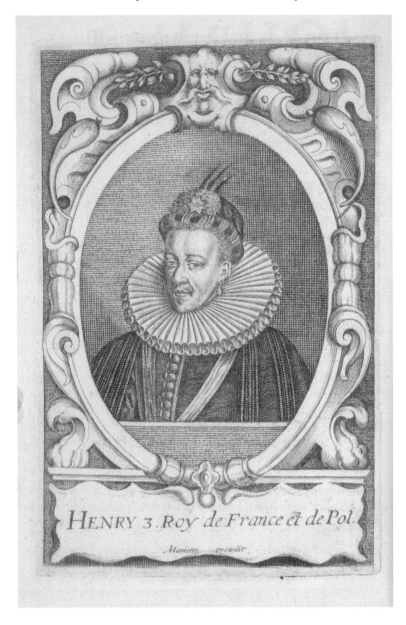

HENRY 3. Roy de France et de Pol.

Figure 7.1   Portrait of Henri III of France, frontispiece from volume 3 of
                  Pierre de l'Estoile's *Journal de Henri III, Roy de France et de
                  Pologne* (Paris: chez la veuve de P. Gandouin, 1744). Courtesy
                  of the Division of Rare and Manuscript Collections, Cornell
                  University Library

(1567) serve not only as sources for Ambroise Paré's treatise on monsters, but as a matrix for political uses of monstrosity and sexuality. Tesserant's second and third stories, the "Histoire de deux enfans Hermaphrodites" ("The Story of Two Hermaphroditic Children") and the "Histoire d'un homme avec des cheveux de femme" ("The Story of a Man with Woman's Hair"), are clearly placed in the context of political upheavals of the time. Most significantly for later propaganda written against Henri III of France, the story of the man with woman's hair hardly touches on the title character, and focuses most intensely on the behavior of Nero and of Heliogabalus. A number of satirical pamphlets compared Henri to one or both of these Roman emperors, and particularly linked his personal life to their perversity.[3] The association of hermaphrodism with bisexuality, and of both with a number of other perversions as well as with random violence, seems of particular concern to Renaissance authors, and most of all to political pamphleteers. Through the links with Nero and Heliogabalus, these ambiguities are seen as politically threatening; thus, a ruler's sexual activities may become a justification for resistance. Disorderly bodies and behavior lead to a disorderly, even chaotic society. Tesserant prepares for this discussion of the relationship between sexual and social disorder in the story of the two hermaphrodites (who are in fact conjoined twins) by declaring the myth of Hermaphroditus to be merely a satire against men overly given to voluptuous pleasure:

> … les Poetes feignent que le premier qui a esté demy homme & demye femme fust fils de Mercure, lequel les Grecs appellent Hermes, & de Venus, laquelle en leur langue est dicte Aphroditis: mais cest fable n'est proprement que contre ceux qui du corps ont toutes les parties de l'homme: mais fussent-ils Mars, ils n'ont le cueur plus viril ne moins lasche que la femme, se rendans serfs des delices & voluptez. (*Quatorze histoires*, p. 224)

> (The Poets pretend that the first to be half-man, half-woman was the son of Mercury, whom the Greeks call Hermes, and of Venus, who is called Aphrodite in their language: but this fable is really against those who are men in every part of their body, but were they Mars himself, they have hearts no more virile nor less cowardly than women, and make themselves slaves to pleasures and sensuality.)

Thus, the figure of the hermaphrodite is used to enforce a certain morality and a certain Gallic lifestyle based on warlike tests of manliness. Tesserant points out that Nero's chariot was drawn by hermaphroditic horses, a sign of his *lascivité* or lustfulness. The monstrous animal signals a monstrous soul, in this case by displacement; this sign serves as a warning to other rulers.

---

3 On this, see Margaret MacGowan, "Les images du pouvoir royal au temps d'Henri III," *Théorie et pratique politiques à la Renaissance* (Colloque Internationale de Tours, 1976–77): 301–20.

The hermaphroditic conjoined twins discussed in this story share this status as a warning. At first, their birth does not seem to be the sign of political upheaval in Germany:

> Car nous lisons que l'an 1486 ... on veid naistre au Palatinat assez pres de Heydelberga en un bourg nommé Rorbachie deux enfans gemeaux s'entretenans & ioincts ensemble dos a dos, desquels l'un & l'autre estoit hermaphrodite, c'est a dire avoit double nature d'homme & de femme ... Pour cest année-là on ne lit pas que du costé d'Alemaigne il soit advenu grand mal .... (*Quatorze histoires*, pp. 224–5)

> (For we read that in the year 1486 ... was seen born in the Palatine near Heidelberg, in a town called Rorbach, two twin infants holding each other and joined together back to back, both of which were hermaphrodites, that is to say that had the sexual organs of man and woman ... For that year, we do not read that any great evil came to pass in Germany.)

But, in conjunction with monsters born in Italy in 1487, they seem to presage civil disorder and plague, particularly in Flanders: "n'estans tels monstres signe non seulement de dissensions civiles ... mais aussi des pestes qui furent presques universelles ..." ("Not only were such monsters a sign of civil unrest ... but also of plagues, which occurred almost everywhere" p. 225). Hermaphrodites in fact seem to be almost common in this period of upheaval:

> Mais c'est assez parlé des monstres qui peuvent apporter quelque esbahissement, voire des Hermaphrodites, veu mesme que ie croy qu'il y a plusieurs personnes qui ont veu tant à la Cour, qu'en ceste ville un ieune homme aagé de 28 ou 30 ans, qui vit encore à present, & se faict voir tantost habillé en homme, tantost en femme, & que l'histoire des Hermaphrodites, qui ont esté decouverts au pays d'Arbigeris depuis sept ans, est assez commune. (*Quatorze histoires*, p. 226)

> (But that is enough about monsters that can cause some astonishment, even Hermaphrodites, although I believe that there are numerous people who have seen at the Court as well as in the city a young man of twenty-eight or thirty years, who is still alive, and who is seen sometimes dressed as a man, sometimes as a woman, and that the tale of the Hermaphrodites who were discovered in the countryside of Arbigeris, seven years ago, is fairly widely known.)

The story of the young Hermaphrodite/transvestite seems to suggest a greater tolerance of such "monstrosities" in the second half of the sixteenth century than in earlier times, at least at the French Court. Tesserant suggests that the hermaphroditic condition should be considered as similar to those with supernumerary digits; they are curiosities, nothing more. Yet he himself has suggested reading them as (politically charged) prodigies. This oscillation between the tolerance conferred by greater scientific understanding of a certain condition, and superstitious horror at that which does not conform to rigid roles of sex, race, or species, follows the model of most of the medical treatises on the subject of monsters and hermaphrodites.

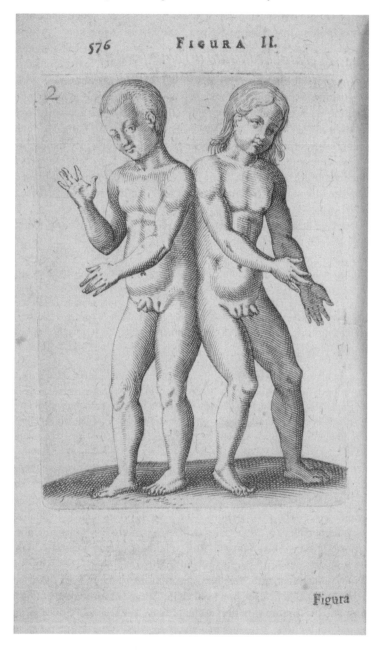

Figure 7.2   Conjoined twin hermaphrodites (male and female), from
                  Bauhin, *De hermaphroditorum* ... . Courtesy of the Division of
                  Rare and Manuscript Collections, Cornell University Library

In his story of the transvestite/ hermaphrodite, Tesserant suggests a link between sexuality and biology that is further explored in his following story: "Histoire d'un homme avec des cheveux de femme" ("The Story of a Man with Woman's Hair"). Tesserant suggests that beyond monsters born naturally, there exist monsters created artificially (p. 227). He cites Livy, Pliny, and Aulus Gellius as sources of stories about women who suddenly become men, and men who have themselves made into women "pour satisfaire à leurs abominables paillardises" (*Quatorze histoires*, pp. 227–8: "to satisfy their abominable lusts"). The transformation from female to male seems to occur naturally, perhaps because, as classical and Renaissance authors believed, the male sex represented perfection, and all things tend towards perfection. Thus it is inconceivable for a man to wish to become a woman, and Tesserant reserves his harshest condemnation for male transsexuals and homosexuals (pp. 228–34), particularly the rulers (*Quatorze histoires*, p. 229: "qui ... devroient estre par l'exemple de leur bonne vie la lumiere de tout leur peuple,"). Tesserant clearly feels that the distinction between the sexes cannot be effaced:

> ... de forcer nature d'estre d'homme, duquel le propre est de commander es armées, tenir les premiers lieux es republiques, & mourir pour leur pays vertueusement, faict femme, de laquelle le plus grand honneur anciennement estoit, comme le tombeau de Claudia le porte, d'aymer son mary & ses enfans, filler la laine & garder la maison: c'est non seulement l'acte, mais aussi l'histoire & memoire la plus prodigeuse. (*Quatorze histoires*, p. 228)

> (To force nature so that a man, whose role is to command armies, to lead republics, and to die virtuously for their country, is made a woman, for whom the greatest honor in ancient times was, as the tomb of Claudia tells us, to love her husband and children, to spin wool and keep the house: it is not only the most marvelous act, but also the most amazing thing told in human memory.)

The contempt for women and their place in society, the urgent need to keep them in that place in order to assure the primacy of masculinity, runs as a barely disguised subtext to this story.

Tesserant concentrates his attention on the stories of Nero and Heliogabalus, whom he calls "fils de putains" (p. 229: "sons of whores"). Nero has "un sien jeune libertin nommé Spore" ("one of his young libertines, named Sporus") castrated because he resembles Poppaea, whom Nero has recently killed. He then lives with Spore, "& l'ayma si impudiquement, qu'il s'en servoit comme de sa femme" (p. 229: "and loved him so shamelessly, that he used him as his wife"), even marrying the young man and parading around his Empire with his partner dressed as Empress. "Spore" is described as a being of "double sexe." Tesserant even claims that Nero "en son propre corps ... voulut estre Androgyne homme & femme sinon de nature, puis qu'elle le luy avoit denié aumoins par la turpitude de sa vie" (p. 229: "wanted to be an Androgyne, male and female, in his own body, if not naturally, because Nature had denied him this, at least in the moral turpitude of his life"). What is apparently most threatening about Nero's behavior, then, is his bisexuality:

> Car comme Spore luy avoit servy abhominablement de femme, aussi voulut il en servir à un sien libertin, lequel Sueton nomme Doriphore, & Dion Pythagoras, auquel il assigna dot, comme les femmes apportent à leurs maris ... il contrefaisoit les plainctes & cris que font les vierges quand on les despucelle. (*Quatorze histoires*, p. 230)

> (For, just as Sporus had served abominably as his wife, so he wanted to be the wife of one of his debauched men, whom Suetonius names Doriphore, and Dio Cassius Pythagoras, to whom he gave a dowry just as women give to their husbands ... he imitated the moans and screams virgins make when they are deflowered.)

This parody of heterosexual behavior, more than any of the vicious cruelty Nero exercised towards his subjects, horrifies the author, who sees it as a destabilizing force for the Empire as a whole:

> Brief il prenoit si grand plaisir à telles lascivetez, qu'il pardonnoit tous les autres crimes à ceux qui confessoient franchement devant luy leurs detestables luxures & paillardises. (*Quatorze histoires*, p. 230)

> (In short, he took such great pleasure in such lasciviousness, that he pardoned all other crimes committed by those who frankly confessed to him their detestable lusts and debaucheries.)

Nero's disordered sexuality is thus at the root of all crimes committed in the Empire, and causes a general chaos in society. This emphasis on "disorderly" sexuality as the root of all other evils does not reflect the Latin sources on Nero, in which this sexuality is seen merely as one symptom of Nero's instability. For Tacitus at least, Nero's random execution of innocent victims, his murdering and casual torture of Roman citizens were far worse crimes.[4] Clearly, sexuality and gender roles had become even more critical issues in sixteenth century French society than they had been in ancient Rome.

In Tesserant's account, Heliogabalus takes this destabilizing sexuality a step further by inscribing it upon his body. Granted, this transgression is linked to other forms of disorder, rather than offered as the cause: "faire tuer un nombre infiny d'hommes" (p. 231: "had an infinite number of men killed"), "jouer des Senateurs Romains" (p. 231: "mock the Roman Senators"), "immoler les enfans pour les sacrifices" (p. 231: "sacrificed children to the gods"). But his sexual transgression is portrayed as the worst

---

4   Tacitus does describe Nero's licentiousness in his *Annals*, trans. Alfred John Church and William Jackson Brodribb (New York: The Modern Library, 1942), bk 13, ch. 25 (pp. 298–9), but devotes his greatest anger to the violence and "wanton bloodshed" caused by the Emperor (bk 16, ch. 16; p. 406) and for the most part discusses only this bloodshed.

of all ("il nageoit en pleine mer ... tout plongé en la paillardise," p. 231: "he swam in a deep ocean of debauchery"). He plays the prostitute: "il se tenoit nud comme les femmes publiques ... il se faisoit payer" (p. 231: "he presented himself naked like the prostitutes, and made men pay him"). He marries one of his serving-men and:

> ... se feit appeller Dame & Royne: il s'addonna à la fillure & tissure de la laine, il portoit quelque fois une coefe, il se fardoit le visage, oignoit ses yeux, faisoit raser son menton & tout le poil, afin de sentir d'avantage sa femme, de la quelle le nom luy plaisoit si fort .... (*Quatorze histoires*, p. 231)

> (He made others call him Lady and Queen; he took up spinning and weaving, he wore a feminine headdress, he put makeup on his face, and around his eyes, he shaved his chin and all of his hair, in order to feel more like a woman, for to be called this pleased him greatly.)

Evidently, it is not merely Heliogabalus' sexual activity that disturbs our author, but the whole game of playing a woman's role, spinning, wearing makeup, shaving off one's beard. His pleasure in these activities is the most destabilizing aspect of all.

Worse still, Heliogabalus has excised that which most clearly defines him as a man:

> Mais i'ay honte de dire le reste ... il aima tant non seulement à porter le nom de femme, mais aussi à l'estre du tout que pour y parvenir il se feit coupper tout ce qu'il avoit d'homme & d'abandonna aux barbiers pour le tailler en telle sorte qu'ils voudroient, pourveu qu'il peut devenir femme entierment, & peust avoir compagnie avec les hommes comme les autres femmes naturellement. Voila le prodige & monstre qu'il voulut faire apparoir en son corps .... (*Quatorze histoires*, p. 232)

> (But, I am ashamed to say the rest ... he loved so much not only to be called a woman, but to be one, that in order to achieve this he had all his male parts cut off, and gave himself over to surgeons to tailor [or cut] him as they wished, provided that he could become entirely a woman, and could keep company with men as other women did naturally. This is the marvel and monster that he wanted to make appear in his own body.)

Heliogabalus becomes a prodigy or sign of his own impending death; having prepared many precious ways to kill himself (a tower above a courtyard paved with gold and precious stones, vials of poison covered with emeralds and sapphires, etc., p. 233), he is cornered in the latrine, killed, beheaded, and his body thrown into the city sewer. His death is an example of the sort of extreme annihilation reserved for those most threatening to the social order, and resembles murders or "executions" that took place during the Wars of Religion, as well as the various massacres that occurred in late sixteenth-century France:

> La teste fut couppee à l'un & à l'autre, & leurs corps despouillez nuds furent premierement trainez par toute la ville ignominieusement, puis le corps de la mere

ayant esté iecté d'un costé, on iecta celuy du fils en une cloaque qui estoit l'esgoust de toutes les ordures de la ville. Mais pour ce que de fortune le trou de la cloaque estoit si petit que le corps ne peut passer, on le traina iusques au Tibre, dedans lequel on le iecta apres luy avoir attaché quelques poids pesans, afin que son corps ne flottast sur l'eau, & qu'il ne fut ensevely. (*Quatorze histoires*, p. 233)

(Both their heads were cut off, and their bodies, stripped naked, were first dragged shamefully everywhere in the city, then, the mother's body having been cast aside, they threw the son's body into a waste pipe which was the sewer for all of the excrement of the city. But because by chance the hole of the pipe was so small that the body couldn't pass through, they dragged it to the Tiber, into which they threw it after attaching some heavy weights to it, so that his body would not float, and so that he would not be buried.)

This "monster" endures much the same treatment as hermaphroditic infants, and is ritually destroyed and humiliated in order to negate his (formerly considerable) powers. The sheer effort made to assure annihilation also signals fear of the monster's potential power, as if he were supernaturally strong; thus the Neoplatonic tradition meets the Aristotelian in this figure.

For Tesserant, it is doubly evil for a ruler to destabilize the sexual hierarchy in this fashion: "il devoit servir de mirouer et d'exemple de vertu à une milliade d'hommes, comme doivent faire tous Princes" (p. 233: "he should have served as a mirror and example of virtue for thousands of men, as should all Princes"). Perhaps he has in mind the current French court, led by the unstable and foppish Charles IX and his mother, Catherine de Medicis, a pairing which reflects that of Heliogabalus and his mother. At any rate, as we shall see in Thomas Artus' novel, *L'Isle des Hermaphrodites*, Heliogabalus becomes a favored figure of the corrupt and self-indulgent Court.

Royal Effeminacy: The *Mignons*

A decade after the publication of the *Histoires prodigieuses*, Henri's sexual "ambiguity" is reduced to a form of asexuality, in which he and the mignons are accused of being "moins que femmes" ("less than women," L'Estoile, vol. 3, p. 50, sonnet 3). Henri himself is linked to Heliogabalus, a pairing that will take on many nuances (see also the following chapter, on Thomas Artus's novel, *L'Isle des Hermaphrodites* ...):

Cest Heliogabal, empereur des Rommains,
Ne se contenta pas de la mere Nature
Qui donne le tetin à toute Creature,
Mais exposa son corps aux Barbiers inhumains,

Affin d'estre changé, par l'oeuvre de leurs mains,
Au sexe Feminin. Ainsi, par la frizure

Des crins blonds et dorés, par le Fard et Teinture,
Lui veulent ressembler nos Damoiseaux mondains,

Qui prennent les habits des folles damoiselles:
Et pourtant servira, et pour eux et pour elles,
Le discours qu'on en fait, puis qu'on ne congnoist plus

Que Gens effeminés en cest pauvre France,
Qui jadis florissoit ornée de prudence,
Et non point de godrons et cheveux crespelus. (L'Estoile, vol. 3, pp. 51–2, sonnet 7)

(This Heliogabalus, emperor of the Romans, / Was not content with mother Nature, / Who gave suck [or teats] to all creatures, / But exposed his body to inhuman barbers, / So that he might be transformed, by the work of their hands, / To the feminine sex. So, by the curling / Of blond and golden hair, by makeup and tinting, / He wanted to resemble our worldly young men, / Who borrow the clothes of light girls: / And nonetheless, one can use the same descriptions / for either one or the other, since we only see / Effeminate types in this poor France, / Which once flourished, crowned by prudence, / And not with collars and curly hair.)

This sonnet seems to indicate that the phallus is granted not merely by Nature (as it is in the first quatrain), but by dress, grooming, and discourse (second quatrain and first tercet). That is, the performative aspect of gender is just as crucial in late sixteenth-century France as any biological sex might be. This poem can be seen as a pendant to Jean Godard's celebration of female transvestism ("A l'heure que Madame en homme se deguise"), discussed in the previous chapter. Whereas the woman's adoption of male garb was seen as playful, here, the male adoption of feminine appearance becomes much more threatening, and is portrayed as a failure of wisdom that disables all of France. A number of themes evoked in this sonnet will recur in other polemical literature against Henri III: the self-destructive nature of the desire to embody femininity; the emphasis not only on dress, but on other surface "treatments," such as hair-curling and make-up, used to transform appearances; the consequent gap between appearance and any possible underlying "reality" or "natural" body.

Sexual ambiguity was not always seen as threatening, but evolved in that direction over the course of the sixteenth century, as the Valois court declined into very visible self-indulgence and excess. The hermaphroditic portrait of François I, attributed by some to Nicolò Belin da Modena and by others to Nicolò dell'Abbate,[5] and painted sometime after 1530, became with its accompanying doggerel a model for later *poetic* portraits of public figures:

---

[5]   Barbara Hochstetler Meyer, "Marguerite de Navarre and the Androgynous Portrait of François 1er," *Renaissance Quarterly* (Summer 1995): 287–325. It is of some significance to my argument that this inscription on the portrait is in fact poetry, not prose, as Meyer states.

Francoys en guerre est un Mars furieux
En paix Minerve et Diane a la chasse
A bien parler Mercure copieux
A bien aymer vray Amour plein de grace
O france heureuse honore donc la face
De ton grand Roy qui surpasse Nature
Car l'honorant tu sers en mesme place
Minerve, Mars, Diane, Amour, Mercure

(François in war is a furious Mars
In peace Minerva and Diana of the hunt,
A well-spoken, copious Mercury,
A much-loving, true Amor full of grace.
O fortunate France, honor this face
Of your great king who surpasses Nature,
For there you will have honored in the same place
Minerva, Mars, Diana, Amor, Mercury.)[6]

There is some disagreement between scholars as to the tone of this presentation. Raymond B. Waddington contends in his article that the tone is somewhat ambiguous. A medal struck to commemorate Henri II's military successes, dated 1552, even though in imitation of this hermaphroditic portrait, displays an unmistakably masculine figure. Waddington links the portrait of François to a certain blurring of gender roles at the court ("Bisexual Portrait," p. 112). He analyzes several representations of the Hercules and Omphale myth of role-reversal (she wears his lion skin, he wears her robes, "Bisexual Portrait," pp. 117–18). Waddington concludes: "In short, the bisexuality of Bellin da Modena's human deity is not the self-sufficient integration of the androgyne but the impotent neutrality of Hermaphroditus" ("Bisexual Portrait," p. 122). Thus, this portrait can be read not only as a glorification of François's achievements, but as an allusion to his foibles.

Barbara Hochstetler Meyer, after a detailed analysis of the portrait, offers a more Neoplatonic interpretation of this androgyny. This interpretation, she argues, is more in keeping with the philosophical interests of François' sister, Marguerite, and also reveals the closeness of their relationship. Meyer thus sees the portrait as more idealizing.

Given the coexistence of the humorous Aristophanic portrayal of the hermaphrodite with more spiritualized Neoplatonic versions of the myth, and given the afterlife of this panegyric poetry, which also cut both ways, both interpretations hold some value, and should be considered mutually enriching, rather than mutually exclusive. While comparison to the gods is a staple of court poetry, the proliferation of gods and goddesses, and the potential for Rabelaisian slippage into comparisons with

---

6   Cited and translated by Raymond B. Waddington, in his article "The Bisexual Portrait of
     Francis I: Fontainebleau, Castiglione, and the Tone of Courtly Mythology," in *Playing
     with Gender: A Renaissance Pursuit*, pp. 99–101.

less palatable gods such as Priapus, lend a certain edge to this ephemeral form. And why shouldn't poetry based on the hermaphrodite be strangely dualistic in nature, offering conflicting possibilities in the same representation, dualities that cannot be reconciled or subsumed into the greater whole, just as the hermaphrodite cannot be made to conform to merely one sex, or even to the general schema of sexual difference? If there is a hermaphroditic rhetoric or poetics, it would be precisely this duality remaining in constant tension with itself, offering at one and the same time, "either/or," "neither/both."

This possibility for slippage from panegyric into satire is evident in poems written about Henri III's *mignons*. Particularly in two poems about the death of Maugeron, one of Henri's favorites, in April of 1578, there are echoes of the "He was a Mars in war, a Venus in love" theme. These poems seem in fact to be a combination of that topos with the theme from the spurious fragment of the Satyricon (see the previous chapter), in which the gods fight for dominion over a mortal:

DU BEAU MAUGERON

Tel qu'un Caesar, il fut grand en courage;
Tel qu'Adonis, il eut beau le visage.
Il pleut à Mars, et eust le coeur espris
De son amour la déesse Cypris.
Mars le dit sien, et Cypris, au contraire,
L'advoue à soi. Mars, outré de colére,
Pour enlaidir un visage aussi beau,
Estaint, cruel, le céleste flambeau
De son bel oeil. Tel acte davantage
De la déesse enflamme le courage.
C'est oeil perdu ne le rend point plus laid:
Ce jeune enfant lui aggrée et lui plaist,
C'est tout son coeur. Maugeron, ce lui semble,
A Cupidon de plus en plus ressemble,
Qui n'a qu'un oeil. Car s'il n'avoit point d'yeux
Car s'il n'avoit point d'yeux,
Qui est celui qui lui sembleroit mieux?
Lors le dieu Mars, troublé de jalousie,
Se resolut de lui oster la vie.
Il mourut donc, pour n'avoir moins esté
Rempli de coeur que rempli de beauté. (L'Estoile, vol. 2, pp. 193–4)

(Like a Caesar, he was great in courage; / Like an Adonis, he had a beautiful face. / He pleased Mars, and Venus's / Heart was consumed with love for him. / Mars said he was his, and Venus, on the contrary, / Claimed him as hers. Mars, outraged, / In order to make such a handsome face ugly, / Cruelly extinguished the divine light / Of his beautiful eye. Such an act / Enflamed the love of the goddess even more. / This lost eye does not make him uglier: / This young child pleases her, / And has all her heart. / Maugeron, it seems to her, / Resembles Cupid more and more, / Since he has but one eye. For if he had no eyes / If he had no eyes / Who would resemble Cupid better? / So the god Mars, wracked with jealousy, / Decides to take away his life. / And so he died, for having / As great a heart as he had beauty.)

The conventional praise does seem somewhat undercut by Maugeron's particular devotion to Venus, and the awkward conceit that the more eyes he loses, the more he will resemble blind Cupid. The constant emphasis on that which is missing, the eye, makes this piece quite awkward. More interesting for our purposes, because more concerned with sexual ambiguity, is the satirical version of this theme, immediately following the serious one in L'Estoile's journal:

Quand ce beau Maugeron prinst naissance ici-bas,
Trois grandes déités pour lui prindrent querelle:
Mars, le dieu de Lampsaque, et Cyprine la belle,
Qui tous diversement se plaisent aux combas.

Juppiter, qui voioit leurs courageux debats,
Son troien eschanson Ganimedes apelle,
Voulant qu'il appaisast ceste noise nouvelle,
Comme competant juge en amoureux esbats.

"Un si beau corps, dist-il, à trois ne peult suffire:
Pour un ce seroit trop; pour deux il bastera:
Vénus son beau devant, et Priapus aura

Le derriere pour soi, qui le devant n'empire."
Mars, frustré de son droit, forcenoit en son ire,
Et qu'il auroit son ame en partage il jura! (L'Estoile, vol. 2, pp. 194–5)

(When handsome Maugeron was born down here, / Three great gods quarreled over him. / Mars, Priapus, and beautiful Venus, / Who all enjoy different sorts of battles. / Juppiter, who saw their brave fights, / Called his Trojan cupbearer, Ganymede, / And wanted him to settle this new quarrel, / As a competent judge of amorous pleasures. / "Such a beautiful body," said he "is not enough for three: / For one it is too much; for two it is enough: / Venus will have his handsome front side, and Priapus will have / The backside for himself, so that he doesn't ruin the front." / Mars, cheated of his rights, raged in anger, / And swore that he would take the soul as his share!)

Here, bisexuality and hermaphrodism are confounded in the double figure of Venus and Priapus (the latter often associated with the figure of the hermaphrodite, Delcourt, *Hermaphrodite*, pp. 77–8). Priapus's penis is sometimes attached to his buttocks (Delcourt, *Hermaphrodite*, p. 77), a fact which would confirm the hermaphroditic aspect of the image. The presence of Ganymede clearly signals the sexual context (as if it were not overt enough in the figure of Priapus), but also renders that sexual context more complex, as Leonard Barkin suggests in relation to that myth:

The exceptional quality of Jupiter's love for Ganymede places the life of the myth in a charged arena of symbolization, an arena in which the taboos concerning homosexuality confront the individual exercise of desire as well as the mores of a particular society, which may permit or even glorify certain homosexual practices while confirming the taboos in respect to ordinary, quotidian behavior. Encounters with this material thus invariably consist of both individual confrontation with a marginalized form of desire and a cultural confrontation with an age in which things were done differently.[7]

It is hard to establish exactly what Henri's sexual practices were; all accounts of his sexuality (and that of his *mignons*) extant to us are from the hands of Huguenot and Catholic enemies. It is clear that he patronized poets who wrote of ambiguous sexual encounters and portrayed themselves in stereotypically feminine roles; it is also clear that alchemy was a current interest among some members of the court. Henri's sexuality cannot in fact be divided from his intellectual interests as a humanist, since all we have are the literary results of that sexuality. Although the word "homosexuality" was not in use at the time; the terms "sodomite" and "bougre" were (the former most frequently designating the active, and the latter the passive, roles). Although it is not always clear whether the author of the satirical poem or pamphlets is criticizing actual sexual practices or the general effeminacy and refinement of the court, some of the works are very graphic and specific. Thus, the various forms of homosexuality became practices that divided one element of society, the court, from the others; the more so because the behaviour of those at the court was not punished (if in fact it did occur), when that of other French men was.

Further complicating this issue is the fact that late sixteenth-century French satirists clearly distinguished homosexuality (itself divided into active and passive)[8] from bisexuality (as the poem cited above makes quite evident); and the latter practice was considered infinitely more dangerous, because somehow destabilizing of the social order. The image of the hermaphrodite becomes a code for bisexuality (as well as for transvestism and effeminacy), just as Ganymede becomes a code for male homosexuality.[9] In fact, Poirier points out that one anagram on Henri's name is *O Crudelis Hyena*, "O Cruel Hyena," which links cruelty to the supposed sexual

---

[7]   Leonard Barkin, "Ganymede Aloft," in *Transuming Passion: Ganymede and the Erotics of Humanism* (Stanford: Stanford University Press, 1991), p. 24.

[8]   As noted above, there are the "sodomites" and the "bougres." The "bougres," those playing what would have been considered the female's role, are more frequently and more vehemently condemned than those engaging in the active role.

[9]   Used again in a 1577 sonnet, cited by L'Estoile (vol. 2, p. 95):

Passer outre Venus, perdre ce qu'on labeure,
Doubler Ganimedès, renverser la nature ....

And again in a 1579 sonnet (vol. 3, p. 49, sonnet 3):

Ganimedès effrontés, impudique canaille ....

instability of that animal, which was believed to be able to transform itself from one sex to the other (*L'homosexualité*, p. 149).

Often, however, the two practices are confounded, for the sake of satiric *amplificatio*. A later piece (1581), labeled both a *pasquil* and a *coq à l'âne*, piles on accusation after accusation of hedonism in various forms:

SUITTE

> Coq, nostre frère et bon ami,
> Je suis infiniment marri
> Que je ne te puis faire entendre
> Ce que j'ai peu ici apprendre.
> Tu ne vis jamais tant de choses
> Qui dedans Paris sont encloses!
> Les dieux, les nimphes, les driades,
> Satyres, tritons et naiades
> Y ont visité nostre Roy,
> Qui avecques ses Ganimèdes
> Les a receus en bel arroy.
> Que ce sont de beaux compagnons
> Que le Roy et tous ses mignons!
> Ils ont le visage un peu palle,
> Mais sont-ils femelle ou masle?
> Car ils servent tous d'un mestier.
> La Valette est bien en quartier,
> Et le plus aimé, ce dit-on;
> Il est un peu bougre et poltron:
> Sont-ce pas belles qualités
> Pour estre entre les déités? (L'Estoile, vol. 3, p. 180)

(Cock, our brother and good friend, / I am so infinitely dismayed / That I cannot make you understand / What I have been able to learn here. / You have never seen so many things / As are enclosed in Paris! / Gods, nymphs, dryads, / Satyrs, Tritons, and Naiads / Have visited our King, / Who, with his Ganymede / Received them in an elegant manner. / What handsome fellows / The King and his *mignons* are! / They seem a little pale, / But are they female or male? / For they seem to serve both roles. / La Valette is well placed, / And the best loved, they say; / He is a bit of a bugger and a coward: / Are these not good qualities / To be among the deities?)

Confusion of gender roles is linked to sexual promiscuity (and not only male homosexuality); Henri is depicted as engaging in various sexual relations (mostly sodomitic) with many in his court (and names are named). La Valette is accused of taking the passive role in these acts (later, this accusation will be leveled against Henri himself). Here, such sexuality is not depicted as a personal, individual choice, but as the common practices of an entire class. Whomever this satire did not implicate in these practices, the previous *pasquil* did, even going so far as to contend that Henri had married La Valette (L'Estoile, vol. 3, p. 171: "Un homme à l'autre se marie,"), although this marriage was disguised by the presence of La Valette's wife.

Thus, the problematic relationship between gender and power is made evident in public representations of the royal person of Henri III of France, who was frequently portrayed as playing ambiguous roles, dressing in attire somewhat feminized from the waist up (a decolletage covered by transparent material, strings of pearls, elaborate headdress, often a rouged and powdered face),[10] acting very emotional (crying and fainting), surrounding himself with similarly attired and mannered *mignons*:

> De cordons emperlez sa chevelure pleine,
> Sous un bonnet sans bord fait à l'italienne,
> Faisoit deux arcs voutez; son menton pinceté,
> Son visage de blanc et de rouge empasté,
> Son chef tout empoudré nous monstrerent ridee,
> En la place d'un Roy, une putain fardee.
> Pensez quel beau spectacle, et comm'il fit bon voir
> Ce prince avec un busc, un corps de satin noir
> Couppé à l'espagnolle, ou, des déchicquetures,
> Sortoyent des passements et des blanches tireures;
> Et, affin que l'habit s'entresuivist de rang,
> Il monstroit des manchons gauffrez de satin blanc,
> D'autres manches encor qui s'estendoyent fendues,
> Et puis jusques aux pieds d'autres manches perdues.
> Pour nouveau parement il porta tout ce jour
> Cet habit monstrueux, pareil à son amour:
> Si qu'au premier abord chacun estoit en peine
> S'il voyoit un Roy femme ou bien un homme Reyne.[11]

(His hair full of ropes [of pearls], under a brimless hat in the Italian style, made two high arcs; his plucked chin, his face plastered with chalk and rouge, his powdered forehead showed us, in the place of a King, a wrinkled whore. Think about what a beautiful spectacle, and how pleasant it was to see this Prince wearing a buskin, a bodice of black satin cut in Spanish style, on which, through slashes, peeked out braidwork and white cords; and, so the costume was consistent with his rank, it displayed little sleeves of quilted white satin, then other sleeves which hung open, and finally other sleeves which reached all the way to the floor. As his new regalia he wore this costume

---

10   André Blum discusses various satirical portraits of the King as hermaphrodite in *L'Estampe satirique en France pendant les Guerres de Religion* (Paris: Giard & Briere, 1917), pp. 255–6, as does Keith Cameron, in his book *Henri III: A Maligned or Malignant King? (Aspects of the Satirical Iconography of Henri de Valois)* (Exeter, England: University of Exeter, 1978), p. 82.

11   Théodore Agrippa d'Aubigné, "Princes," *Les Tragiques*, in *Oeuvres*, ed. Henri Weber (Paris: Gallimard, 1969), ll. 779–94.

all that day, a costume similar to his love: so that at first glance, everyone had some difficulty distinguishing whether he saw a female King or a male Queen.)

A passage from Pierre de L'Estoile's journal for 1577 seems to confirm d'Aubigné's portrait:

> Ce pendant le Roy faisoit jouxtes, tournois, ballets et force masquarades, où il se trouvoit ordinairement habillé en femme, ouvroit son pourpoint et descouvroit sa gorge, y portant un collier de perles et trois collets de toile, deux à fraize et un renversé, ainsi que alors les portoient les dames de sa cour. (vol. 2, p. 104)

> (At this time, the King held jousts, tournaments, ballets, and many masques at which he was ordinarily to be found dressed as a woman, his jacket opened and his chest uncovered, wearing a pearl necklace and three cloth collars, two ruffled and one reversed, just as the women of his court wore them at that time.)

This account is echoed in a 1579 passage: "aiant ordinairement son pourpoint ouvert, et la gorge nue et descouverte, comme les femmes, dans laquelle il portoit souvent (comme elles) un collier de Perles, chose effeminée" (L'Estoile, vol. 3, p. 63: "usually having his vest open, and his chest naked and uncovered, like the women, on which he often wore [like them] a pearl necklace, an effeminate thing"), and elsewhere in the journal, suggesting that this practice was not exceptional. This passage places heavy emphasis on the femininity of Henri's attire, repeating feminine nouns and pronouns with some insistence. This parody of feminine court behavior and dress caused many to question his suitability as king. Nonetheless, these sources for understanding Henri III have been skewed by the campaign of political propaganda mounted against him by the Catholic League.[12] Furthermore, that any *perceived* ambiguity was taken as a threat to the fabric of society is evidence of a problematic sense of the gender roles informing social structures such as monarchy or marriage. Like Aristippus in Sextus's example, the French would not have felt threatened by signs of effeminacy if masculinity had been an established and unquestioned fact rather than a social role.

Questioning of such social roles as gender evidently implied a questioning of the social hierarchy itself, and a weakening of the established orders of French society. Masculinity is used as a metaphor for political power, even as it is used in the political propaganda to justify that power. For example, Théodore Agrippa D'Aubigné accuses Henri III of homosexuality in his *Histoire Universelle*.[13] At first, he designates this behavior as unspeakable, since it is outside of the realm of accepted social discourse: "Ces mignons, car c'est le terme du siècle, avoyent des familiaritez avec leur maistre

---

[12] For detailed analysis of this campaign, see the article by David A. Bell, "Unmasking a King," pp. 371–86; as well as the studies by Elie Barnavi, *Le Parti de Dieu: Etude sociale et politique des chefs de la Ligue parisienne, 1585–1594* (Louvain: Nauwelaerts, 1980), and by Frederic Baumgartner, *Radical Reactionaries: The Political Thought of the French Catholic League* (Geneva: Droz, 1975), as well as that of Keith Cameron, cited above.

[13] André Thierry, ed. (Geneva: Droz, 1992), vol. 6.

que je ne veux ni ne peux exprimer" (*Histoire universelle*, bk 9, ch. 15, p. 70: "The *mignons*, since that was the word used at the time, were familiar with their master in a manner I do not wish to, and cannot, express"). But later, he makes himself perfectly clear, and links the King's sexual behavior to issues of political power:

> Vous oyiez dire tout haut, que depuis que ce prince s'estoit prostitué à l'amour contre nature, mesme avoit tourné ses voluptez à patir au lieu d'agir, on cottoit la perte du courage qu'on avoit veu à Monsieur avant la naissance de telles énormitez. (*Histoire universelle*, bk 10, ch. 12, p. 208)

> (You have heard it said aloud that, since this prince had prostituted himself to the love against nature, and had even turned his pleasures to those of submission[14] (or inaction) rather than those of action, people [*on*] noted the measurable loss of that courage which they had seen in *Monsieur* before the birth of such monstrosities.)

Here, it becomes somewhat clearer that Henri III is accused of taking the passive (considered at the time feminine) role (*patir*) instead of the active (masculine) one (*agir*) in his sexual relations. As in Roman times, such passivity denoted servitude, a lowering of personal status and power.[15] D'Aubigné makes clear that this is in fact the result of Henri III's effeminate behavior – he is shamed and scorned, and loses power with his prestige. D'Aubigné associates Henri's passive sexuality with attempts on his life, attempts to dethrone and cloister him, and with the ascension of the Duc de Guise to popular acclaim and effective power. Thus effeminacy becomes a metaphor for powerlessness, even as it is used to justify this demotion. The association of passivity and powerlessness with the feminine was common in Renaissance France (and elsewhere) as Waddington points out: "It may be no oversimplification to conclude that, for Cinquecento culture, the behavioral antimonies of active versus passive and dominant versus subordinate can be subsumed into the categories of masculine and feminine."[16] In the Renaissance, many authors on the subject of sexual difference (male

---

[14] Here, d'Aubigné seems to be using *patir* in its latinate sense, from *patior*, "to submit to someone else's lust" (Charlton T. Lewis and Charles Short, *A Latin Dictionary*, Oxford: Clarendon Press, 1975).

[15] See Paul Veyne, "Homosexuality in Ancient Rome," in *Western Sexuality: Practice and Precept in Past and Present Times*, eds Philippe Ariès and André Béjin, trans. Anthony Forster (Oxford: Basil Blackwell, 1985), pp. 26–35.

[16] "A Bisexual Portrait of Francis I," p. 120. In fact, from Roman times, active sexuality was deemed the domain of upper-class men, and women, as well as men of lesser prestige, were doomed to passivity (one need only read a few poems by Catullus to realize this fact – he condemns unworthy politicians as *pathicus* and vaunts his own ability to sodomize others). The political/cultural interface which reflects this stereotypical gender division (male/active – female/passive) is explored by Linda L. Carroll in her article "Who's on Top? Gender as Societal Power Configuration in Italian Renaissance Drama" (*Sixteenth Century Journal* 20, 1989): 531–58 and by Natalie Davis in her article "Women on Top" (in *Society*

and female anatomy) considered women to be merely internalized (i.e., imperfect) men. There was only one sex, and all beings were placed in the social hierarchy according to how closely they approximate this ideal sex.

But this singular version of sex, which fits in so well with the other "unities" of French society ("une foi, une loi, un roi," "one faith, one law, one king"), is thrown into question by Henri III's apparent bisexuality. And this is the true monstrosity of his behavior, as depicted in the satirical portrait of him that often accompanies the first edition of *L'Isle des Hermaphrodites*:

> Je ne suis masle ny femelle
> Et sy je suis bien en cervelle
> Lequel des deux je doibs choysir
> Mais qu'importe à qui on ressamble
> Il vault mieux les avoir ensemble
> On en reçoit double plaisir.

> (I am neither male nor female, and if I were sane, I would have to choose one of the two. But who cares which I resemble, it is better to have the two together, since one then gets double pleasure.)[17]

In the land of one sex, the hermaphrodite destroys the unitary hierarchy, by setting two beings in suspension. Such a suspension dissolves the possibility of there being only one sex. If females were merely deficient males, then the hermaphrodite would be a male (perhaps a weakened male, as in Ovid's story of Hermaphroditus, but nonetheless male). The coexistence of the two, male and female, as discrete entities in one person, argues for a two-sex theory of human physiology.

The accusations of homosexuality against Henri III seem to begin around 1575, that is, shortly after his coronation. One "Sonnet Courtizan," in which a sister accuses her brother of submitting to the King, appears in L'Estoile's May entry for that year (vol. 1, p. 166). The timing of this poem suggests the political purpose of such

---

and Culture in Early Modern France), pp. 124–51. Davis in particular links transvestism to social upheaval. Men dressed as women in the Ancien Régime in order to foment riots and revolts with impunity, since women had limited legal status and responsibility.

17   Thomas Artus, *Description de l'Isle des Hermaphrodites, nouvellement descouverte* (n.p., 1605), frontispiece. The Hermaphrodite is a paradox, an impossibility, in the land of one gender, or even in a binary system, as Butler points out in relation to Foucault's edition of the journals of Herculine Barbin: "Herculine is not an 'identity,' but the sexual impossibility of an identity ... The linguistic conventions that produce intelligible gendered selves find their limit in Herculine precisely because she/he occasions a convergence and disorganization of the rules that govern sex/gender/desire. Herculine deploys and redistributes the terms of a binary system, but that very redistribution disrupts and proliferates those terms outside the binary itself" (*Gender Trouble: Feminism and the Subversion of Identity* (New York: Routledge, 1990), p. 23).

satire; it is followed shortly in the journal by numerous poems railing at Catherine de Medicis' power (July, 1575; L'Estoile, vol. 1, pp. 178–93). This group of poems contains references to Catherine's castrating power: "Mais, nous, qui sommes Francs, devenons misérables/ D'une femme asservis" (L'Estoile, vol. 1, p. 184: "And we, who are Francs [free], become wretched in the service of a woman"). The Italians at court are called sodomites: "Les faits que leurs ayeuls aprirent à Sodome / Et qu'au aceu d'un chacun exercent dedans Romme" (L'Estoile, vol. 1, p. 183: "The deeds that their ancestors learned in Sodom/ And with everyone's knowledge they practice at Rome"). Sodomy and female power are seen as foreign practices, to be expelled. Sexual innuendo against Catherine and against the men at court is conflated into the myth of Cybele:

> Quid mirum Gallos instructos grandibus olim
> Testibus, Eunuchos nunc evasisse vietos!
> Foemina magna Deum Mater, peregrina, profusa,
> Altera nunc Cybele, magnas invecta per urbes,
> Sublimisque in equis, Gallos, gentem omnipotentem
> Olim, castratos hodiè atque virilibus orbos
> Membris, esse sibi famulos, mollesque ministros
> Atque Sacerdotes, sine mente et mentula inertes,
> Cogit. Sic Galli, servato nomine, sed re
> Amissâ, Cybelen Galli, Eunuchique sequuntur. (L'Estoile, vol. 1, p. 189)

(What a wonder that the Gauls, once instructed by great men (testes = testicles; also witnesses), now are wasted and withered Eunuchs! A woman, the Great Mother to God, a foreigner, extravagant, now another Cybele, is carried through (or invading) the great cities on high horses, and the Gauls, once an all-powerful (potent) people, are today castrated and deprived of their male members; she forces them to be her servants, soft attendants and priests, indolent without minds and without members. So the Gauls retain their name, while the thing itself is lost, and the Gauls as Eunuchs follow their Cybele.)[18]

Catherine is called a *virago* in another poem (also L'Estoile, vol. 1, p. 189). Some poems rail about a hen (*gallina*) ruling the Gauls or cocks (*gallos*; L'Estoile, vol. 1, p. 190). The reversal of male and female roles was not taken lightly in this period; and the fear of symbolic castration, in the form of loss of power, is vehemently expressed.

---

[18]   For analysis of this and similar polemical works against Catherine, see Stephen Murphy, "Catherine, Cybele, and Ronsard's Witnesses," in *High Anxiety: Masculinity in Crisis in Early Modern France*, ed. Kathleen Long (Kirksville, MO: Truman State University Press, 2002), pp. 55–70.

Transgressive Sexuality and the Demonization of Henri III

L'Estoile's collection of political material (pamphlets, poems circulated about Paris, popular songs, etc.) indicates a very swift, negative reaction to Henri's reign and to Catherine's involvement in the government of France. The accusations of sodomy recur, but are less frequent after the first few years of Henri's reign. More significant are the poems lamenting a "world turned upside-down" ("Le serf commande, et la femme conseille," L'Estoile, vol. 2, p. 96, sonnet 16), in which gender and social hierarchy are closely linked. Also frequent are the satirical attacks against foreigners, particularly Italians.[19] Apparently, the fear of sexual otherness is linked to fears of various forms of difference (religious and national).[20]

Nonetheless, there continue to be accusations of homosexual behavior, as well. Yet another sonnet cited by L'Estoile accuses Saint-Luc of being a "bougre" ("Tu ne peux, bougeron, petit bougre Saint-Luc," vol. 3, p. 55, sonnet 10), as does the "pasquil" which follows it (vol. 3, pp. 56–62). In the same "pasquil," Henri is called a "poulle couronnée" ("a crowned hen"). Yet, at the same time, he is being accused of assaulting nuns (L'Estoile, vol. 3, p. 62).

Accusations of sodomy recur when Henri institutes a confraternity called "Les Pénitents" (April, 1583), the members of which parade around town, flagellating themselves. A series of epigrams and other satirical pieces circulates around Paris:

II
Ils sont accouplés deux à deux
D'une assez dévote manière:
Mais je les trouve vicieux,
Quand ils s'enfilent par derrière.

III
Ils sont advisés et bien sages
D'ainsi se couvrir les visages;
Car on verroit, entre les bons,
Les bougres et les bougerons. (L'Estoile, vol. 4, p. 80)

(They are coupled two by two / In a fairly devout fashion: / But I think that they are nasty, / When they couple from behind. / They are wise and well advised / To cover

---

[19]   L'Estoile, vol. 2, p. 189–90, "Vaudeville sur le combat des mignons," in which the "seed of Florence" is blamed for the impending ruin of France; vol. 2, pp. 211–12 ("A Messire Poltron …"). In this poem, the Italians are called *bougrins*, thus linking that nationality with homosexual practices (a frequent accusation in French satirical poetry of the period). Anti-Italian sentiment recurs frequently in the works cited by L'Estoile.

[20]   Another sonnet cited by L'Estoile links religious difference to sexuality by means of its unknown narrator declaring that "la plus grand part du monde est héretique" and refusing to join in this heresy in the phrase "J'abhorre d'estre bougre" (3.52, sonnet 8).

their faces this way; / Because you would see, among the good men, / The buggers and their little friends.)

Another stanza plays on the words *fouteurs* and *fouettés* (L'Estoile, vol. 4, p. 82).

Finally, the murders of the Duke of Guise and his brother the Cardinal of Lorraine (23 and 24 December, 1588), give rise to many poems and pamphlets recapitulating the various sins of which Henri was accused over the course of his reign:

Chérir les Huguenots, les Chrestiens mespriser,
Sçavoir dissimuler, bien faire l'hipocrite;
Faire le pénitent, faire le saint hermite;
Or' de rouge son corps, or' de blanc, tapisser;

Apauvrir ses subjets et leur mort pourchasser;
Enrichir un Gascon d'une façon maudite;
Violer les nonnains [et], ô chose inaudite!
En bougre sodomit' les hommes embrasser;

Jurer dessus son Dieu de maintenir l'Eglise
Et son plus ferme appui, qu'est la maison de Guise,
Les tuer à l'instant; menasser les Docteurs,

S'ils disent vérité chasser cil qui [ne l'aime],
Pour meurtrir du grand Dieu les plus grands zélateurs,
Sont les rares vertus de Roy Henri Troisiesme! (L'Estoile, vol. 6, pp. 178–9)

(To cherish Huguenots and despise Christians, / To know how to lie, to play the hypocrite well; / To pretend penitence, to feign being a saintly hermit; / Then to paint his body with red, then white; / To impoverish his subjects, and seek their death; / To enrich a Gascon in a damnable way; / To rape nuns, and – an unheard of thing! / As a sodomitical bugger to embrace men. / To swear to God to uphold the Church / And then to kill instantly its strongest support, / That is the house of Guise; to menace Professors / If they tell the truth, to exile those who do not like him, / To kill the most zealous supporters of God, / These are the rare virtues of King Henri the Third!)

Again, bisexuality is associated with a world turned upside-down, with toleration of the Huguenots, and with the general social disorder in France. There is an escalation in the number and severity of accusations from the earliest moments of Henri's reign to his assassination. The first accusations are of effeminacy, then of homosexuality, later of bisexuality, then of murder, and finally of Satanism. Thus, the whole range of transgressions against society and religion are explored, and are almost always linked to sexuality.

Bisexuality is associated with this Satanism or magic in another late pamphlet, *Les Choses horribles contenues en une Lettre envoyée à Henri de Valois par un Enfant de Paris, le 28e janvier 1589.*[21] In this piece, the Duc d'Espernon, Jean de Nogaret, is called Teragon and described as a demon:

> Vous sçavez bien que, pour passer plus outre vostre malignité, avez contraint iceux sorciers et enchanteurs de transmuer leur esprit en figure d'homme naturel, ce qu'ils trouvèrent fort estrange, et neanmoins avec leur art diabolique ont accordé ceste requeste et … on fit sortir un Diable d'Enfer, figuré en homme. Et de la région où il fut premier apparu, ce fut en Gascongne, d'un nommé Nogenne, où il prist le nom de Nogaret, ou Teragon … la nuit suivante, il coucha dans vostre chambre, seul avec vous dans vostre lit. Vous sçavez bien que, toute la nuict, il tinst sur vostre ventre, droit au nombril, un anneau et sa main liée dans la vostre; et fut, le matin, vostre main trouvée comme toute cuite … et ce matin il monstra que, dans la pierre de son anneau, estoit là vostre âme figurée … L'on tient que cedit Teragon eust affaire à une fille de joye en la chambre secrète de quoi elle cuida mourir, certifiant que ledit Nogaret n'est point un homme naturel, pource que son corps est trop chaud et bruslant. (*Choses horribles*, pp. 37–8)

> (You know well that, to surpass your previous evils, you forced these wizards and enchanters to transmute their spirits into a natural man, which they found very strange, and nonetheless with their diabolical art they granted this request and made a Devil come out of Hell in the form of a man. And from the region where he first appeared, which was in Gascony, a place named Nogenne, he took the name of Nogaret or Teragon … the following night he slept in your room, alone with you in your bed. You know well that all night he held a ring on your stomach, right on your navel, and his hand in yours; and your hand was found the next morning to be as if it were all cooked … and that morning he showed you that your soul was trapped in the stone of his ring. They say that this Teragon slept with a prostitute in the secret room, from which she thought she would die, swearing later that Nogaret was not a natural man, because his body was too hot and burning.)

Another pamphlet cited by L'Estoile, *La grande Diablerie de Jean Vallette, dit de Nogaret, par la grace du Roy, duc d'Esparnon, Grand Amiral de France et Bourgeois d'Angoulesme, sur son département de la Court* (*The Great Devilry of Jean Vallette, named de Nogaret, by the grace of the King, Duke d'Epernon, Grand Admiral of France and Burgher of Angoulême, on his departure from the Court*), details the satanic practices of the Duke.[22] This linking of bisexuality with sorcery and satanism

---

21 (Paris: Jacques Grégoire, 1589), from the collection, *Les Belles Figures et drolleries de la Ligue*, also edited as part of Pierre de L'Estoile's journal (Paris: Librairie des Bibliophiles, 1886), vol. 4, pp. 36–8.

22 *Belles Figures de la Ligue*, vol. 4, p. 47; this piece is echoed by several others, *La Sorcellerie de Jean d'Espernon*, also vol. 4, p. 102; *Pourtrait des charmes et caractères de Sorcellerie de Henry de Valoys, IIIe du nom* (a placard cited by L'Estoile, vol. 4, pp. 115–19); and by *Les Sorcelleries de Henri de Valois et les oblations qu'il faisoit au Diable dans le Bois de Vincennes* (Paris: Didier Millot, 1589). See also *La Vie et faits notables de Henri de Valois, maintenant tout au long, sans rien requérir: où sont contenues les trahisons,*

(and in the most grotesque possible fashion), demonstrates more clearly than any of the other poems, the irrationality of this fear of a practice that called into question a social order based on rigidly constructed gender roles. The man had to penetrate, be active, in order to justify and confirm his domination; the woman had to let herself be penetrated; and any other form of behavior was seen as a threat. The issues of satanism, sexual difference, and politics seem to unite in an engraving from the *Adjournement fait a Henry de Valois pour assister aux Etats tenus aux Enfers* (*The Invitation made to Henri de Valois to attend the Estates General in Hell*) reprinted by André Blum in his study, *L'Estampe satirique en France pendant les Guerres de Religion*.[23] The "huissier infernal" is a creature with a cow's head, bird's feet, fur-covered legs, and quite evident breasts; thus monstrous in both genus and sex. Thus, even in the realm of political discourse, the hermaphrodite effaces all manner of boundaries, between human and animal, male and female, good and evil. It is the threat of this loss of boundaries that renders Henri's behavior so horrifying, as if the shaking of one aspect of the edifice of society would bring the rest of culture tumbling down with it. This intense and disturbing reaction to any form of difference seems to suggest just how fragile the French felt this edifice to be.

Although hermaphrodism is overtly linked with bisexuality in only one of these works cited (the satirical sonnet on Maugeron, discussed above); many of these works hover around the question of duality or discuss concerns related to those raised in other domains by hermaphrodism. Homosexuality, bisexuality, and transvestism all lead to the question of what is male, what female; and Henri de Valois seemed to embody these ambiguities in a very effective (that is, menacing) manner:

> Sardanapale n'eust de masle qu'une image,
> Et de femme l'esprit, le vouloir et les faicts:
> Ce Roy, homme de nom, en ses plaisirs infects
> Devient putain de coeur, et de geste et d'usage.[24]

(Sardanapalus was only male in appearance, / In spirit, will, and deeds a woman: / This King, a man in name, and his pestilential pleasures / Has become a whore in his heart, in deed, and in practice.)

D'Aubigné clearly associates homosexual activity with monstrosity, and with catastrophic events:

> Des monstres avortez, bastards de la Nature
> Nos peres presagoient quelque gauche malheur,

---

perfidies, sacrileges, exactions, cruautés & hontes de cet hypocrite, ennemi de la Religion Catholique (Paris: Didier Millot, 1589).

23   (Paris: Giard & Briere, n.d.), p. 272. The pamphlet itself is reprinted in the 1886 edition of the *Belles figures* (vol. 4, pp. 128–31).

24   Théodore Agrippa d'Aubigné, *Oeuvres*, "Sonnets épigrammatiques," 10 (p. 339).

Changement de l'Empire ou bien de l'Empereur,

…

Le chimere à trois corps, trois vices mis en un.
Ainsi que le forfaict à Sodome commun,
Nous promettent aussy une commune peine. (*Oeuvres*, p. 340, sonnet 11)

(From aborted monsters, Nature's bastards / Our fathers predicted some evil disaster, /
A change of empire or emperor, / … The chimera with three bodies, three vices in one.
/ So the sin in common with Sodom, / Promises us a similar punishment.)

The "Roy/femme, homme/Reyne" (the female King, male Queen) of "Princes" elicited violent criticism from all quarters, Huguenot and Catholic, nobility and bourgeoisie; this criticism is virtually always accompanied by a strong expression of the desire to maintain the current social order, and a fear of a nation turned topsy-turvy by the King's "unnatural vices." The violent expulsion of the King, first from the public regard (as early as 1575), then from Paris (May, 1588), and then from this world (August, 1589), reflects a society dependent on rigid categorization in all aspects of life, private as well as public, a society for which the private and public are not easily distinguished from each other. Rigid regulation of gender roles is called for by those publishing all manner of works, literary or political, scientific or philosophical. This regulation is in turn maintained by those very works. It is clear that by the end of the sixteenth century, sodomy laws were being enforced, and the sexual ambiguity so prevalent in the court of François I, although welcome in the court of Henri III as well, was not welcomed by his subjects. No longer was the hermaphrodite a figure of spiritual refinement, regarded with awe (or at worst, amusement); it had become once more a monster, an object of ridicule or even horror, in an era of extreme political upheaval.

Chapter 8

Hermaphrodites Newly Discovered: The Cultural Monsters of Early Modern France

Skeptical Philosophy, Sex, and Gender

In the late sixteenth century, panegyric devolved into satire in the course of the League's campaign to destroy Henri III. The figure of the hermaphrodite had completed its downward spiral into the depths of shame, thus returning to the Roman representations of it as a horrifying portent of doom, to be annihilated for the good of society. Strangely, however, the more playful aspect of the hermaphrodite, as a figure that does not quite fit into social norms but does not seem to threaten them, either, as a sort of aesthetic or epistemological puzzle concerning our knowledge of sex and identity in all its forms, concerning appearances and ever-elusive reality, remained attached to the more vehemently negative view, as a sort of parasitic twin. Nowhere is this conjunction of the threatening and the amusing more evident than in the novel, *Description de l'Isle des Hermaphrodites, nouvellement découverte* (*Description of the Island of Hermaphrodites, Newly Discovered*), written shortly after 1598[1] by a Thomas Artus.[2]

---

[1] The first edition of this work, published around 1605, contains no information on publisher, place of publication, or date, but rather is inaugurated by an intricate engraving of Henri III as a hermaphrodite, with doggerel verse beneath it. Copies of this original edition are very rare. Many editions of this work were published in the eighteenth century as supplements to Pierre de L'Estoile's *Journal de Henri III*, as was the edition I have used (Paris: La Veuve de Pierre Gandouin, 1744). This is an expanded version of the Duchat edition. All references to the *Isle des Hermaphrodites* in this chapter are to this edition (except the doggerel from the frontispiece of the original edition).

[2] There has been some discussion of the author's name, which, to my mind, is still unclear. Claude Gilbert-Dubois, in his edition of *L'Isle des Hermaphrodites* (Geneva: Droz, 1996), uses Artus Thomas, as does Poirier, in *L'homosexualité*, and Lise Leibacher-Ouvrard in her article "Decadent Dandies and Dystopian Gender-Bending: Artus Thomas's *L'Isle des Hermaphrodites*," *Utopian Studies* 11 (2000): 124–31. But works published in his own lifetime and shortly after alternate between Thomas Artus and Artus Thomas. *L'histoire de la décadence de l'empire grec*, published in Paris in 1650, lists him as Thomas Artus (repeated editions of this list him as Thomas Artus; although a continuation of this work is listed under Artus Thomas); his work on another project by Blaise de Vigenère is credited

Recent works on the figure of the hermaphrodite, especially as manifested in early modern France, have concentrated on the medical and legal bases for its depiction.[3] When philosophical sources are explored, Platonic and Neoplatonic sources are emphasized.[4] Thus, the hermaphrodite becomes either a figure of menace or of divine completion and wisdom. These views evade many of the epistemological, theological and political problems raised by sexual ambiguity, problems currently discussed in modern gender theory, but already known to Renaissance audiences well versed in skepticism. The ambiguities played out in the court of Henri III of France were as much the result of the revolution brought about by the revival of the works of Sextus Empiricus as of any Platonic or medical theories. More than an expression of the desire for spiritual wholeness, these ambiguous roles also represent a subversion of social norms. Evidence of this subversion surfaces in Artus's novel, published decades after Henri's death.

Throughout his satirical novel about the court of Henri de Valois, Artus seems obsessed with the cultural signs of gender – clothing, gesture, language, public behavior – rather than bodily marks of sex or reproductive questions. The barely described hermaphroditic body is pushed, prodded and primped into its dualistic form. This outward appearance in turn *creates* the hermaphroditic identity, rather than echoing some inherent quality. Thus, although his book is meant to be a conservative critique of the fashionable court and moderate politics of Henri III, in the end, Artus seems to question normative views of sex (and by extension of other social issues) without restoring any solid epistemological grounding for these views which he seems at first to support: his narrative takes place in a realm of pure signification. By these means, Artus brings into question virtually all of the structures of the society in which he lives, structures which he links continually to the question of sexual difference.

These doubts are closely linked to philosophical issues that dominated the cultural context of late sixteenth-century France. In 1562, Henri Estienne had published a Latin edition of Sextus Empiricus's *Outlines of Pyrrhonism*. As Richard Popkin points out, "Sextus Empiricus ... came to have a dramatic role in the formation of modern

---

to Artus Thomas (*Les images ou tableaux de Platte peinture des deux Philostrates ... avec des Epigrammes ... par Artus Thomas*; Paris: Guillemot, 1637). Dubois cites L'Estoile as calling him Arthus Thomas (pp. 14–15). I will keep to Thomas Artus, because of Pierre Bayle's entry on him in the *Dictionnaire historique et critique* (Rotterdam, 1697), but I recognize that the name is still unclear.

3   For example, Thomas Laqueur's book *Making Sex*; Julia Epstein, "Either/Or – Neither/ Both: Sexual Ambiguity and the Ideology of Gender," pp. 99–142. Ann Rosalind Jones and Peter Stallybrass do analyze cultural constructs of the hermaphrodite, including a brief consideration of Artus's novel, in their essay "Fetishizing Gender: Constructing the Hermaphrodite in Renaissance Europe," pp. 80–111.

4   In this case, Constance Jordan's chapter on "Sex and Gender" in her book *Renaissance Feminism: Literary Texts and Political Models*, pp. 134–247, is exemplary (especially pp. 136–7).

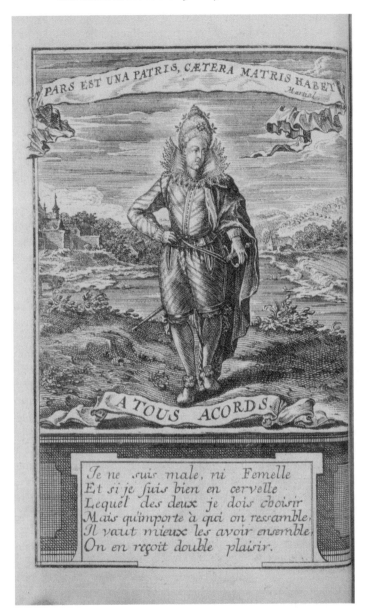

Figure 8.1   Portrait of Henri III of France as a hermaphrodite. The
frontispiece from Thomas Artus, *Description de l'Isle des
hermaphrodites, nouvellement descouverte* (Cologne: Demen,
1724). Courtesy of the Division of Rare and Manuscript
Collections, Cornell University Library

thought."[5] Sextus argues that apprehension of meaning is mediated by the senses or by language, and that direct knowledge may therefore not be possible: "nothing can be apprehended [known] through itself" (that is, the signified cannot signify itself); but, by logical extension of the first rule "nothing can be apprehended through another thing."[6] That other thing would itself have to be established, in relation either to the first thing or to yet another thing, and thus "If that through which an object is apprehended must always itself be apprehended through some other thing, one is involved in a process of circular reasoning or in regress *ad infinitum*" (*Outlines*, bk 1, ch. 16, p. 179). Circular reasoning, for Sextus, is the constant referral from one to the other element of a definition, and back again to the first. Regress *ad infinitum*, similar but not identical to the Derridean notion of the supplement,[7] is the constant replacement of one element used to define another by yet a third (and the third by a fourth, and so on) in infinite and linear fashion. These two skeptical concepts create a potential basis for questioning cultural constructs of gender in early modern Europe, for the definition of "female" purely in relation to the concept "male" (what Laqueur calls the "one sex model")[8] calls either for circular reasoning or infinite regress in the search for some form of foundational identity.

Once intellectual dogmatism is put into doubt, all ground is taken out from under any proposition. This groundlessness leads to the skeptical ideal, suspension of judgment, often expressed as "to every argument an equal argument is opposed" (*Outlines*, bk 1, ch. 27, p. 202). This suspension of judgment, achieved by accepting the impossibility of apprehension of a thing in itself or through another thing, can be linked to the problematic nature of gender roles. Thus suspension also echoes, even while it surpasses, the refusal of distinctions in Academic philosophy (delineated in Cicero's *Academica*), distinctions between subject and object, true and false, real and unreal, alike and different, self and other. These distinctions are impossible to affirm because of the inherent subjectivity and variability in the presumed subjects and/or objects. The list of forms of variability consitute Sextus's Ten Modes. These Modes not only put into question the possibility of accurate representation or perception; they put into doubt the possibility of existence of stable objects of perception or representation. In short, all of our "knowledge" is based on appearances (our perceptions), which vary constantly in relation to a number of factors, and therefore may or may not be linked to any higher truth. What we declare to be the "true" nature of something is simply whatever is apparent to us, a sign rather than the thing itself. For this reason, nothing

---

5 *The History of Scepticism from Erasmus to Spinoza* (Berkeley, CA: The University of California Press, 1979), p. 19.

6 *Outlines of Pyrrhonism*, trans. R.G. Bury (Cambridge, MA: Harvard University Press, Loeb Classical Library, 1976), bk 1, ch. 16, pp. 178 seq.

7 See *De la grammatologie* (Paris: Seuil, 1967), ch. 2, "Ce dangereux supplément ..." pp. 203–34.

8 In *Making Sex*, "Destiny is Anatomy," pp. 25–62; and "New Science, Once Flesh," pp. 63–113.

can be established as foundational, and the skeptical philosopher, in contemplating this regress, achieves suspension of judgment by balancing the multiple possibilities.

The majority of Sextus's examples in his list of Ten Modes are drawn from sexuality or gender; these examples are most important in his discussion of cultural relativism (the Tenth Mode). In particular, he mentions the custom among Persian men of wearing long robes: "while the Persians think it seemly to wear a brightly dyed dress reaching to the feet, we think it unseemly" (*Outlines*, bk 1, ch. 148, p. 87). Shortly after, he discusses the Persian acceptance of homosexuality and incest, and links it to different forms of dress and to religious beliefs (*Outlines*, bk 1, chs. 152–5, pp. 89–91). Sextus tests the limits of cultural relativism in this passage, linking divergent views of cannibalism and religion to diverse forms of sexuality. The link between sexuality and religious matters becomes tighter when Sextus alludes to portrayals of the gods "as committing adultery and practising intercourse with males; whereas the law with us forbids such actions." Sextus links this question of divine sexuality to those of incest and divine impassivity (*Outlines*, bk 1, chs. 159–62, pp. 91–3). This catalogue of diverse customs concerning transvestism, incest, cannibalism, adultery, patricide and homicide is repeated in the third book. The lesson of this catalogue can be read in a paradoxical fashion: either all of these practices are indifferent, and attitudes towards them merely dictated by culture rather than nature; or these certain practices are abhorrent, and cultures based upon them are inherently self-destructive (cannibalism). Just when the reader seems poised to choose the more conservative reading, Sextus adds an example of moral relativism within the Greco-Roman culture: homicide is punished by law, yet gladiators who kill are rewarded (*Outlines*, bk 3, ch. 212, p. 469). Not only are moral and sexual codes variable, but they seem so arbitrarily imposed by societies that no "true" code could be said to exist at all. Identities based on such codes are fragile indeed.

Sextus discusses cultural relativism in relation to dress, sexual behavior, religious practice, and legal or moral codes. But all of these practices, and indeed most of our experiences, are mediated by language or sign systems, and so he devotes his most careful criticism to the use of such signs. Sextus separates out suggestive signs from indicative ones. Suggestive signs are habitually associated with phenomena; for example, smoke suggests the presence of fire, or a scar suggests the former existence of a wound. Indicative signs are chosen to designate the thing signified, but do not invariably accompany the signified; language is composed entirely of indicative signs (*Outlines*, bk 2, ch. 10, pp. 212–17, for example). Sextus's argument in the first book that nothing can be apprehended by means of another thing argues against the efficacy of language. Invariably, language becomes an empty signifier, a shell divorced from the thing it is used to represent.[9]

---

[9]   For an assessment of early modern semiotics and skepticism, see Marie-Luce Demonet, *A plaisir: Sémiotique et scepticisme chez Montaigne* (Orléans: Paradigme, 2002).

Sextus's thought offers a significant source of ideas and examples for Artus, who cleverly makes his hermaphrodites "embody" these skeptical theorems. In turn, this philosophical context casts a skeptical light on the purported conservative program of the *Isle des Hermaphrodites*. First, the hermaphrodites are only the appearance of human beings, recognizable only by speech, costume, gesture, and the laws they create – all socially dictated, that is appearance-oriented and performative, aspects of identity. They also embody the suspension of judgment, in that they are neither male nor female (also not entirely French or alien, not entirely fact or fiction). When the instability of their sexual or gendered identity is recognized, then all other forms of identity, such as familial origins, social rank, and religious faith, are swept away as well. In the end, the emptiness of their identity is grounded in their strange use of language, floating free from any potential signification.

At first, Artus seems to portray cultural, religious, and sexual diversity as the sources of all of France's woes. In particular, he castigates the political moderates of the time, known as the *politiques*, for their insistence on toleration of religious difference, accusing them of abolishing all religion in France because it seems too harsh to them. This religious tolerance is associated with the general degeneration of morals at the Court. The reign of the *politiques*/hermaphrodites has trivialized everything, from the law, through language, even to questions of faith. The accommodating spirit of the *politiques* is equated here with a sort of early libertine movement, and thus with hypocritical atheism. And Artus encourages the perception of the dishonesty of the *politiques* by insisting on the dual nature of the hermaphrodite – who seems like a woman, but is also a man; seems religious, but is not; says one thing, but means another. This hypocrisy leads to laws that bend to the mutable wills of the most criminal elements in society, as incest and all conceivable forms of murder are not only permitted, but even encouraged in the realm of the hermaphrodites (*L'Isle des Hermaphrodites*, pp. 57–61). At least upon first reading, the monstrous hermaphrodite seems to be the figure of a disordered society in which traditional laws and values have been set aside in favor of a feigned moderation, which reveals itself to be excess.

What seems to menace dogmatically ordered French society is the acceptance that there may be more than one perspective on any issue. Acceptance of Protestantism puts the "truth" of Catholicism into doubt – two religious truths cannot exist at one and the same time. If one tolerates the existence of both, one achieves only suspension of judgment, which dissolves hierarchical orderings based on a supposedly foundational truth. Both religions cannot contradict each other and still be true, yet this is purportedly what the *politiques* want to believe. Similarly, given the coexistence of two sexes in one person, the notion of one sex as the "true" sex is canceled out. If the sexes are only defined in relation to each other, as they are in the one-sex system, then we are left with a mise-en-abime in any attempt to categorize sexes.

Without any foundational truth, the subject is left only with appearances by which to judge sexes. These appearances are culturally imposed acts or signs: "Gender is the repeated stylization of the body, a set of repeated acts within a highly rigid regulatory frame that congeal over time to produce the appearance of substance, of a natural sort of being."[10] Further, this stylization, also in circular fashion, is dictated by power relations and in turn confirms those power relations: "The body gains meaning within discourse only in the context of power relations. Sexuality is an historically specific organization of power, discourse, bodies, and affectivity" (Butler, *Gender Trouble*, p. 92). Thus, bisexuality, transvestism, and hermaphrodism, all situations in which two different signs of gender ("male" and "female" desire; male and female clothing and gesture; male and female genitalia) coexist in problematic relation, both render the artificial or culturally imposed nature of gender evident and undercut the power relations that inform and are informed by gender. Artus is fascinated with the signs of gender and with the disorder that confusion or suspension of these signs can create in society. And, in spite of his proclaimed conservatism, Artus offers no foundational truth to counter these signs. Rather, he creates a proliferation of parodic signs that seems to indicate pleasure in the act of subverting dogmatic society.

Novelty, Gender, and Transgressive Signs

Artus begins his account with a reference to the New World, a discovery which itself shattered the illusion of unity or uniqueness which cradled the old for millenia (*L 'Isle des Hermaphrodites*, pp. 4–5). In this, he echoes travel accounts that flooded France in the second half of the sixteenth century, alluding especially to narratives such as that of René Goulaine de Laudonnière's *Histoire notable de la Floride*, in which the author claims that hermaphrodites are common in the "New World":

> Il y a en tout ce pays grande quantité d'Hermaphrodites, lesquels ont tout le plus grand travail, mesmes ils portent leurs vivres quand ils vont à la guerre. Ils se peignent fort le visage ....[11]

> (There is throughout this whole country a large quantity of hermaphrodites, who do the most onerous work, they even carry the victuals when they go to war. They paint their faces heavily ....)

Theodor de Bry takes up this account, and extends it in his compilation, *America* (*Brevis narratio eorum quae in Florida americae provincia Gallis acciderent ... 1591*; *A Brief narration of the events which occurred in Florida, an American province of France*).[12] Plate 17 shows "hermaphroditic" natives carrying the wounded from the field of battle, and describes other duties that are assigned to them. We now know that these "hermaphrodites" were probably berdaches, men in some Native American populations who choose to live as women, but who in fact have a special status in the

---

10 Judith Butler, *Gender Trouble*, p. 33.
11 Paris: Auvray, 1586, A5.
12 Frankfurt, 1597.

tribe, as Judith Lorber, among others, has pointed out: "Berdaches educate children, sing and dance at tribal events, tend the ill, carry provisions for war parties, and have special ritual functions."[13] This special role is incomprehensible to European eyes, so authors translate it into hermaphrodism; these men can only take on feminine roles because, in some essential biological way, they are feminine. Once again, European culture absorbs that which is different by translating it into its own language, making it conform to European rules. This use of the hermaphrodite signals the extent to which Europe cannot even recognize difference, let alone accept it.

Artus himself deplores the rush to novelty and change that disturbs the presumed stability of the Old World. Yet he contradicts himself a few lines later, mentioning "the continual upheavals which have occurred in Europe for so many years" (*L'Isle des Hermaphrodites*, p. 5). One is left with the question of whether these explorers are searching for social novelty or escaping social upheaval. The narrator himself voyages in order to avoid participation in murderous strife (*L'Isle des Hermaphrodites*, p. 5). He wanders throughout the world until he hears of the treaty of Vervins (1598). In his attempt to return home, he lands on a sort of anti-utopian island governed by hermaphrodites, one which resembles the court of Henri de Valois (Henri III). This island is not anchored, but floats about in the ocean (*L'Isle des Hermaphrodites*, p. 8). The narrator underscores the unreality of the island: "nous vîmes par tout si fertile & florissant que nous croyons la Fable des *Champs Elisées* être une pure vérité" (*L'Isle des Hermaphrodites*, p. 9: "we saw this island everywhere so fertile and flowering that we thought the fable of the Elysian Fields to be absolute truth in comparison"). First placed in evidence is the most immediately visible sign of power, that is, elaborate architecture. The palace is characterized by its "diversity": "l'oeil qui peut voir tant de choses en un instant, n'étoit pas assez suffisant pour comprendre tout le contenu de ce beau Palais" (*L'Isle des Hermaphrodites*, p. 9: "The eye that can see everything in an instant was not sufficient to take in all that was contained in this beautiful Palace"). The multiplicity of signs apparent in this palace defies comprehension. Notably, it is at this point that the voyagers discover this is the land of hermaphrodites.

Significantly, the narrator's first encounter with a hermaphrodite results not in a view of that mysterious being, but rather of its elaborately described clothing: "un petit manteau de satin blanc chamarré de clinquant, doublé d'une étoffe ressemblant à la pane de soye" (*L'Isle des Hermaphrodites*, p. 13: "a small coat of white satin edged with metallic fringe, lined in a material that resembled silk plush"). Note that even the lining (*doublure*) only resembles plush, rather than being it. Reality is at two removes from this material, since silk plush was used as a sort of fake fur. Thus, this "pane de soye" is an imitation of a fake. Similarly, the creatures themselves exist removed from direct observation. There is a cloth covering a mask which lies on the hermaphrodite's face, so that any (bodily) "reality" is unavailable to public view. The narrator also describes the food eaten by this creature, but never the hermaphrodite's

---

[13]   *Paradoxes of Gender*, p. 90.

body or face, as if it is the accoutrements of this being that create its identity, rather than some foundational essence. When the narrator observes what he believes to be a scene of torture, in which the hermaphrodites' hair is pulled by red-hot pincers, he realizes the gap between appearance and reality (and that the hermaphrodites are simply having their hair done).

The hermaphroditic body is constructed by means of makeup, prosthetic devices, and clothing; it is alternately built up and carved out, and becomes a sort of early modern cyborg.[14] The voyager watches these hermaphrodites being primped, powdered, and tweezed into form. They are rouged, bleached, their beards are thinned and cheeks filled out (by means of bones attached inside the mouth). They are dressed in silk *chausses* (trousers) and their feet are jammed into tiny shoes. This forcing of the foot into a too-small space could be seen as a parody of the narrow sexual and social roles imposed upon men and women and expressed by means of clothing.[15]

> Un autre vint incontinent après, apporter une petite paire de souliers fort étroits & mignonnement découpés. Je me mocquois en moi-même de voir si petite chaussure, & ne pouvois comprendre à la verité comme un grand & gros pied pouvoit entrer dans un si petit soulier, puisque la regle naturelle veut que le contenant soit plus grand que le contenu, & toutesfois c'étoit ici le contraire .... (*L'Isle des Hermaphrodites*, p. 20)

> (Another arrived immediately after, to carry in a small pair of shoes, very narrow and cut out in cute fashion. I laughed to myself when I saw such small shoes, and could not understand, in truth, how a large, fat foot could enter into such a small shoe, since the natural rule wills that that which contains be larger than that which is contained, and nonetheless it was the contrary in this case ....)

In this image, the hermaphrodites seem to take on a parodic force of their own, and one begins to wonder whether Artus is criticizing them or French society. The notion of restriction, whether in costume or in behavior is often repeated in the novel. Thus, when Artus seems to allude to "natural law" ("la regle naturelle"), his critique seems to expand from that of transgressive dressing to that of any cultural repression of natural drives or states of being. The elaborate ritual of dressing itself is infinitely multiplied: "ils ne laissent pas de changer ainsi en ce pays-là de jour & de nuit" (*L'Isle des Hermaphrodites*, p. 21: "They never left off changing [their clothes] in

---

14   Donna Haraway, "A Cyborg Manifesto: Science, Technology, and Socialist-Feminism in the Late Twentieth Century," *Simians, Cyborgs, and Women*, p. 149: "A cyborg is a cybernetic organism, a hybrid of machine and organism, a creature of social reality as well as a creature of fiction. Social reality is lived social relations, our most important political construction, a world-changing fiction," and p. 150: "The cyborg is a condensed image of both imagination and material reality."

15   The restrictive potential of clothing is expressed in the "discours de la vieille" in the *Roman de la Rose* (Jean de Meun), ed. Daniel Poirion (Paris: Garnier-Flammarion, 1974), ll. 13319–50.

this country, either day or night"). Thus, while the hermaphrodites seem to submit to extreme restrictions, they also escape such limitations by the infinite parodic repetitions of such restrictive behavior.

Artus emphasizes the ornamental aspects of gender distinction, and links these aspects to the notion of instability by means of the hermaphrodites' shaky mode of walking, prized as aesthetically superior to a firm step. He (and the hermaphrodite is actually designated by the pronoun *il*, even though he is called a "demi-femme," p. 24) is perfumed and gloved and handed little candies to put in his pocket. He carries a fan, and walks mostly off-balance (*L'Isle des Hermaphrodites*, p. 27). Even the hermaphrodite's movement is dictated by social norms, in spite of the inconvenience of this mode of propulsion. Utility, and any possible "natural" behavior is overwhelmed by artificial marks of gender, just as the body of the hermaphrodite is overwhelmed by clothing in the frame narrative.

As if to emphasize this artificiality, Artus creates the world of the hermaphrodites as a tissue of textual references, artistic embellishment, and theatrics. Musicians sing airs based on Petronius' *Satyricon*, and the bedchamber of the next, apparently even more important, hermaphrodite is decorated with scenes of mutable sexuality from Ovid's *Metamorphoses,* that of Caeneus in particular (*L'Isle des Hermaphrodites*, p. 30).[16] Dominated by this artificial context, the narrator notices a statue of a man in the middle of the bed, and this statue is or becomes confused with the hermaphrodite himself: "Le visage étoit si blanc, si luisant & d'un rouge si éclatant, qu'on voyoit bien qu'il y avoit plus d'artifice que de nature; ce qui me faisoit aisément croire que ce n'étoit que peinture" (*L'Isle des Hermaphrodites*, p. 31: "The face was so white, so bright, and of a red so striking that one saw clearly that there was more artifice than nature involved; which easily made me believe that this was nothing more than paint [or a painting]"). Distinctions between real and artificial, fact and fiction are easily blurred in this realm of indistinct genders. Again, the bed, the room, the clothing – even the surface of the hermaphrodite's skin (or at least the makeup on it) – are described, but no sense of essential identity is apparent.

It is at this point, when the statue is confused with the powerful Hermaphrodite by means of the word *idole*, that language becomes an issue in the narrative and is inextricably linked to the basic problems of gender and identity that have been suggested so far:

> En cette ruelle allerent les trois personnes ... & commencerent à invoquer cette idole par des noms qui ne se peuvent pas bien représenter en notre langue, d'autant que tout le langage & tous les termes des *Hermaphrodites* sont de même que ceux que les Grammairiens appellent du genre commun, & tiennent autant du mâle que de la femelle:

---

[16]　Ovid, *Metamorphoses*, bk 12, ll. 168–535. Artus confuses Caeneus, who does not return to female form, with both Tiresias (who changes into a woman and back again, bk 3, ll. 316–38) and Erysichthon's unnamed daughter, to whom Neptune has given the power to change her form at will (bk 8, ll. 850–74).

toutefois desirant sçavoir quels discours ils tenoient-là; un de leur suite, de qui je m'étois accosté & qui entendoit bien l'*Italien*, me dit .... (*L'Isle des Hermaphrodites*, p. 31)

(The three people went to this bedside ... and began to invoke this idol by names which have no equivalent in our language, inasmuch as the entire language and all of the terms of the *Hermaphrodites* are of that same sort which Grammarians call the "common" gender, and take as much from the male as from the female. Nonetheless, wishing to know what subjects they were discussing, one of their retinue, whom I had approached and who understood Italian, said to me ....)

The idol (or statue, although the word is also related to *idea*) is designated by various names, none of which can be translated into French. The problem is that the French language does not have a common gender, one that serves as both masculine and feminine. Still, the narrator manages to elicit an approximative translation of the *discours* from someone who understands Italian.[17] This problematic being can only be represented in the most indirect fashion. The arbitrary imposition of signs of identity extends to language itself, which does not have any necessary relation to the thing being observed, and which in fact cannot express that thing.

Using *cette idole* as the antecedent in this long sentence, the text designates the hermaphrodite by the pronoun *elle*, thus achieving a sort of oscillation between masculine and feminine. The narrative also uses *ce que* (that which) to indicate the hermaphrodite, thus achieving a sort of neuter: "mais aussi-tôt ce que j'avois tenu pour muet & sans vie, commença à parler" (*L'Isle des Hermaphrodites*, p. 32: "but immediately that which I had held to be mute and without life, began to speak"). Ambiguous identity is thus mirrored by unstable or vague language.

The Palace of the Hermaphrodites begins at this point to resemble a series of Chinese boxes. The narrator moves on to another room, richer than the first (*L'Isle des Hermaphrodites*, pp. 32–3). Obviously, this next hermaphrodite is even more important than the previous one, yet it resembles the other fairly closely (p. 33). This succession of "important" hermaphrodites becomes nightmarish; all sense of order or hierarchy is destroyed, and no one seems to be in charge, although this second "important" hermaphrodite does go into a council-room purportedly to discuss the business of state. This secret room is called "something like" the wardrobe: "Ils appelloient cela d'un nom, pareil à celui que nous disons ici la garde-robe ..." (*L'Isle des Hermaphrodites*, p. 34: "They called this some name, similar to what we call a wardrobe in France"). Although actually a great deal of state business was conducted

---

17   This can be read as a reference to the speculation during Henri's reign that he acquired his sexual preferences in Venice (the French liked to think that homosexuality was an Italian speciality), as well as to Henri's love of Latin letters (seen as a form of corruption). This latter accusation of hyper-intellectualism echoes that made by Jean Boucher, in his treatise *De Iusta Henrici tertii abdicatione e Francorum regno* (*On the Just Renunciation of Henry the Third by the People of France*; Lyon: Ioannem Pillehotte, 1591), pp. 327–43.

in the King's dressing-room, Artus seems to suggest that the most important business of *this* state *is* the wardrobe itself. Clothing is part of the performative nature of power and of gender:

> The effect of gender [or power] is produced through the stylization of the body and, hence, must be understood as the mundane way in which bodily gestures, movements, and styles of various kinds constitute the illusion of an abiding gendered self. This formulation moves the conception of gender off the ground of a substantial model of identity to one that requires a conception of gender as a constituted *social temporality* … Gender is also a norm that can never be fully internalized; "the internal" is a surface signification, and gender norms are finally phantasmatic, impossible to embody. (Butler, *Gender Trouble*, p. 141)

According to Butler, then, that which many consider essential sexual identity is created by signs that are inscribed on the surface of the body over the course of time by repeated actions that are themselves dictated by social norms. Such are the signs enumerated by Artus.

Artus plays with every aspect of sexuality in his work: he is fascinated by transvestism, by laws governing sexual mores, by the confusion language can create in the expressions of gender and sexuality. The problematic nature of signs of gender is linked to the problematic nature of signs in general in the two representative figures of hermaphrodism. After wandering the halls of this Palace and admiring the numerous art-works, the narrator comes across statues of the Island's heroes; particularly prominent among them are those of Hermaphroditus and Heliogabalus. These figures seem to represent the two extremes of hermaphrodism. Hermaphroditus embodies both male and female characteristics, whereas Heliogabalus, according to the tapestries in the Hermaphrodites' Palace, which depict his castration, embodies neither. Heliogabalus is neuter, neither male nor female, an empty cipher. Hermaphroditus is both male and female, and thus a self-contradictory being (at least in the context of social norms). Since the book of laws is found next to these statues, and the laws categorize various signs of identity (particularly those related to gender), one could link Heliogabalus to Sextus Empiricus's skeptical aphasia (occuring when the impossibility of distinction and categorization leads to silence, *Outlines*, bk 1, ch. 20, pp. 110–13) and Hermaphroditus to skeptical suspension of judgment (occuring when multiple possibilities are allowed to coexist without any choice being made, *Outlines*, bk 1, ch. 22, pp. 114–15). Thus, these figures create a transition to a long discussion of laws and language which dominates the novel.

The Laws of the Hermaphrodites

Most of the remaining narration consists of this book of laws of conduct and governance of the island, laws which create and confirm the ambiguity of hermaphrodism and connect gender ambiguity to moral and epistemological confusion. For the most part, Artus connects gender ambiguity to religious diversity in the section "Ordonnances sur le fait de la Religion" ("Ordinances on Religious Matters"). This diversity leads to the virtual annihilation of religion (and in this, Artus echoes and mocks the nascent atheism of the *libertins*):

> Les cérémonies de *Bacchus*, & de *Cupidon* & de *Venus*, soient ici continuellement & religieusement observées; toute autre religion en soit bannie à perpétuité, si ce n'est pour plus grande volupté. Toutesfois nous n'empêchons de s'accommoder avec les autres Religions, pourvu que ce ne soit qu'en apparence, & non par croyance. (*L'Isle des Hermaphrodites*, pp. 43–4)

> (The ceremonies of Bacchus, and of Cupid, and of Venus, must be continually and religiously observed in this realm; all other religions are hereby banished in perpetuity, unless they contribute to sensual pleasures. Nonetheless, we will not prevent accommodation with other Religions, provided that this is only in appearance, and not because of any belief.)

As mentioned before, this is not merely a criticism of Henri III, but of the entire *politique* faction at court, the moderates who realized that the Wars of Religion, gone unchecked, would simply destroy France rather than restore Catholicism as the sole religion.

For the most part, the laws of the hermaphrodites are redefinitions of social norms: "La plus grande volupté soit tenuë par tout cet Empire pour la plus grande sainteté" (*L'Isle des Hermaphrodites*, p. 44: "The greatest sensuality will be held throughout this Empire as the greatest sanctity"). Similarly, cowardice is redefined as worthiness; "presumptuous vanity" becomes "a perfect knowledge of oneself" (*L'Isle des Hermaphrodites*, p. 44). This last quality borders on narcissism, which would probably be an appropriate form of love for a hermaphrodite, who is at once him/herself and an other. Such narcissism is suggested throughout the laws ("La volonté par tout cetui notre Empire soit tenuë pour raison … à peine d'être tenu pour ennemi de soi-même," *L'Isle des Hermaphrodites*, p. 46: "Personal desires will be held to be Reason itself throughout this our Empire … otherwise, one will be thought to be an enemy to himself"). "Effrontery" becomes its opposite "gentillesse" ("kindness"). The hermaphrodites create this sort of strange mirror world of French society. This mirror opposition is achieved by the use of paradox, a turning of language upon itself.

The paradoxical definitions of moral values are echoed by a self-contradiction in presentation of these values; hypocrisy thus becomes the ideal hermaphroditic behavior. This hypocrisy again privileges language as the supreme expression of hermaphroditic identity. "Nous conseillons à tous nos Sujets, quand ils se rencontreront avec ceux qui font cas de la piété, ce qui doit être fort rarement, de discourir avec beaucoup de zele de la dévotion" (*L'Isle des Hermaphrodites*, p. 45, law 3: "We advise all of our subjects, when they encounter those who consider piety important, an event which should be avoided as much as possible, to discourse about matters of faith with great zeal"). This hypocrisy extends to every aspect of culture; for example, the hermaphrodites should use brave words around genuinely courageous military men (*L'Isle des Hermaphrodites*, p. 45, law 3 continued). Thus, the hypocrisy of the hermaphrodites creates a gap between word and deed (signifier and signified) that becomes almost absolute opposition. Those who speak of bravery are not brave; thus, the words supplement the missing deed, but this supplement also stands in opposition also to the actual cowardice of the hermaphrodites. Similarly, words that are considered to be of great "substance" in French culture are shown to be empty in hermaphrodite culture: "Nous voulons & entendons que tous ces mots de conscience, tempérance, repentance, & autres de pareil sujet, soient tenus tant en la substance qu'aux termes, pour choses vaines & frivoles" (*L'Isle des Hermaphrodites*, p. 45, law 4: "We wish and intend that all those words of conscience, temperance, repentance, and others of similar meaning, be held as empty and frivolous things, the substance as well as the words themselves"). In other words, not only do libertine terms replace chivalric ones in a reversal of cultural norms, but a gap is created between what the laws call *substance* and what they call *termes*. The *substance* is then emptied from these terms, and only the signifying surface of the term remains. But a word divorced from the potential of meaning becomes merely a series of letters, not only a mask or shell, but a logical impossibility. A signifier torn from its signifying aspect is nothing. This emphasis upon the signifier divorced of any meaning is then linked to the question of appearance and therefore of clothing and toilette, the two elements which dominated the introductory section of the novel:

> Nous réputons la bonne mine & l'apparence en toutes choses que ce soit, beaucoup plus que l'action, d'autant qu'elle cache beaucoup d'effets avec moins de peine. C'est pourquoi nous exhortons tous nos sujets, de quelque état, qualité ou condition qu'ils soient, de l'acquérir, autant dissimulée que faire se pourra & de la préférer à toute autre vertu. (*L'Isle des Hermaphrodites*, pp. 45–6, law 6)

> (We respect good looks and appearance at all times, much more than action, since looks get more results with much less difficulty. This is why we encourage our subjects, of whatever class, quality, or condition they may be, to acquire good looks, as artificial as they can possibly be, and to prefer this appearance to any other virtue.

Not only is appearance valued above action, but this appearance must be cultivated to be as divorced from any "essential" or "natural" being as possible. This cultivation of sign systems devoid of meaning makes the hermaphrodites themselves unreadable. It could be argued that this undecipherable quality gives the hermaphrodites a sort of hermetic power over the reader.

The hermaphrodites not only lack respect for the established symbols of culture, but they replace them with their own system of signs, or give new signification to whatever symbols they appropriate; thus, the church is more suitable for the "misteres véneriens" (*L'Isle des Hermaphrodites*, p. 48, law 11: "mysteries of Venus") than for the mysteries of the Catholic mass (this sentiment is echoed in the fourteenth law, *L'Isle des Hermaphrodites*, p. 49). Entertainment becomes the hermaphrodites' preferred form of worship, understandably so, since entertainment would involve masks and role-playing. Singers, dancers, actors, and comics become the ministers of the Temple, and the most lascivious poets are the preachers (*L'Isle des Hermaphrodites*, p. 51, law 18). Sexuality is thus linked to this role-playing, this entertainment, rather than being portrayed as some inherently necessary part of society. This role-playing is portrayed as bisexual, and therefore most threatening to the social (sexual) hierarchy: "Qui aura quelque Maîtresse ou quelque ami les pourront entretenir aux Eglises ..." (*L'Isle des Hermaphrodites*, p. 47, law 11: "Whoever has some Mistress, or some male friend, can converse with them [support them][18] in the Churches"). A person playing both the passive (then considered feminine) and active (masculine) roles is essentially annihilating hierarchy and putting into doubt these value-ridden designations of passive and active.

The favored authors of the hermaphrodites are those who have contended with questions of sexual ambiguity and the relationship between power and sex. In the case of Ovid, sexual and gender ambiguity, in the forms of hermaphrodism,[19] transsexuality,[20] and transvestism,[21] are dealt with frequently. Catullan lyric deals with various forms of sexuality, clearly linking passive and active roles to the social and power structures of Rome.[22] Thus, literature plays a crucial role in the realm of the hermaphrodites; even the hymns are taken from collections of erotic poetry ("Mignardises, Follâtreries & Gayetés," *L'Isle des Hermaphrodites*, p. 51, law 20). The reading or singing of these lascivious poems seems to be the primary religious and cultural activity of the kingdom; in fact, discussion of sexuality seems far more important than the sexuality itself. Again, the signifier seems to dominate the realm.

If there is no stable or foundational meaning, no one true sex, no one true religion, then the hermaphrodites are protean beings who change to suit their circumstances. Thus, not only are they of dual nature, they are beings who can infinitely multiply their roles. They are self-supplementing creatures who have refused to accept the basic premises that buttress French society, and thus are free to reinvent themselves constantly. They

---

[18] Note that the laws of the hermaphrodites are written in *double-entendres*; *entretenir* means both converse with and support (presumably the hermaphrodites could give their lovers *bénéfices ecclésiastiques* as rewards and means of living, as well as to mock the vows of celibacy).

[19] See the story of Salmacis and Hermaphroditus, *Metamorphoses*, bk 4, ll. 285–388.

[20] In the stories of Tiresias (bk 3, ll. 316–38); Erysichthon's daughter (bk 8, ll. 850–74); of Iphis (bk 9, ll. 666–797); and of Caeneus (bk 11, ll. 168–535).

[21] In the stories of Iphis (see above); and of Vertumnus and Pomona (bk 14, ll. 622–97). Vertumnus disguises himself as an elderly woman in order to seduce Pomona.

[22] In particular, poems 16 and 25, in which imposition of one's own sexuality upon others is seen as a means of revenge and of degradation of one's enemies. Catullus portrays his ability to assault others as a form of personal power in poems 21 and 37, and clearly links sexual appetite and victimization of others to abuse of political power in poems 28, 29, 47, 57 (*Catullus: The Poems*, ed. Kenneth Quinn, London: Macmillan, 1973).

define themselves by their roles, thus demonstrating a recognition of the performative power of social roles and liberating themselves by this recognition. This liberation can be read as irresponsibility that might lead to social chaos, but this conservative view is belied by the already chaotic conditions created by dogmatic repression of differences in early modern France, conditions mentioned at the opening of Artus's narrative.

A further example of the delicate balance between the perceived threat of pluralism caused by the denial of dogmatism, and the violent religious extremism which threatened the very existence of France can be seen in the articles of faith of the hermaphrodites:

> Nous ignorons la création, rédemption, justification, & damnation, si ce n'est en bonne mine & en paroles ...
>
> Nous ignorons s'il y a aucune temporalité, ou éternité au monde, ni s'il doit avoir un jour quelque fin, de crainte que cela ne nous trouble l'esprit, & nous cause de la frayeur. (*L'Isle des Hermaphrodites*, p. 55, articles 1 and 2)
>
> (We know nothing of the creation, or of redemption, justification [by faith], and damnation, unless it is all achieved with good looks and clever words ....
>
> We do not know if there is any temporality or eternity in the world, nor if there must be an end some day, for fear that this might trouble our spirits and cause us a fright.)

Obviously, the hermaphrodites trivialize numerous religious beliefs, and to some extent trivialize themselves by refusing any form of ethics or ideals (other than parodic forms).

But the force of this parody is undeniable in the face of insistent dogmatic categorization of every aspect of religious life. The proliferation of doctrine, the minuteness of detail expected in every person's understanding of such doctrine, renders religious belief almost absurd – albeit with tragic consequences. One need only compare the hermaphrodites' articles to parts of the deadly serious "Confession de Bordeaux," which Huguenots were forced to repeat publicly if they did not wish to be executed (this following the massacre of Saint Bartholomew's Day):

> I believe that in the Holy Sacrament of the Altar are present the true body and natural blood of our Lord by means of divine Transsubstantiation, and that we receive this bodily and spiritually. And I confess most of all, that it is a true sacrifice, not to supplement or repeat the unique and very sufficient sacrifice of the Cross ....[23]

---

[23] Article 14: "Je croi qu'au S. Sacrement de l'Autel sont presens le vrai corps et naturel sang de nostre Seigneur par la divine Transsubstantiation, et que nous le recevons corporellement et spirituellement. Et confesse premierement, que c'est un vrai sacrifice, non pour suppleer ou repeter l'unique et tres suffisant sacrifice de la Croix ...." Cited by Théodore Agrippa d'Aubigné in his *Histoire Universelle*, vol. 1, p. 134.

The demand is for belief in something non-evident, even paradoxical within itself. The nature of the sacrifice is blurred by the insistence on accumulation of definitions: it is *a* true sacrifice, but not *the* true sacrifice.

In the case of categorizations of sin, the distinction between mortal and venial, although declared clear by the Church, is in effect unclear:

> I confess that the sins are distinct, according to the transgression, some mortal, such as the desire for debauchery, others venial, such as the feeling of debauchery which is void of desire and consent.[24]

Since the words *feeling* and *desire* are not defined, the difference between these two terms, and thus between the two forms of sin, remains blurred. Furthermore, all of doctrine becomes based on terminology rather than any form of essential belief, and the terms themselves are neither defined nor used in a consistent fashion. Because of this dependence on language, the instability of language undermines doctrine. This form of forced belief, on incredibly detailed questions of doctrine which seem to have no foundation in the experiential world, seems no more rational to the modern eye than the skepticism of the hermaphrodites.[25]

Yet one begins to wonder while reading their laws if the hermaphrodites are so revolutionary after all, or if they are not merely the logical extension of an overly codified society, one in which identity is clearly and repressively defined in every possible detail. Thus, the hermaphrodites create "unrules" that negate this codification: "Nous ignorons une providence supérieure aux choses humaines, & croyons que tout se conduit à l'aventure." (*L'Isle des Hermaphrodites*, p. 56, article 4: "We know nothing of a providence superior to human matters, and believe that everything occurs purely by chance") In fact, they believe in nothing, and so their articles are articles of unfaith, rather than of faith. They refuse to accept mere faith as a basis for action: "Nous ignorons toute autre vie que la présente" (*L'Isle des Hermaphrodites*, p. 56, article 6: "We know nothing of any other life than the present one"). They believe only in the performative, not the pedagogic or foundational, aspect of society.

Thus, the laws of *Justice* ring strangely in the reader's ear when they speak of murder and mayhem in the land of hermaphrodites. For example, homicide is only a crime if it is committed in self-defense, in the course of a fair fight (*L'Isle des Hermaphrodites*, p. 57, article 2). Although this is one of the signs of cultural relativism offered by Sextus Empiricus, there must have been an immediacy to this example for

---

24 Article 36, again cited by d'Aubigné: "Je confesse les pechés estres distincts, selon la transgression, les uns mortels, comme desir de paillarder, les autres veniels, comme l'esmotion à paillardise, sans le desir et consentement," p. 138.

25 One might argue that these articles were not written for the modern eye, but early skeptics and *politiques* would see the detailed and Inquisitional imposition of this doctrine as cruelly absurd in the face of the ignorance of the average Catholic. See Montaigne, "Des Cannibales," in the *Essais*, vol. 1, p. 209.

readers in late sixteenth-century France that overrode skeptical bemusement. Similarly, the law that states that "Patricides, matricides, fratricides, and other such actions will not be punished if committed by our people, as long as they use these crimes to increase their wealth" (*L'Isle des Hermaphrodites*, p. 58, article 4), rings all too true when one considers that many were killed in the Saint Bartholomew's Day massacre for their money rather than for questions of religion.[26] Thus, Artus deflects the skeptical example away from the *politiques* to crimes committed by extremist Catholics.[27] In truly skeptical fashion, Artus sees cultural relativism operating in all societies and in all members of society, not merely among skeptics or libertines.

Marriage also is recognized as a performative, rather than foundational role, and therefore adultery is not only condoned, but encouraged: "Voulons aussi que ce que nos contraires nomment adultere soit en vogue, en honneur & réputation par tout cetui notre Empire" (*L'Isle des Hermaphrodites*, p. 59, article 6: "We also wish that that which our opposition calls adultery be in fashion, in honor, and in good repute throughout our Empire"). Even the negative sign used by society to designate this behavior is denied. Similarly, incest is allowed:

> Pour le regard des incestes du pere avec la fille, du frere avec la soeur, du gendre avec la belle mere & autres, que les fols & mal avisés tiennent à si grand crime, nous voulons & entendons qu'on en puisse user avec toute franchise & liberté .... (*L'Isle des Hermaphrodites*, p. 61, article 11).

> (In regard to incest between father and daughter, brother and sister, son-in-law and mother-in-law, and others, which foolish and ill-advised people think is such a great crime: we desire and expect that all can engage in these acts in all freedom and liberty ....)

Echoing Sextus, the hermaphrodites dismantle all the fundamental relations which drive society; but most of all, they attack marriage and the family. The incest taboo is considered by anthropologists to be one of the bases of social interaction, and therefore of social identity, in that it both "distinguishes and binds" families (Butler, *Gender Trouble*, 39). Without the laws that constitute identity (and all of the hermaphrodites rules are basically anti-laws that undo all current laws and taboos), society disintegrates: "Nous n'entendons point qu'il y ait parmi nos Sujets aucuns dégrés de consanguinité ... C'est pourquoi nous abolissons dé-maintenant & pour toujours ces noms de pere, mere, frere, soeur & autres, ains voulons qu'on use seulement ceux de *Monsieur, Madame*" (*L'Isle des Hermaphrodites*, pp. 62–3: "We wish to eliminate all

---

26 For example, Bussy d'Amboise took advantage of the occasion to kill some cousins and seize their property. See Théodore Agrippa d'Aubigné, *Sa Vie à ses enfants*, ed. Gilbert Schrenck (Paris: Champion, 1988), p. 71, n. 78.

27 This was a not uncommon practice of the extremist Catholic League. As Elie Barnavi points out in his study, *Le Parti de Dieu*, pp. 184–5, the League was involved in a good deal of surreptitious violence itself, and left quite a few bodies in the Seine.

degrees of consanguinity among our Subjects ... It is for this reason that we abolish from this moment forward those names of father, mother, brother, sister, and others, and so wish that only those of *Monsieur* and *Madame* be used"). The hermaphrodites are now flatly rejecting the signifiers that create identity, whereas previously they simply parodied such social roles; in this light, it is ironic that they retain the gender distinctions implied by the words *Monsieur* and *Madame*.

This freedom from rigid roles is expressed at every level of signification, for example in the clothing, which is freed from hierarchical constraints:

> Chacun pourra s'habiller à sa fantaisie, pourvu que ce soit bravement, superbement & sans aucune distinction ni considération de sa qualité ou faculté ... Aussi tenons-nous pour une regle presque générale parmi nous, que tels accoûtrements honorent plutôt qu'ils ne sont honorés: car en cette Isle l'habit fait le moine, & non pas au contraire. (*L'Isle des Hermaphrodites*, pp. 79–80, article 13)

> (Each one may dress according to his/her whims, provided that this is done elegantly, proudly, and without any distinction of or consideration for rank or privilege ... We also held as an almost general rule among ourselves, that such garb brings honor more than it reflects honor: for on this Island, the clothes make the man, and not the other way around.)

Recognition of the artificial nature of social roles brings on the breakdown of those roles, and of the hierarchy supported by those roles. The dissolution of class hierarchy is accompanied by that of gender: "Les accoûtrements qui approcheront plus de ceux de la femme, soit en l'étoffe ou en la façon, seront tenus parmi les nôtres pour les plus riches & mieux séans, comme les plus convenables aux moeurs, inclinations & coûtumes de ceux de cette Isle" (*L'Isle des Hermaphrodites*, p. 80: "The garb which most closely resembles that of a woman, either in its material or in its style, will be considered by our people to be the most rich and appropriate, as being the most suited to the morals, inclinations, and customs of the inhabitants of this Island"). Here again, Artus reveals the artificiality of gender roles by means of the changeable nature of fashion; but he links also gender to other social roles, familial, class-oriented, and religious. Clothing becomes a means of linking social roles to more general issues of signification and knowledge, issues which inevitably return to the primacy of language.

Hermaphroditic Language

Artus devotes an entire section of his novel to "Entregent," in particular to conversation and etiquette. The language of the hermaphrodites is at once a richly abundant and inventive self-supplement, and a sort of annihilating anti-supplement:

> Leurs discours seront le plus souvent de choses controuvées, sans verité, ni sans aucune apparence de raison, & l'ornement de leur langage sera de renier & de blasphémer

posément, & avec gravité faire plusieurs imprécations & malédictions, & autres fleurs de notre Réthorique pour soutenir ou pour persuader le mensonge, & lorsqu'ils voudront persuader une chose fausse, ils commenceront par ces mots: La verité est. (*L'Isle des Hermaphrodites*, p. 91, article 4)

(Their conversations will consist most often of wholly invented matters, without any truth or appearance of reason, and the proper embellishment of their language shall be to abjure (renounce) and blaspheme calmly and to curse and swear with gravity, and other such flowers of Rhetoric used to support or give credence to a lie. Whenever they wish to persuade someone of an utter falsity, they will begin with the words: "The truth is ....")

But here, in this reversal of "truth," the reader falls upon a basic paradox: if the basic mode of speech of the hermaphrodites is a lie, then are they telling the truth when they write this law about lying? Such a paradox calls into question the very nature of "truth."

The hermaphrodites use language to oppose what has been accepted as normal society, urging their subjects to lose a good friend rather than a *bon mot* (*L'Isle des Hermaphrodites*, p. 92, article 7), to mix blasphemy into their conversation (*L'Isle des Hermaphrodites*, p. 93, article 9), to slander (*médire*, to mispeak) without regard for family, society or friendship (*L'Isle des Hermaphrodites*, p. 93, article 10). Language is their means of opposition, their way of rendering social norms absurd by revealing their factitious nature. By opposing the "truths"of society with "untruths," the hermaphrodites reveal *truth* to be a signifier without stable meaning. When language is divorced from meaning, or when the accidental nature of its relationship to meaning is revealed, then "truth" becomes a problematized word, shifting ground with every changing circumstance. When face to face with the King: "Commandons aussi à tous les nôtres de ne dire jamais à leur Prince que choses plaisantes" (*L'Isle des Hermaphrodites*, p. 95, article 13: "We order our people to say only pleasant things to their Prince"). Yet in his absence, his subjects' language can be quite different indeed: "Lesdits Officiers permettront aussi tous discours & libelles diffamatoires contre l'honneur du Prince, & de son Etat ..." (*L'Isle des Hermaphrodites*, p. 73, article 2: "These above-mentioned Officers will permit all sorts of slanderous sermons and libellous pamphlets against the honor of the Prince and of his State ..."). Language itself is perpetually reinvented, since there is no fixed relation between signifier and signified:

Par grace et privilege spécial nous voulons aussi qu'il soit permis à nos Sujets d'inventer les termes, & les mots nécessaires pour la civile conversation, lesquels sont ordinairement à deux ententes: l'une presentant à la lettre ce qu'ils auront envie de dire: l'autre un sens mystique de voluptés, qui ne sera entendu que de leurs semblables .... (*L'Isle des Hermaphrodites*, p. 94, article 12)

(By special grace and privilege we wish also that our Subjects be permitted to invent the terms and words necessary for civil conversation, which words ordinarily have two senses: one presenting to the letter whatever they wish to say: the other a mystical meaning of sensuality, which will only be understood by those who resemble them [their equals] ....)

The question remains, if words have two meanings, then what does a hermaphrodite *mean* to say when it uses these words? Foundational meaning is dissolved merely by these dual possibilities. Language breaks down almost entirely through its constant reinvention:

> Nous leur avons permis & permettons d'avoir dès maintenant, & à toujours quelque langue, ou jargon composé à leur fantaisie qu'ils nommeront de quelque nom étrange, comme *Mésapotamique, Pantagruelique*, & autres. Useront aussi de signes au lieu de paroles, afin d'être entendus en leurs pensées plus secrettes, par leurs consçachans, & sans être découverts. (*L'Isle des Hermaphrodites*, p. 95, article 14)

> (We have permitted and will continue to permit them to have now and forever some language or jargon invented according to their whim [or by their imagination], to which they will give some strange name like *Mesopotamian, Pantagruelian*, or some other such name. They will also use signs instead of words, in order to make even their most secret thoughts understood.)

This dissolution of language, even at the level of gesture, mirrors the dissolution of a society driven by performative repetition of externally imposed roles. By permitting the infinite multiplication of sign systems according to individual whim or imagination, the Hermaphrodites recreate not only language but themselves. Heteroglossia becomes a form of self-determination.[28] If identity is revealed only through such signs as costume, language (title or name), and behavior (deportment – *entregent*), then how can it be established that identity is not created by these outward signs? Once this doubt is raised, it cannot simply be dismissed, for any attempt to define a person other than by outward signs leads merely to aphasia. No essence of identity is available to us. Thus Artus, in raising the issue of the relationship between sign systems and identity formation, enters into a revolutionary discourse, even though he disguises such subversion by his use of the supposedly normative form of satire.

---

[28] This view is echoed by Donna Haraway in her "Cyborg Manifesto," p. 181: "Cyborg imagery can suggest a way out of the maze of dualisms in which we have explained our bodies and our tools to ourselves. This is a dream not of a common language, but of a powerful infidel heteroglossia." Haraway, like Artus, uses language metonymically to designate all of the sign systems which are used to construct culture.

Conclusion

Although it had faded in importance by the end of the preceding century, the figure of the hermaphrodite did not entirely disappear from seventeenth century European culture. Particularly in French and German alchemical treatises, the figure persists as a crucial stage in the processes of sublimation. Works by Jamsthaler[1] and Mylius[2] contain emblems of the hermaphroditic rebis as Sol and Luna, King and Queen.[3] Annibal Barlet designates Mercury as the mystic hermaphrodite.[4] Gabriel de Foigny's *La terre australe connue* (1676)[5] continues the tradition of the *utopie hermaphrodite*, as Ronzeaud labels it,[6] although following in the slightly more traditional satirical footsteps of Bishop Joseph Hall's *Mundus alter et idem*[7] rather than the more subversive traces of Thomas Artus.

These works are not without their complexity. Barlet associates the hermaphrodism of Mercury both with monstrosity and with generation, thus linking the spiritual with the physiological, and common biological processes with that which is designated as

---

[1] Herbrandt Jamsthaler, *Viatorium spagyricum. Das ist: Ein gebenedeyter spagyrischer Wegweiser* (Frankfurt: 1625).

[2] Johann Daniel Mylius, *Philosophia reformata* (Frankfurt: 1622).

[3] See Jung, *Psychology and Alchemy*, figures 125 and 199.

[4] Annibal Barlet, *Le Vray et methodique cours de la physique resolutive, vulgairement dite "Chymie." Representé par figures generales & particulieres. Pour connoistre la theotechnie ergocosmique, c'est à dire, l'art de Dieu, en l'ouvrage de l'univers* (Paris: N. Charles, 1653), p. 266.

[5] In an impressive edition by Pierre Ronzeaud (Paris: Société des testes français modernes, 1990).

[6] In his study *L'Utopie hermaphrodite: La Terre Australe Connue de Gabriel de Foigny* (Marseille: Publications de C.M.R., 17, 1981).

[7] See Chapter 6 of the second book, "Hermaphroditica Island," from *Another World and Yet the Same: Bishop Joseph Hall's "Mundus alter et idem,"* trans. and ed. John Millar Wands (New Haven: Yale University Press, 1981), pp. 62–3. This little world is fruitful and seemingly ideal, full of trees laden with hyrid fruit. Yet Bishop Hall does apply some heavy moralization to the scene: "Adolescents and whoever cannot both generate and give birth serve the rest. If they discover anyone of our people of a single nature among them they display the person as a great monstrosity and show exactly the same astonishment as we do when we see offspring with two heads, or mutilated, or lacking their private parts. They boast that they are the perfect offspring of nature ... With these and with other abominable arguments these quite clever people are accustomed to defend themselves ... (p. 63). These lines are echoed in the opening of the fifth chapter of Foigny's work.

abnormal. In this, he is merely echoing the medical treatises of the previous centuries as he combines Aristotelian hierarchization according to norms and Augustine's more benevolent tolerance of monstrous difference:

> ... Pareillement que cette mesme varieté compose le monde, le fait subsister, luy donne sa force, & cause sa beauté; sans laquelle ce ne seroit qu'une masse déplaisante, & de condition inferieure au cahos premier ... En quoy paroist non seulement l'excellence de l'ordre, qui rend son lustre à toutes choses, & nous en donne leur parfaite cognoissance; mais encore leur particuliere distinction, qui les fait telles qu'elles sont.
>
> IV. Auquel subiect Mercure chés les Hermetiques, parlant de soy-mesme, & disant qu'il est hermaphrodite; c'est à dire indifferent de sexe, fait voir ouvertement, que bien que l'Artiste le specifie philosophiquement, imitant en partie la nature; si faut-il neanmoins qu'il le determine plutost à l'un qu'à l'autre sexe metallique, estant trop libre & vagabond .... (Barlet, *Le Vray ... cours*, p. 266)

> (Just as this same variety creates the world, keeps it alive, gives it its strength, and is the cause of its beauty; without which it would only be an unpleasant mass, and of inferior condition to the original chaos ... In which we can see not only the excellence of the order, which lends its brightness to all things, and gives us perfect knowledge of them; but even their particular distinction, that makes them what they are. / IV. On this subject, Mercury, in the works of the Hermetic philosophers, speaking of himself, and saying that he is a hermaphrodite; that is to say of indistinct sex, shows openly, that even though the Artist categorizes him philosophically, imitating in part nature, nonetheless he must determine one metallic sex over the other, otherwise he would be too free and vagabond.)

Clearly, the notions of hermaphrodism as a spiritual state and of the beauty of variety (even monstrous variety) are being made subject to the necessity for order and stability; one senses the triumph of absolutism in the very language of this treatise. Barlet even echoes the commandment issued by Boaistuau (himself echoing legal pronouncements on the subject) and repeated by Paré, that the hermaphrodite must choose one or the other sex, in order to achieve stability, which is perceived as perfection. This is quite distant from the alchemical works of the *Rosarium*, of Clovis Hesteau de Nuysement, of Trismosin, and of Michael Maier, who portray the process of abjection and dissolution as crucial to alchemical and spiritual sublimation.

Similarly, Foigny's *Terre australe* is hardly as subversive as Artus' *Isle des Hermaphrodites* (yet he was condemned for it, whereas Artus was not).[8] In fact, in many ways, whereas Artus' hermaphrodites cleverly destabilize every aspect of

---

8   A sign of the times, or more likely of the place. Henri IV allowed Artus to go unscathed, in spite of a strict ban on political propaganda (see Pierre de l'Estoile, *Mémoires-journaux: Journal de Henri IV* (Paris: Alphonse Lemerre, 1888), p. 180). Foigny was condemned by the Council of Geneva, the city where he had taken refuge (see Ronzeaud's introduction to *La Terre australe*, xviii-xx). Certainly seventeenth-century Geneva could not be considered a safe harbor even for the mildest of libertines.

society as thoroughly as they can, Foigny's characters merely create an inverted hierarchy based on Western European culture. They destroy as monsters any single-sexed child which is born, just as ancient Romans destroyed any hermaphrodite: "Tous les Australiens ont les deux sexes: & s'il arrive qu'un enfant naisse avec un seul, ils l'etouffent comme un monstre" (*Terre australe*, p. 83: "All Australians are of both sexes, and if it happens that an infant is born with just one, they suffocate it as a monster"). Although Foigny offers some amusing details about their anatomy, he is quite modest in his description (or lack thereof) of their sexuality:

> Ils sont obligez de presenter au moins un enfant au Heb: mais ils les produisent d'une façon si secrete, que c'est un crime entre eux de parler "de conjonction" de l'un avec l'autre à cet effet: & jamais je n'ay pu connêtre comme la generation s'y fait. (*Terre australe*, p. 85)

> (They are obliged to present at least one child to Heb: but they produce it in such a secret fashion, that it is a crime among them to speak of the "conjunction" of one with the other to this end; and I could never find out how children were generated.)

True, in his critique of Aristotelian arguments about the primacy of the father in generation ("le mot de 'pere' est inconnu entre les Australiens," p. 96: "the word 'father' is unknown among the Australians"), the old "Australian" sage does efface the bases for sexual hierarchy. But again, he establishes another reverse hierarchy in arguing for the primacy of the mother (*Terre australe*, pp. 96–7). The narrator recognizes this reversal: "bien que je ne peusse consentir à ses raisons qui renversoient toutes nos loix" (*Terre australe*, p. 98: "even though I could never consent to his reasoning, which reverses all our laws"). But he is nonetheless shaken by this argument, and decries the tyranny of men over women, leaving the validity of this hierarchy in some doubt.

The Australians themselves strive to reject all hierarchy, except perhaps a vague form of order based on merit: "nous faisons profession d'être égaux en tous: nôtre gloire consiste à parêtre les mêmes" (*Terre australe*, p. 101: "we make it our goal to be equal in everything: our glory consists in seeming the same"). The Australian sage rejects the imposition of culture or custom as if it were essential nature: "la coutume faisoit tant d'effort sur nos esprits, qu'on croyoit necessaire, ce qu'on pratiquoit de naissance" (*Terre australe*, p. 102: "custom had such an effect on our spirits, that we felt that what we had practiced from birth was in fact necessary"). Thus, Foigny does echo Artus in his anti-essentialist critique of culture, here seeming almost as deeply subversive as his predecessor.

But the Australians are true inhabitants of utopia, exceptionally virtuous. They are not affected by avarice, and thus: "leur vie peut passer pour une veritable image de la beatitude naturelle" (*Terre australe*, p. 107: "their life could pass as a truthful image of natural beatitude"). They live without ambition, do not subject other men to servitude, and believe in equality for all (p. 107). There is a certain uniformity and conformism in this society; because all hermaphrodites are intellectually perfect, they all think alike (p. 108). This is certainly a far cry from the inventive and almost seductive disorder of Artus' hermaphrodites.

Like Artus, Foigny discusses the religious beliefs of this utopian society, although with somewhat more circumspection: "C'est le sujet le plus delicat & le plus caché qui soit parmy les Australiens que celuy de la Religion. C'est un crime inouy d'en parler" (*Terre australe*, p. 113: "Religion is the most delicate and hidden subject among the Australians. It is an unheard of crime to speak of it."). Nonetheless, he does reveal some of the Australians beliefs, in an exposition that recalls portions of Montaigne's "Apologie de Raimond Sebond."[9] The division of religion into various battling sects merely demonstrates that man is not capable of knowing the divine truth; thus, it is better if God is not profaned by human discussion of His qualities and nature: "... il faut étre infiny comme luy pour pouvoir en parler également, par ce que nous supposons qu'il est Incomprehensible ... C'est la raison qui nous oblige de n'en point parler, parce que nous sommes persuadez qu'on n'en sauroit parler sans faillir" ("one must be infinite like him in order to speak as an equal, because we suppose that he is incomprehensible ... that is the reason which obliges us not to speak of it, because we are persuaded that we could not speak of it without making a mistake", p. 119).[10] Unlike Artus' characters, Foigny's Australians are not atheists who mock religion by parodying its rules, but skeptical humanists intent on man's insufficiency in matters of religion. Of course, Foigny's fervent argument in favor of complete freedom of religious thought ("laisser un chacun dans la liberté d'en penser ce que son esprit lui en suggere," *Terre australe*, pp. 119–20: "to leave each in liberty to think whatever his spirit suggests about it") would not have been favored by Catholics or Protestants.

Foigny's utopian society seems like a constructive revision of Artus' destructive hermaphrodites. Artus' characters, containing diversity of gender within each person, represented the effacement of established social distinctions and cultural norms; Foigny's Australians demonstrate the human dignity and richness that can be gained through toleration of such diversity and through recognition of the autonomy of each individual. The place of the individual in the larger social whole is not nearly as important as the obligation society has incurred to protect the individual as a separate entity. Whereas Artus' hermaphrodites had to deconstruct society in order to reveal

---

9   *Essais*, vol. 2, essay 12.
10 Compare this to Montaigne's skepticism about man's capacity for knowing God: "Si ce rayon de la divinité nous touchoit aucunement, il y paroistroit par tout: non seulement nos parolles, mais encore nos operations en porteroient la lueur et le lustre. Tout ce qui partiroit de nous, on le verroit illuminé de cette noble clarté. Nous devrions avoir honte qu'és sectes humaines il ne fust jamais partisan ..." ("If this ray of divinity touched us at all, it would appear everywhere, not only in our words, but even our acts would carry its glow and its luster. Everything which came from us, one would see illuminated by this noble clarity. We should be ashamed that he was never a partisan of any of our human sects," vol. 2, essay 12, p. 442).

the nature (good and bad) of individualism, Foigny's characters construct from the basis of this individualism in order to establish a new, more humane, society.

For all the revolutionary programs and complexity of Foigny's text, it was an isolated and quickly suppressed instance of the exploration of the political, spiritual, and epistemological ramifications of sexual difference. Certainly issues of sex and gender did not disappear in the seventeenth century (transvestism in particular seems to have maintained some hold on court society and the popular imagination);[11] but the hermaphrodite does not hold center stage as it did in the previous century. Ambiguity of gender is expressed through isolated acts of subversion, not problematic states of being. It can even be argued that these acts, tolerated by the state (in the case of the Abbé de Choisy) and controlled by the theatrical gaze that limits their efficacity, are not in fact subversive at all, but merely entertaining diversions, much as the *carnaval* was conceived as a diversion that enforced social norms by the very means of mocking those norms.[12] Nonetheless, these limited acts of subversion can also be read as rehearsals for more substantive acts, or as reminders of the problematic nature of social roles.

The pre-revolutionary eighteenth century is the chief beneficiary of Renaissance and Baroque discussions of sex and gender. Thomas Artus' novel is reprinted frequently in this century, either by itself or as part of Pierre de l'Estoile's journals.[13] The transvestite Chevalier d'Eon intrigued both French and English society by means of a deliberate confusion of gender roles.[14] Resurgence of interest in and publication of alchemical treatises in France and Germany resulted in the production of such works as the *Hermaphroditisches Sonn- und Mondskind. Das ist: Des Sohns deren Philosophen naturlich-ubernaturliche Gebahrung, Zerstorung und Regenerierung* (*The Hermaphroditic Son of the Sun and the Moon. That is: the Son of the Philosophical Birth, Destruction, and Regeneration*) and the *Figurarum Aegyptiorum secretarum*

---

11   See in particular Marjorie Garber's discussion of the Abbé de Choisy in her book *Vested Interests: Cross-Dressing and Cultural Anxiety* (New York: Routledge, 1992), "Phantoms of the Opera: Actor, Diplomat, Transvestite, Spy," pp. 256–9.

12   See Natalie Zemon Davis, "The Reasons of Misrule," in *Society and Culture*, pp. 97–123.

13   It is reprinted in Brussels by H. Demen in 1724; as a part of l'Estoile journals in Paris by Duchat in the same year, and in 1744 by La Veuve de Pierre Gandouin (also in Paris). Each of these latter two editions ran through several printings.

14   For a thorough exploration of the problematics of the Chevalier d'Eon's projections of gender ambiguity, see Gary Kates, "D'Eon Returns to France: Gender and Power in 1777," in *Body Guards*, pp. 167–94. See also Kates' book-length study, *Monsier d'Eon is a Woman: A Tale of Political Intrigue and Masquerade* (Baltimore, MD: Johns Hopkins University Press, 2001). See also Marjorie Garber, *Vested Interests*, pp. 259–66. Garber hints at the "political" nature of d'Eon's subversion: "It seems likely that the King and his ministers saw this "fixing" of d'Eon's gender identity as a way of containing his/her anarchic impulses" (p. 263).

(*Explication des figures hiéroglifiques des Aegyptiens; An Explanation of the Hieroglyphic Figures of the Egyptians*), with its images of an ambiguous Mercury, alternately male and female.[15] Medical and legal examination of the physiology and status of the hermaphrodite were transmitted to the seventeenth century in the influential work of Paolo Zacchia.[16] But the eighteenth century saw new developments in medical theories about hermaphrodism, establishing the condition as a "natural medical anomaly" (Epstein, "Either/Or," p. 117), which further undermined the notion of women as merely defective men.[17] Although enforced by legal and social structures even today, the neatly drawn hierarchical order of gender(s) was largely discredited in the realm of physiology by the end of the eighteenth century.

In short, the Renaissance hermaphrodite embodies the very issues so central to gender studies today, even if only in embryonic form. For example, Bauhin's discussion of hermaphrodites reveals unease about forms of distinction crucial to his society; not only those of sex, but of race and species as well. As he reassures himself and his reader of the insuperable gap between male and female, whereby a male can never become female (although the reverse might well be possible, as it is for Duval), his examples of hermaphrodites problematize that distinction and render the Aristotelian hierarchy of the sexes null and void. The gap between the Western European race and those of the Western Hemisphere is expressed as a fundamental difference of sex; hermaphrodites are omnipresent in the latter region, whereas they are anomalous in Europe. Yet this assumption that sexual difference does not follow one universal model undermines the notion of "natural" sex. Similarly, the notion of hermaphrodism as "natural" to some species, linked to the presumption of human superiority, destabilizes the notion of human physiology as the ideal model for nature. As Anne Fausto-Sterling has admirably demonstrated in her book, *Sexing the Body*, the "science" of physiology seems more a fiction created to satisfy political or social exigencies; the scientific investigator begins with the presumption of certain social givens, and seeks to justify these cultural creations by finding them in nature. But the self-contradictory aspects of this investigation reveal it to be factitious. These issues, touched upon but certainly not explored by Bauhin, are raised again and discussed in detail by Donna Haraway,

---

[15]   Both are cited by Jung in *Psychology and Alchemy*. See especially figures 123, 157, 164. The manuscript of the *Explication des figures hiéroglifiques* is to be found in the Bibliothèque de l'Arsénal (MS. 973).

[16]   These questions are examined in his *Questionum medico-legalium* (Basel: 1653), cited by Laqueur in *Making Sex*, pp. 140–42. But, as Laqueur, Lorraine Daston and Katharine Park point out, Zacchia is in large part repeating Bauhin's discussions (see Park and Daston, "Unnatural Conceptions: The Study of Monsters in France and England," *Past and Present* 92 (1981): 20–54.

[17]   For a fuller discussion of the medical, legal, and epistemological ramifications of developments in eighteenth-century teratology or developmental science, see Epstein, "Either/Or," pp. 113–18. See also Laqueur's chapter on the "Discovery of the Sexes," in *Making Sex*, pp. 149–92.

in her two studies *Primate Visions: Gender, Race, and Nature in the World of Modern Science* and *Simians, Cyborgs, and Women: The Reinvention of Nature.*

Thomas Artus's devastatingly amusing critique of the politics and epistemology of gender is echoed by contemporary critics such as Jonathan Dollimore (*Sexual Dissidence*) and Judith Butler (*Gender Trouble*). The constantly self-inventing and re-inventing hermaphrodites are the ultimate sexual dissidents; they refuse any identity, in favor of costumes which at once express and efface their "natures." They represent gender as a cultural construct, and proceed to deconstruct culture by erasing gender distinctions. Artus' novel is perhaps the most revolutionary of the early modern works examined in this study, profoundly skeptical as it is about any culture's attempts to understand, define, or control nature. To a large extent, his hermaphrodites embrace polymorphous perversity, a lack of essential sex, as their foundational nature.

Of course, early modern figures of the hermaphrodite did not always invoke innovation or revolution in matters of sexual difference. The lyrical hermaphrodism of such poets as Agrippa d'Aubigné and Philippe Desportes seems to arise from a desire to embody, but also to efface or replace, the feminine. This engulfing of the feminine within the masculine is strikingly consonant with the conservative use of the hermaphroditic figure in political pamphlets, where sexual ambiguity is linked to the feminine and both are condemned as degenerate and therefore ruinous to French society. Aristotle's notions of sex and generation continued to dominate many aspects of European culture. It was primarily in the realms of medicine and alchemy, the physiological and spiritual branches of early science, that ancient assessments of gender roles were questioned.

Alchemy in particular was unusually innovative in its glorification of the effacement of difference by means of conjunction. That which was condemned as abject by society, the feminine, the monstrous, the putrid or sickly, was recognized as crucial to existence itself. Certain alchemical treatises, particularly those of Clovis Hesteau de Nuysement and Michael Maier, came closest to assessing the hermaphrodite in its own terms, not as masculine or feminine, gay or straight, monstrous or divine, but as a being that oscillates between identity and difference, self and other, subject and object. In alchemical texts, the hermaphrodite remains pre-social and pre-linguistic, a rebis or thing which defies categorization, resembling Kristeva's abject, at once that upon which language, identity, and culture are founded and that which must be rejected by these constructs in order to justify their existence. The return of this repressed abject threatens these forms of categorization upon which society is founded, and thus society itself, by revealing them as man-made, circular and self-justifying constructs rather than essential and natural elements of being. Artus, Nuysement, even Bauhin recognized this problematic aspect of the hermaphrodite, and their presentations of this protean being call for further theoretical exploration of its "nature."

Bibliography

Primary Sources

Aldrovandi, Ulisse. *Monstrorum historia*. Bononia: N. Tebaldini, 1642.

Aneau, Barthélemy. *Imagination poétique*. Lyon: Macé Bonhomme, 1552.

Aristotle. *On the Generation of Animals*. In *The Complete Works of Aristotle*. Jonathan Barnes, ed. Princeton: Princeton University Press, Bollingen Series, 1984. Vol. 1, 1111–218.

Artus, Thomas. *Description de l'Isle des Hermaphrodites, nouvellemement descouverte*. Claude Gilbert Dubois, ed. Geneva: Droz: 1996.

Aubigné, Théodore Agrippa de. *Oeuvres*. H. Weber, ed. Paris: Gallimard, 1969.

———. *Le Printemps: Stances et Odes*. Eugénie Droz, ed. Geneva: Droz, 1973.

———. *Histoire universelle*. André Thierry, ed. Geneva: Droz, 1980–99.

———. *Histoire universelle*. André Thierry, ed. Geneva: Droz, 1985.

———. *Sa Vie à ses enfants*. Gilbert Schrenck, ed. Paris: Nizet, 1986.

Augustine. *The City of God*. Henry Bettenson, trans. London: Penguin, 1976.

Barlet, Annibal. *Le Vray et methodique cours de la physique resolutive, vulgairement dite "Chymie." Representé par figures generales & particulieres. Pour connoistre la theotechnie ergocosmique, c'est à dire, l'art de Dieu, en l'ouvrage de l'univers*. Paris: N. Charles, 1653.

Bauhin, Caspar. *De corporis humani partibus externis tractatus*. Basel, 1588.

———. *Institutiones anatomicae corporis virilis et muliebris historiam exhibentes*. Bern: Ioannes le Preux, 1604.

———. *Theatrum anatomicum*. Frankfurt: de Bry, 1605.

———. *De hermaphroditorum monstrosorumque partuum natura ex Theologorum, Jureconsultorumque, Medicorum, Philosophorum, et Rabbinorum sententia libri duo*. Oppenheim: Galleri, De Bry, 1614 (reprint of the 1600 Frankfurt edition).

———. *Vivae imagines partium corporis humani aeneis formis expressae et ex theatro anat.* Frankfurt: de Bry, 1620.

———. *Catalogus plantarum circa Basileam sponte nascentium*. Basel, 1622.

———. *Pinax theatri botanici*. Basel, 1623.

Les Belles Figures et drolleries de la Ligue. Paris: Librairie des Bibliophiles, 1886.

Boaistuau, Pierre. *Histoires prodigieuses les plus memorables qui ayent esté observes depuis la nativité de Jesus Christ, jusques à notre siecle*. Paris: Vincent Sertenas, 1560.

Boucher, Jean. *De Iusta Henrici tertii abdicatione e Francorum regno*. Loudun: Ioannem Pillehotte, 1591.

Boursier, Louise (Bourgeois). *Apologie de Louyse Bourgeois dite Bourcier Sage femme de la Royne Mere du Roy, et de feu Madame. Contre le Rapport des Medecins.* (Paris: 1627).

———. *Récit veritable de la naissance de Messeigneurs et Dames les enfans de France* .... François Rouget, ed. (Geneva: Droz, 2000).

Bry, Theodor de. *America* (*Brevis narratio eorum quae in Florida americae provincia Gallis acciderunt* ... 1591).

Catullus. *The Poems.* Kenneth Quinn, ed. London: Macmillan, 1973.

Desportes, Philippe. *Cartels et masquarades. Epitaphes.* Victor Graham, ed. Geneva: Droz, 1958.

———. *Les Amours de Diane.* Victor Graham, ed. Geneva: Droz, 1959.

———. *Les Amours d'Hippolyte.* Victor Graham, ed. Geneva: Droz, 1960.

Discours merveilleux de la vie, actions et deportements de Catherine de Médicis, Royne-mère. Nicole Cazauran, ed. Geneva: Droz, 1995.

Dorn, Gerard. *Congeries Paracelsicae chemicae de transmutationibus metallorum. Theatrum Chemicum, praecipuos selectorum auctorum tractatus ... continens.* Ursel, 1602.

Duval, Jacques. *Des Hermaphrodits, accouchemens de femmes, et traitement qui est requis pour les relever en santé.* Rouen: David Geuffroy, 1612.

Eros baroque: Anthologie thématique de la poésie amoureuse. Gisèle Mathieu-Castellani, ed. Paris: Nizet, 1986.

Etienne, Henri, ed. *Fragmenta poetarum veterum latinorum, quorum opera non extant: Eunii, Accii, Lucilii, Laberii, Pacuvii, Afranii, Naevii, Caecilii aliorumque multorum.* N.p.: Fuggeri, 1563.

Etienne, Henri, ed. *Petronii Arbitri Massiliensis Satyrici Fragmenta Restituta et aucta.* Antwerp: Plantini, 1565.

Eusebius. *Chronicon.* Paris: H. Estienne, 1512.

Explication des figures hiéroglifiques. Bibliothèque de l'Arsénal MS. 973.

Ficino, Marsilio. *Sur le Banquet de Platon ou de l'Amour.* Raymond Marcel, trans. and ed. Paris: Les Belles Lettres, 1956.

Foigny, Gabriel de. *La Terre Australe Connue.* Pierre Ronzeaud, ed. Paris: Société des textes français modernes, 1990.

The Fugger News-letters: Being a Selection of Unpublished letters from the Correspondents of the House of Fugger during the Years 1568–1605. Victor von Klarwill, ed. Pauline de Chary, trans. London: John Lane, 1924.

Hall, Joseph. *Another World and Yet the Same: Bishop Joseph Hall's "Mundus alter et idem.* John Millar Wands, trans. and ed. New Haven: Yale University Press, 1981.

Hippocrates, *On Generation. The Hippocratic Treatises.* Iain M. Lonie, ed. Berlin: Walter de Gruyter, 1981.

Jamsthaler, Herbrandt. *Viatorium spagyricum. Das ist: Ein gebenedeyter spagyrischer Wegweiser.* Frankfurt: 1625.

Kramer, Heinrich and James Sprenger. *The Malleus maleficarum.* New York: Dover, 1971.

Laudonnière, René Goulain de. *L'Histoire notable de la Floride*. Paris: Auvray, 1586.

Leone Ebreo (Leo Hebraeus). *The Philosophy of Love*. Trans. F. Friedeberg-Seeley and Jean H. Barnes. London: The Soncino Press, 1937.

L'Estoile, Pierre de. *Registre-Journal du Regne de Henri III*. Madeleine Lazard and Gilbert Schrenck, eds. Geneva: Droz, 1992–2003. 6 vols.

Livy. *Historia*. Book 27. Frank Gardner Moore, trans. Cambridge, MA: Harvard University Press, Loeb Classical Library, 1963.

Livy. *Historia*. Book 31. Evan T. Sage, trans. Cambridge, MA: Harvard University Press, Loeb Classical Library, 1961.

Lorris, Guillaume de and Jean de Meun. *Roman de la Rose*. Daniel Poirion, ed. Paris: Garnier-Flammarion, 1974.

Loyer, Pierre le. *Les Oeuvres et meslanges poetiques de Pierre Le Loyer, Angevin*. Paris: Jean Poupy, 1579.

Maier, Michael. *Atalanta fugiens*. Frankfurt, 1617.

———. *Atalanta fugiens*. Kassel: Bärenreiter, 1964.

———. *Atalanta fugiens*. Joscelyn Godwin, trans. Grand Rapids, MI: Phanes Press, 1989.

Monstres prodigeux advenus en la Turquie, depuis l'année de la Comette, iusqu'en l'an present 1624. Menaçans la fin, & entiere ruyne de l'Empire turquesque .... Paris: Jean de Bordeaux, 1624.

Montaigne, Michel de. *Les Essais*. Pierre Villey, ed. Paris: Presses Universitaires de France, 1978.

Mylius, Johann Daniel. *Philosophia reformata*. Frankfurt: 1622.

Nuysement, Clovis Hesteau. *Poème philosophic de la verité de la phisique minéralle ou sont refutees les objections que peuvent faire les incredules & ennemis de cet art*. Paris: Jeremie Perier & Abdias Buisard, 1620.

———. *Traittez de l'Harmonie et constitution generalle du vray sel secret des philosophes, & de l'Esprit universelle du Monde....* Paris: Jeremie Perier et Abdias Buisard, 1621.

———. *Traictez du vray sel secret des philosophes et de l'esprit général du monde. Les Visions hermétiques*. Sylvain Matton, ed. Paris: Bibliotheca hermetica, 1974.

———. *Les Oeuvres poétiques, livres I et II*. Roland Guillot, ed. Geneva: Droz, 1994.

Ovidius Naso, Publius. *Metamorphoses*. William S. Anderson, ed. Leipzig: Teubner, 1985.

Palissy, Bernard de. *Recepte véritable*. Keith Cameron, ed. Geneva: Droz, 1988.

Paracelsus (Theophrastus Bombast von Hohenheim). *Concerning the Nature of Things (De Natura rerum)*. Arthur Edward Waite, trans. *The Hermetic and Alchemical Writings of Aureolus Philippus Theophrastus Bombast of Hohenheim, called Paracelsus the Great*. London: James Elliott and Co., 1894.

———. *Theophrast von Hohenheim, Samtliche Werke*. Karl Sudhoff, ed. Munich and Berlin: R. Oldenbourg, 1928.

Paré, Ambroise. *Des Monstres et prodiges*. Jean Céard, ed. Geneva: Droz, 1971.

————. *On Monsters and Marvels*. Janis L. Pallister, trans. Chicago: University of Chicago Press, 1982.

Petronius. *Petronii Arbitri Satyricon*. Paris: Pithou, 1587.

————. *The Satyricon*. Evan T. Sage and Brady B. Gilleland, eds. New York: Irvington, 1982.

Plato, *Symposium*, trans. Michael Joyce. *The Collected Dialogues of Plato*, ed. Edith Hamilton and Huntington Cairns. Princeton: Princeton University Press, Bollingen Series, 1963.

Riolan, Jean. *Discours sur les hermaphrodits, où il est démontré contre l'opinion commune, qu'il n'y a point de vray hermaphrodits*. Paris: Ramier, 1614.

Rosarium philosophorum. Joachim Telle, ed. Weinheim, VCH. 1992. Facsimile of the first edition, Frankfurt, 1550.

Rosarium philosophorum: Le Rosaire des philosophes . Etienne Perrot, trans. Paris: Librairie de Medicis, 1973.

Rueff, Jacob. *De conceptu et generatione hominis*. Frankfurt, 1580.

Sextus Empiricus. *Outlines of Pyrrhonism*. R.G. Bury, trans. Cambridge, MA: Harvard University Press, Loeb Classical Library, 1976.

Les Sorcelleries de Henri de Valois et les oblations qu'il faisoit au Diable dans le Bois de Vincennes. Paris: Didier Millot, 1589.

Tacitus. *Annals*. Alfred John Church and William Jackson Brodribb, trans. New York: The Modern Library, 1942.

Tesserant, Claude de. *Histoires prodigieuses*. Paris: Jean de Bordeaux, 1567.

The Theological and Philosophical Works of Hermes Trismegistus, Christian Neoplatonist. Edinburgh: T. & T. Clark, 1882.

Thou, Jacques-Auguste de. *Historiarum sui temporis ...*. London: Buckley, 1733.

Trismosin, Salomon. *La Toyson d'or*. Paris: Charles Sevestre, 1612.

————. *Splendor Solis*. Joscelyn Godwin, trans. Grand Rapids: Phanes Press, 1991.

Verville, Béroalde de. *Les Recherches de la pierre philosophale*. Paris: T. Jouan, 1584.

————. *Le Moyen de Parvenir*. C. Royer, ed. Geneva: Droz, 1970.

La Vie et faits notables de Henri de Valois, maintenant tout au long, sans rien requérir: où sont contenues les trahisons, perfidies, sacrileges, exactions, cruautés & hontes de cet hypocrite, ennemi de la Religion Catholique. Paris: Didier Millot, 1589.

Secondary Sources

Allen, D.C. *Mysteriously Meant: The Rediscovery of Pagan Symbolism and Allegorical Interpretation in the Renaissance*. Baltimore: Johns Hopkins University Press, 1970.

Barkin, Leonard. *Transuming Passion: Ganymede and the Erotics of Humanism.* Stanford: Stanford University Press, 1991.

Barnavi, Elie. *Le Parti de Dieu: Etude sociale et politique des chefs de la Ligue parisienne, 1585–1594.* Brussels: Nauwelaerts, 1980.

Baumgartner, Frederic. *Radical Reactionaries: The Political Thought of the French Catholic League.* Geneva: Droz, 1975.

Bell, David A. "Unmasking a King: The Political Uses of Popular Literature Under the French Catholic League, 1588–89." *The Sixteenth Century Journal.* 20 (1989): 371–86.

Berriot-Salvadore, Evelyne. *Un corps, un destin. La femme dans la medicine de la Renaissance.* Paris: Champion, 1993.

Berthelot, M. *Les Origines de l'alchimie.* Paris: Steinheil, 1885.

————. *Collection des anciens alchimistes grecs.* Osnabruck: Otto Zeller, 1967.

Blanchard, André. *La Poésie baroque et precieuse.* Paris: Seghers, 1985.

Blum, André. *L'Estampe satirique en France pendant les Guerres de Religion.* Paris: Giard & Briere, 1917.

Boswell, John. *Christianity, Social Tolerance, and Homosexuality. Gay People in Western Europe from the Beginning of the Christian Era to the Fourteenth Century.* Chicago: University of Chicago Press, 1980.

Brundage, James A. *Law, Sex, and Christian Society in Medieval Europe.* Chicago: University of Chicago Press, 1987.

Bredbeck, Gregory W. *Sodomy and Interpretation, Marlowe to Milton.* Ithaca: Cornell University Press, 1991.

Bullough, Vern L. *Sexual Variance in Society and History.* New York: John Wiley & Sons, 1976.

Butler, Judith. *Gender Trouble: Feminism and the Subversion of Identity.* New York: Routledge, 1990.

Bynum, Caroline Walker. *Jesus as Mother. Studies in the Spirituality of the High Middle Ages.* Berkeley: University of California Press, 1982.

Cameron, Keith. *Henri III: A Maligned or Malignant King? (Aspects of the Satirical Iconography of Henri de Valois).* Exeter, England: University of Exeter, 1978.

Carroll, Linda L. "Who's on Top? Gender as Societal Power Configuration in Italian Renaissance Drama." *Sixteenth Century Journal.* 20 (1989): 531–58.

Céard, Jean. *La Nature et les prodiges.* Geneva: Droz, 1975.

Daston, Lorraine. "Marvelous Facts and Miraculous Evidence in Early Modern Europe," *Critical Inquiry.* 18 (1991): 93–124. Reprinted in *Wonders, Marvels, and Monsters in Early Modern Culture.* Peter Platt, ed., pp. 76–104. Newark, DE: University of Delaware Press, 1999.

Daston, Lorraine and Katharine Park. "Unnatural Conceptions: The Study of Monsters in France and England." *Past and Present.* 92 (1981): 20–54.

————. "Hermaphrodites in Renaissance France." *Critical Matrix.* 1 (1985): 1–19.

————. "The Hermaphrodite and the Orders of Nature: Sexual Ambiguity in Early Modern France." *Gay and Lesbian Quarterly.* 1 (1995): 419–38.

Davis, Natalie Zemon. *Society and Culture in Early Modern France.* Stanford: Stanford University Press, 1975.

De Certeau, Michel. "Montaigne's 'Of Cannibals': The Savage 'I'." *Heterologies: Discourse on the Other.* Brian Massumi, trans., pp. 67–79. Minneapolis: University of Minnesota Press, 1986.

Debus, Allen G. *The Chemical Philosophy: Paracelsian Science and Medicine in the Sixteenth and Seventeenth Centuries.* New York: Science History Publications, 1977.

Delcourt, Marie. *Hermaphrodite: Mythes et rites de la bisexualité dans l'antiquité classique.* Paris: Presses Universitaires de France, 1958.

Demerson, Guy. *La Mythologie classique dans l'oeuvre lyrique de la "Pléiade".* Geneva: Droz, 1972.

Demonet, Marie-Luce. *A plaisir: Sémiotique et scepticism chez Montaigne.* Orléans: Paradigme, 2002.

Derrida, Jacques. *De la grammatologie.* Paris: Seuil, 1967.

————. *La dissemination.* Paris: Seuil, 1972.

Dollimore, Jonathan. *Sexual Dissidence: Augustine to Wilde, Freud to Foucault.* Oxford: Oxford University Press, 1991.

Dubois, Claude Gilbert. *L'Utopie hermaphrodite: La Terre Australe Connue de Gabriel de Foigny.* Marseille: Publications de C.M.R., 17, 1981.

Epstein, Julia and Kristina Straub, eds. *Body Guards: The Cultural Politics of Gender Ambiguity.* New York: Routledge, 1991.

Epstein, Julia. "Either/Or – Neither/Both: Sexual Ambiguity and the Ideology of Gender." *Genders.* 7 (1990): 99–142.

Faludi, Susan. *Backlash: The Undeclared War Against American Women.* New York: Crown Publishers, 1991.

Fausto-Sterling, Anne. *Sexing the Body: Gender Politics and the Construction of Sexuality.* New York: Basic Books, 2000.

Federmann, Reinhard. *The Royal Art of Alchemy.* Philadelphia: Chilton, 1969.

Garber, Marjorie. *Vested Interests: Cross-Dressing and Cultural Anxiety.* New York: Routledge, 1992.

Gatens, Moira. *Imaginary Bodies: Ethics, Power and Corporeality.* London: Routledge, 1996.

Gélis, Jacques. *History of Childbirth: Fertility, Pregnancy, and Birth in Early Modern Europe.* Rosemary Morris, trans. Boston: Northeastern University Press, 1991.

Gilbert, Ruth. *Early Modern Hermaphrodites: Sex and Other Stories.* New York: Palgrave, 2002.

Givry, Grillot de. *Witchcraft, Magic, and Alchemy.* J. Courtenay Locke, trans. New York: Dover, 1971.

Graves, Robert. *The Greek Myths.* Harmondsworth: Penguin, 1957.

Gray, Floyd. *Gender, Rhetoric and Print Culture in Renaissance Writing.* Cambridge: Cambridge University Press, 2000.

Greenblatt, Stephen. "Fiction and Friction." *Twelfth Night*. R.S. White, ed., pp. 99–128. New York: St Martin's Press, 1996.

Grosz, Elizabeth. *Volatile Bodies: Toward a Corporeal Feminism*. Bloomington: Indiana University Press, 1994.

Haraway, Donna. *Primate Visions: Gender, Race, and Nature in the World of Modern Science*. New York: Routledge, 1989.

————. *Simians, Cyborgs, and Women*. New York: Routledge, 1991.

Huet, Marie-Hélène. *Monstrous Imagination*. Cambridge, MA: Harvard University Press, 1993.

Jacquart, Danielle and Claude Thomasset. *Sexuality and Medicine in the Middle Ages*. Princeton: Princeton University Press, 1988.

Jordan, Constance. *Renaissance Feminism: Literary Texts and Political Models*. Ithaca, New York: Cornell University Press, 1990.

Jung, C.G. *Mysterium Coniunctionis*. Princeton: Princeton University Press, 1977.

————. *Psychology and Alchemy*. Princeton: Bollingen, 1980.

Kates, Gary. *Monsieur d'Eon is a Woman: A Tale of Political Intrigue and Sexual Masquerade*. Baltimore: Johns Hopkins University Press, 2001.

Kessler, Suzanne J. *Lessons from the Intersexed*. New Brunswick, NJ: Rutgers University Press, 1998.

————. "The Medical Construction of Gender: Case Management of Intersexed Infants." *Signs*. 16 (1990): 3–26.

Kristeva, Julia. *Pouvoirs de l'horreur*. Paris: Seuil, 1980.

Laqueur, Thomas. *Making Sex: The Body and Gender from the Greeks to Freud*. Cambridge, MA: Harvard University Press, 1990.

Leibacher-Ouvrard, Lise. "Tribades et gynanthropes (1612–1614): Fictions et fonctions de l'anatomie travesti." *Papers on French Seventeenth Century Literature* 24 (1997): 519–36.

Long, Kathleen Perry. "Salomon Trismosin and Clovis Hesteau de Nuysement: The Sexual Politics of Alchemy in Early Modern France." *L'Esprit Créateur. Writing about Sex: The Discourses of Eroticism in Seventeenth-Century France*. Abby Zanger, ed., 35 (1995): 9–21.

Lonie, Iain M. "The 'Paris Hippocratics': Teaching and Research in Paris in the Second Half of the Sixteenth Century." *The Medical Renaissance of the Sixteenth Century*. A. Wear, R.K. French, I.M. Lonie, eds, pp. 155–74. Cambridge: Cambridge University Press, 1985.

Lorber, Judith. *Paradoxes of Gender*. New Haven: Yale University Press, 1994.

MacGowan, Margaret. "Les images du pouvoir royal au temps d'Henri III." *Théorie et pratique politiques à la Renaissance*. Colloque internationale de Tours, 1976–77, pp. 301–20.

Maclean, Ian. *The Renaissance Notion of Woman: A Study in the Fortunes of Scholasticism and Medical Science in European Intellectual Life*. Cambridge: Cambridge University Press, 1980.

Mathieu-Castellani, Gisèle. *Les Thèmes amoureux dans la poésie française, 1570–1600*. Paris: Klincksieck, 1975.

Meyer, Barbara Hochstetler. "Marguerite de Navarre and the Androgynous Portrait of François 1er." *Renaissance Quarterly*. (Summer 1995): 287–325.

Miquel, Pierre. *Les Guerres de Religion*. Paris: Fayard, 1980.

Moran, Bruce T. *The Alchemical World of the German Court: Occult Philosophy and Chemical Medicine in the Circle of Moritz of Hessen (1572–1632)*. Stuttgart: Franz Steiner Verlag, 1991.

Murphy, Stephen. "Catherine, Cybele, and Ronsard's Witnesses." *High Anxiety: Masculinity in Crisis in Early Modern France*. Kathleen Long, ed., pp. 55–70. Kirksville, MO: Truman State University Press, 2002.

Newman, Karen. *Fetal Positions: Individualism, Science, Visuality*. Stanford: Stanford University Press, 1996.

Niccoli, Ottavia. *Prophecy and People in Renaissance Italy*. Princeton, NJ: Princeton University Press, 1990.

Perkins, Wendy. *Midwifery and Medicine in Early Modern France: Louise Bourgeois*. Exeter: University of Exeter Press, 1996.

Poirier, Guy. *L'Homosexualité dans l'imaginaire de la Renaissance*. Paris: Champion, 1996.

Popkin, Richard. *The History of Scepticism from Erasmus to Spinoza*. Berkeley, California: University of California Press, 1979.

Rabelais, François. *Gargantua*. V.L. Saulnier, ed. Geneva: Droz, 1970.

Randall, Catharine. *(Em)bodying the Word: Textual Ressurections in the Martyrological Narratives of Foxe, Crespin, de Bèze and d'Aubigné*. New York: Peter Lang, 1992.

———. "A Surplus of Significance: Hermaphrodites in Early Modern France." *French Forum*. 19 (1994): 17–35.

Reeser, Todd. "Fracturing the Male Androgyne in the Heptaméron." *Romance Quarterly*. 51 (Winter 2004): 15–29.

Richlin, Amy. "The Meaning of *irrumare* in Catullus and Martial." *Classical Philology*. 76 (1981): 40–46.

———. *The Garden of Priapus: Sex and Aggression in Roman Humor*. New Haven: Yale University Press, 1983.

Rigolot, François. "Quel 'genre' d'amour pour Louise Labé?," *Poétique*. 55. Paris: Seuil, 1983, pp. 303–17.

———. "Gender vs. Sex Difference in Louise Labé's Grammar of Love." *Rewriting the Renaissance: The Discourses of Sexual Difference in Early Modern Europe*. Margaret Ferguson, Maureen Quilligan, and Nancy Vickers, eds, pp. 287–98. Chicago: University of Chicago Press, 1986.

Roberts, Gareth. *The Mirror of Alchemy: Alchemical Ideas and Images in Manuscripts and Books*. Toronto: Toronto University Press, 1994.

Rothstein, Marian. "Mutations of the Androgyne: Its Functions in Early Modern French Literature." *Sixteenth Century Journal*. 34 (2): 409–38.

Schleiner, Winifred. "Early Modern Controversies about the One Sex Model." *Renaissance Quarterly*. 53.1 (Spring 2000): 180–91.

Schwartz, Jerome. "Scatology and Eschatology in Gargantua's Androgyne Device." *Etudes rabelaisiennes*. 14 (1977): 272–74.

Seguin, Jean-Pierre. *L'Information en France avant la periodique*. Paris: Maisonneuve et Larose, 1964.

Shephard, Simon. "What's so Funny about Ladies' Tailors? A Survey of Some Male (Homo)sexual Types in the Renaissance." *Textual Practice*. 6 (1992): 17–30.

Veyne, Paul. "Homosexuality in Ancient Rome." *Western Sexuality: Practice and Precept in Past and Present Times*. Philippe Ariès and André Béjin, eds, Anthony Forster, trans., pp. 26–35. Oxford: Basil Blackwell, 1985.

Waddington, Raymond B. "The Bisexual Portrait of Francis I: Fontainebleau, Castiglione, and the Tone of Courtly Mythology." *Playing with Gender: A Renaissance Pursuit*. Jean Brink, Maryanne C. Horowitz, and Allison Coudert, eds, pp. 99–132. Urbana and Chicago: University of Illinois Press, 1991.

Wear, Andrew. "Medicine in Early Modern Europe, 1500–1700." *The Western Medical Tradition, 800 BC to AD 1800*. Lawrence Conrad, et al., eds, pp. 234–5. Cambridge: Cambridge University Press, 1995.

Wind, Edgar. *Pagan Mysteries in the Renaissance*. New York: Norton, 1958.

Wiseman, T.P. *Catullus and his World: A Reappraisal*. Cambridge: Cambridge University Press, 1985.

Wollfhart, Conrad. *Prodigiorum ac ostentorum chronicon*. Basel: H. Petri, 1557.

Yates, Frances. *The Rosicrucian Enlightenment*. London: Routledge and Kegan Paul, 1972.

Yavneh, Naomi. "The Spiritual Eroticism of Leone's Hermaphrodite." *Playing with Gender: A Renaissance Pursuit*. Jean Brink, Maryanne C. Horowitz, and Allison Coudert, eds, pp. 85–98. Urbana and Chicago: University of Illinois Press, 1991.

Index

Page references in italic are to illustrations.